6 Ways to Design a Face

Corrective Jaw Surgery to Optimize Bite, Airway, and Facial Balance

Library of Congress Cataloging-in-Publication Data

Names: Coceancig, Paul, author.
Title: 6ways to design a face : corrective jaw surgery to optimize bite,
    airway, and facial balance / Paul Coceancig.
Other titles: 6 ways to design a face
Description: Batavia, IL : Quintessence Publishing Co, Inc, [2021] |
    Includes bibliographical references and index. | Summary: "This book
    details the author's 6Ways to design a face: IMDO, GenioPaully, BIMAX,
    SuperBIMAX, custom PEEK, and SARME. All of these corrective jaw surgery
    procedures address functional issues, primarily the small mandible, to
    maximize the patient's airway, occlusion, and facial esthetics"--
    Provided by publisher.
Identifiers: LCCN 2020035755 | ISBN 9780867159660 (hardcover)
Subjects: MESH: Orthognathic Surgical Procedures--methods | Reconstructive
    Surgical Procedures--methods
Classification: LCC RK529 | NLM WU 600 | DDC 617.5/22059--dc23
LC record available at https://lccn.loc.gov/2020035755

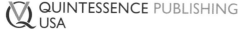

© 2021 Quintessence Publishing Co, Inc

Quintessence Publishing Co, Inc
411 N Raddant Road
Batavia, IL 60510
www.quintpub.com

5 4 3 2 1

Editor: Leah Huffman
Design: Sue Zubek
Production: Sarah Minor

Printed in the USA

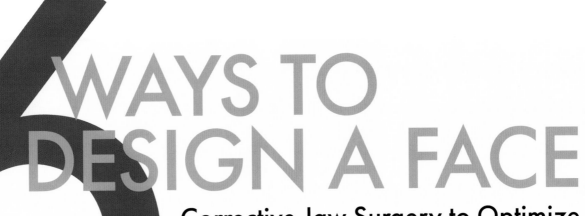

6 WAYS TO DESIGN A FACE

Corrective Jaw Surgery to Optimize Bite, Airway, and Facial Balance

Paul Coceancig, BDS, MDS-OMS, MB, ChB, FDSRCS, FRACDS-OMS

Specialist Facial Reconstruction Surgeon
Private Practice
Sydney, Australia

Illustrated by

Evan M. Stacey (Australia)   Paul Coceancig (Australia)
Angela P. Marty (Australia)   Pieter-Jan Belmans (Belgium)
Alessandra Coceancig (Italy)   Francisco Medina Guerra (Mexico)

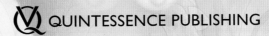 QUINTESSENCE PUBLISHING

Berlin | Chicago | Tokyo
Barcelona | London | Milan | Mexico City | Moscow | Paris | Prague | Seoul | Warsaw
Beijing | Istanbul | Sao Paulo | Zagreb

contents

foreword

Paul Coceancig is not the first dentist to correlate small jaws in adolescents with bad bites and crooked teeth, but his ideas about how to treat this condition—which seems to be rampant in Western society—depart significantly from established views.

Based on his extensive professional training and experience, and to some extent on the abysmal failure of his own orthodontic treatment as a teenager and again during dental school, Coceancig rejects the basic tenets of mainstream orthodontics, with its focus on the occlusion and its reliance on tooth extraction to make the teeth fit in the jaws. The long-term ramifications of this treatment approach—a disproportionate face, a collapsing tongue, and a compromised airway—are widespread and devastating to the overall health of patients.

Coceancig presents and argues very convincingly in favor of an alternative, holistic approach to correcting bad bites and crooked teeth that he has developed over many years, based on the premise that having 32 functional teeth is the natural and ideal state of every adult human. In his view, abnormal states of facial profile and bad bite fall on a spectrum, yet they all have exactly the same etiology—a small mandible. Furthermore, the most efficient way to permanently change a small jaw into one that is more proportionate to the rest of the face is through corrective jaw surgery, using simple distraction techniques that Coceancig has refined over many years with excellent results, as demonstrated by the dozens of well-documented cases he presents throughout his book.

By adopting Coceancig's philosophy and surgical protocol, oral and maxillofacial surgeons can reverse the cosmetic effects and correct for the orthodontic consequences of the small jaw in their adolescent patients. In addition, a variation of this surgery is highly effective in reversing the destructive consequences of a constricted airway on older people who have already developed obstructive sleep apnea (OSA) as a result of their small mandibles. By curing people of breathing difficulties, such as snoring, or of the risk or presence of OSA through corrective jaw surgery, the oral and maxillofacial surgeon is also helping to prevent a range of other diseases that are commonly associated with OSA.

Arun K. Garg, DMD
Miami, Florida

INTRODUCTION

For over a decade my wife has been persistently asking me to write a book about corrective facial skeletal surgery. I resisted for a while, thinking the process to be too big, too elaborate, and too broad. After all, the writing process is very introspective, which for me is very isolating, and requires significant time and dedicated sustained concentration. As my wife can attest, to successfully write a book comes at the sacrifice of children, parents, friends, referrers, business associates, and patients.

Over the course of my career up to this point, certain commonly held philosophies, tenets, and basic ideas concerning what is a face, what is abnormality, and what is considered corrective have all needed alteration. These questions and their evolving answers have shaped my thinking and conceptualization of the necessary solutions.

I suppose, in formulating a basis for what follows in this book, I first need to introduce who I am, where I came from, and what made me.

MY STORY

I began dentistry when I was 17 at the University of Sydney in Australia. The Australian profession was then, as it is now, extremely conservative. The professors all hailed from the Commonwealth, so we students became an ordered, intellectualized, and socially privileged group focused on the community benefit of uniformly applied oral health care. Australian style.

At 23, and newly graduated as a "dental surgeon," I took a job at the local public dental hospital, and while my classmates were entering private practice and buying new cars and homes, I learned to extract teeth and started my fellowship studies with the Royal Australasian College of Dental Surgeons, which opened the door to specialist training positions in oral surgery. This led me to meet Professor John Edgar deBurgh Norman AO, Associate Professor Geoffrey McKellar, and Drs Alf Coren and Peter Vickers, independently brilliant people who would take me into their hospitals and show me orthognathic surgery. I held a retractor and listened while they talked; they advised me to forget about extracting teeth and formed my intellectual connection to orthognathic surgery. Their confidence and mentorship supported an offer for me to enroll in a 5-year specialty oral and maxillofacial surgery (OMS) program across the Tasman Sea in New Zealand. I was the only applicant.

So at 25 I flew to Otago University in Dunedin, where I was enrolled in a shortened medical degree program and also started a combined 3-year specialty degree in oral surgery. I was transferred to the Christchurch Medical School the following year, and with my new girlfriend (now wife) beside me, over the next 4 years I continued to study undergraduate medicine part-time and extracted a lot of teeth, fixed broken jaws, and learned the Kiwi public hospital version of surgically working alongside orthodontists. New Zealand style.

I was 29 when I eventually graduated from both programs. I was a dental surgeon, I was a medical doctor, and now I was a Kiwi version of an oral and maxillofacial surgeon. I was also now married to a Kiwi and had a firstborn Kiwi daughter.

I wanted to return to Australia, so we packed up and headed home. After 2 years of certifying my New Zealand medical degree in Australia, I knew I needed just a couple more years of dedicated jaw surgery mentorship. Not wanting to pursue further training in the United Kingdom, luckily I received an offer from the Singapore General Hospital to work in a private-public capacity under Dr Raymond Peck Hong Lian, a British-trained maxillofacial surgeon. He was to become my final teacher. After almost 2 years of constant operating in this vestige of England surrounded by Asia, I came to practically learn everything there was then to know about corrective jaw surgery. Singapore style.

Sixteen years after starting my training in dentistry, I had completed my Australian specialty qualification in maxillofacial surgery (the FRACDS-OMS) and opened my private specialty office shortly thereafter in Newcastle, Australia. Mostly I extracted diseased teeth for dentists and perfectly good teeth for orthodontists. As it is for most maxillofacial surgeons worldwide, the majority of those teeth were crowded premolars and impacted third molars. Slowly, as confidence grew among my referring orthodontists, a small trickle of corrective jaw surgery cases came through my doors too.

Today my private practice is almost entirely derived from corrective jaw surgery. I now rarely extract teeth.

REFERRAL MODEL FOR CORRECTIVE JAW SURGERY

Because orthognathic surgery is rare, and because it is basically used only following failed specialist orthodontics, the general professional dental view of orthognathic surgery is mostly negative. There is little dental understanding of what corrective jaw surgery is. Rather than seeing orthognathic surgery as being therapeutic, medical, necessary, or something of high reliability or functionality, a referral for orthognathic surgery is often discouraged by the dentist as an unnecessary and highly risky extreme. This pervasive dental view that reduces all forms of jaw surgery to a limited role of only removing teeth means that orthognathic surgery is extremely rare. In all practicality, and regardless of training, most oral and maxillofacial surgeons are reduced only to the role of an oral surgeon.

Few private surgeons practically or routinely offer corrective jaw surgery procedures because orthognathic surgery is seen as secondary to orthodontics. The teeth are always corrected first, followed reluctantly by the jaws.

In all of my training, I was taught that orthognathic surgery was based upon a pragmatic premise of performing to what

Rather than seeing orthognathic surgery as being therapeutic, medical, necessary, or something of high reliability or functionality, a referral for orthognathic surgery is often discouraged by the dentist as an unnecessary and highly risky extreme.

an orthodontist wanted. There was simply no other source of referral. And to an enormous degree, this repeat stream of action-reaction generated a master-servant relationship. Orthodontists literally fed oral surgery practices, albeit with dental extractions and mostly impacted third molars, and to a much smaller degree with remedial orthognathic surgery when extraction-based orthodontics simply didn't work. To run a successful surgical business, I had to fundamentally believe in the orthodontic interpretation of everything to do with impacted and crowded teeth and in the primacy of orthodontists being the first to treat, examine, and interpret.

The major problem with this model, however, is that it traditionally ignores the face and the airway.

MY FIRST ORTHODONTIC EXPERIENCE

When I was 13 years old, my impacted canine tooth erupted extremely high behind my upper lip, and my mother recognized that it would never spontaneously be normal. In 1957, her 14-year-old sister had had an impacted and badly erupted canine removed on the advice of her orthodontist, and at 76 years old my Aunty Pam still complains bitterly of its effects on the symmetry and attractiveness of her face. As a surgical nurse trained at Sydney Hospital in Macquarie Street, my mother resolved in 1982 that her sister's fate would not also befall me, so she took me to a highly recommended Macquarie Street orthodontic specialist in Sydney.

He advised against my mother's proposal that expanding my maxilla would allow enough room to easily fit all my crooked teeth. He also said it was fanciful to believe that stimulating my maxilla to expand would somehow correct the underbite I was developing. He believed her proposal very controversial, impractical, and unfeasible. He further explained that I had a very flat middle face, that my cheekbones were naturally small, and that extracting the canine would indeed be a terrible idea and make the whole appearance of my face worse. I remember feeling very ugly.

My father was very skeptical about removing four perfectly good premolar teeth in order to orthodontically bring down a single impacted canine tooth. It was at this point that my mother asked if there was any way to surgically bring my maxilla forward. She suggested that this would improve my facial proportions and possibly make my nasal breathing better.

You see it was no coincidence that on this same famous Sydney street worked my allergist, who every month would give me a needle against my dust mite allergy. Further down in another building was my respiratory specialist who treated my chronic asthma. Next door to that was the ENT surgeon who had removed my tonsils when I was 4 years old. And of course there was also my pediatrician who tried to help me grow normally despite my early recurrent croup, ongoing throat infections, stuffy nose, bad bite, crooked teeth, low energy, chronic snoring, and everything else.

The blank look, slight facial twitch, and total quiet of the orthodontist spoke everything in his mind about that horrible suggestion. His considered reply, confident and calm and practiced, was to explain that my mandible was too big, and when I was old enough I could have it broken surgically to bring it backward. He commented that this operation was horrible and full of risks; it sounded dreadful. It was obvious that extracting some premolars was the infinitely lesser of two evils. He said it would give me a perfect smile. He had dental models that explained the logic of it all. A lateral cephalometric radiograph explained his mathematics. He gave examples. He gave prices. He was a highly regarded dental specialist.

My father wanted another opinion, but my mother wanted to go ahead. In the end they said it was my decision, and my 13-year-old brain certainly didn't want my jaw broken, and I certainly didn't like my underbite or the look of my impacted canine, and I certainly didn't want to look like my flat-faced aunty either. So I decided it was best to remove my premolars. Two visits, two needles, and two teeth on each side. They put them in a jar for me to take home. My mother cried.

My orthodontic appliances were placed a month later, and when they were eventually taken off 2 years later when I was 15, it was not the pretty smile result my parents or I had expected. Even my schoolteachers expressed dismay at the cosmetic result. Four on the floor, braces in 24. All my school friends had had it too. We all had the same straight-teeth, flat-face look. And so too did every other school kid

on the Sydney train network. One treatment fitted all. The famous Sydney smile was everywhere. I hadn't escaped my aunty's fate.

The orthodontic retainer was very hard to wear. My teeth moved; they became crooked again. The positive over-bite the orthodontist had struggled to gain by pulling my mandibular anterior teeth backward and maxillary anterior teeth forward gradually, relentlessly became edge-to-edge. Eventually I had a reverse bite again. My troublesome canine popped out of alignment. I saw my orthodontist every 6 months for follow-up, and every time he just told me to keep wearing my retainer. It was unbearable.

When I finished school and started university, I started experiencing jaw pain. After fabricating my own bite splint, which turned out to be useless, I visited my orthodontist, telling him that I was now a dental student. Essentially I was asking him as a mentor now to help me put all the random problems together, to help me fix them, to fix me. He smiled, said he was proud of me, said I must be stressed from all the study, and promptly referred me to an oral surgeon down the street to have my third molars removed.

When I turned up, the oral surgeon simply filled out a Sydney Hospital booking form. When I asked why I had to get my third molars removed, he told me that my parents had paid for braces and the orthodontist had asked, and of course because of the tooth crowding that came from not wearing my retainer. He wasn't interested in my jaw pain, saying it would clear up after the third molars were removed anyway. The fact that he was too busy and important to look at me for all the 5 minutes I was in his office made me start to doubt these people. All of them. The dentists who taught me. The dentists who treated me. The science that surrounded everything to do with how faces and bites developed and how they developed together. No one ever really explained anything to me, either as a patient or as a dental student. It was all a complete and illogical mystery to me. Why did everyone need braces for crowded teeth? Why did every kid I know have to have their premolars and third molars removed? Why did everyone need their tonsils out? Why did everyone have allergies, asthma, stress, and jaw pain? Here I was surrounded by books and people and institutions that should have been able to explain it all logically and coherently and scientifically, but they didn't. I kept wondering how I could have all of these unrelatable separate diseases affecting me? It was like one diagnosis per doctor. Damn was I unlucky.

I decided not to get my third molars removed, and they erupted normally (and I still have them). My jaw pain resolved by simply not chewing anything, my nasal allergies cleared up when I moved out of my parent's home and into a series of new student houses, and coincidentally I discovered a love for lap swimming, which also saw my allergic rhinitis, atopic eczema, and chronic asthma all miraculously clear up. It seemed all I had to do was escape Macquarie Street and my mum's insistence on the perfection of a Macquarie Street medical mind.

MY SECOND ORTHODONTIC EXPERIENCE

After moving to New Zealand and talking with many surgeons about what jaw surgery really was, I was still too afraid of it for myself. There was just so little known about it, and the jaw surgeons I worked with in training were mostly operating on syndromal kids and car accident victims. Besides, pushing my mandible backward simply to get a better bite seemed the opposite of what I needed, and my surgical mentors agreed. I was convinced it would surely choke me too, wouldn't it? No one seemed to agree with me on the potential breathing issues, but nonetheless I thought it was my maxilla that needed to be brought forward, which supported my mother's original, though very radical suggestion some 12 years previously. In the meantime I had orthodontic appliances put back on to see if I could achieve at least a stable bite and a smile I could live with.

In 1995 my new orthodontist was adamant that the science and predictability of maxillary surgery was still a long way off. The SARME (surgically assisted rapid maxillary expansion) operation was just getting a foothold in the United States, Professor Maurice Mommaerts in Belgium was still 5 years away from developing his bone-borne palatal expansion device, jaw distraction technology was just starting (and badly), routine jaw correction surgery was just beginning a radical renaissance via Bill Arnett in the United States, and custom titanium plates for midfacial surgery wouldn't be developed in France for another 20 years.

My new orthodontist was convinced he could "grow" my small maxilla with a slower treatment cycle and edgewise brackets. I decided to believe him, and I endured another 2 years of orthodontic appliances, which didn't manage to grow anything of course. Silly me. I still had a flat midface, a too-big mandible, and a weird smile. And I snored. But I did have straight front teeth in a barely normal positive overbite.

SELF-REFLECTION AND FRUSTRATION

What this repeat orthodontic experience did for me was point out that I could not explain my own face to myself. I could not form a rational argument with an orthodontist. I could not see how all of my component layers and the interrelated parts fitted together three dimensionally. I could not see how my teeth sat in my dental bone, or how the dental bone sat in my jawbones, or how my jawbones sat in my face. I could hardly dissect myself. I could not see where my symmetry or proportionality or bite issues began or ended. And if I couldn't see them or simply describe them, how could I direct myself to seek the treatment that I needed or understand or critically examine the orthodontic advice I was receiving? And how could I seek to describe anyone's bite or jaw problems or aim to surgically treat what was evidentially a complex interrelational set of anatomical issues involving many medical and dental and cosmetic themes?

In the 1980s and 1990s there was very little known about how anyone could dynamically see inside a person. There were radiographs of course, but these produced flat 2D views. What I wanted to know was how to construct a whole face, how teeth sat three dimensionally in the pattern of the midface, and how that related to all the structures inside it and outside of it.

Having maintained a schoolboy interest in optics and physics and mathematics, I wanted to build a stereoscopic device to create 3D radiographic images so that I could demonstrate to my teachers my ruminative concepts on volumetric facial radiology. Eventually I made a simple 3D radiographic model of a face. With it I could effectively demonstrate the acquisition and diagnostic simplicity of volumetric imaging. This thing seemed real. It shimmered just in front of the viewer and showed everything in perfect fidelity and accuracy; behind to front, side to side. It was very dramatic when I first saw it, and for everyone since that has seen it too.

After contacting a German engineering scientist who had written on a similar concept decades earlier, soon enough I had a couple of German employees of Siemens visit me in New Zealand to see my setup. I used my physical model as a visual means of explaining the mental image of the future of maxillofacial surgery that I had. I explained that digitizing a series of plain radiographs from a rotating x-ray machine, assigning numerical values to the grayness of the pixels in the image, and then cross-referencing the values to adjacent images obtained in a circle and traveling around an object would enable a suitably powerful computer algorithm to build up the pixels (now voxels) into a 3D space. The Germans were developing this same idea for use in cardiothoracic and arterial imaging using the 1984 work of Feldkamp, Davis, and Kress. While I had no idea how to develop an algorithm to accurately 3D fix the gray value points, I was adamant that the technology, if developed, would be extremely useful in dentistry and for maxillofacial surgery in particular.

I was sure that a dentist could have a unit in the office no bigger than an orthopantomogram machine and three dimensionally image things as fine as a tooth's root canal system or see entire dental arches and bites.

For me, all I wanted was a simply acquired means of explaining that the face, teeth, jaws, and everything else were part of one complex 3D object. I wanted to be able to see into, expand, revolve, and better imagine facial growth disorders and the corrective jaw surgery steps needed to manage them. Once I had that, I could then describe the symmetry and proportions of the skeleton and dentition of a face. And then I could scan many people and compare them, and see patterns, and maybe move on from there. But I never heard from the German Siemens scientists again.

Many years later, I ran into my old boss, Leslie Snape, at a conference. He told me he still has my invention sitting on a bench in a closed room somewhere in the bowels of Christchurch Hospital. He calls it the original cone beam. I just laugh. I call it a Kiwi version of cone beam. If it can't be made with pantyhose and sheep-fencing wire, it's not worth calling it a practical invention. (That's a Kiwi joke.)

PUTTING IT ALL TOGETHER

Today of course, we have software applications much more sophisticated than cone beam that can accurately duplicate the entire head, segmentalize it, and separate the component parts. It's upon this digital version of the patient that we can replicate real-life surgery and the volume changes affecting tongues, airways, faces, temporomandibular joints, and bites. One of the best things about digital imagery is that you can start explaining complex things to your patients. It means that I can reduce a compound anatomical narrative to the common language of the visual medium. I still need a certain kind of intellectual ability on the part of my patients, but increasingly the patients who do independently find me are naturally skilled in broad research and innate logic.

Over the years my jaw surgery practice has naturally divided itself between two broad arms.

The first is that I am providing some form of remedial surgical treatment, usually well after orthodontics has come and gone, and usually only in adults who are deliberately seeking my direct care. The majority of these people snore or have health or lifestyle issues related in some way to their ease of breathing. These people find me because they researched their personal symptoms, asked themselves logical questions, and sought a means to explain everything that has and is happening in their lives as one set of interrelated health issues. These people are generally free of an orthodontist referral.

> In effect, I offer two ends of a stick. One is a simple end where I use a simple operation to prevent bigger problems, and the other is a complex end where I treat really big problems using really big operations.

The second arm usually involves young adolescents who are accompanied by parents, who have first brought their child to an orthodontist, usually for an overbite correction. These patients usually have an orthodontist's referral. They are usually the hardest to treat, firstly because they did not independently seek me, secondly because they require a complex and seemingly contrived explanation they do not really want to hear, and thirdly because parents naturally see jaw correction surgery as incredibly invasive.

The ironic thing is that IMDO (intermolar mandibular distraction osteogenesis) is the simplest surgical operation that I offer. It is even simpler than third molar removal, and it usually helps avoid the third molar surgery that is part and parcel of normal orthodontics for overbite correction (not to mention it helps avoid everything else too). But the greatest benefit of IMDO in this second practice arm is that it prevents these adolescent patients from becoming patients in the first practice arm—the adults who come to me for snoring or other problems that lead to jaw surgery remediation through remedial BIMAX (advancement of both jaws).

In effect, I offer two ends of a stick. One is a simple end where I use a simple operation to prevent bigger problems, and the other is a complex end where I treat really big problems using really big operations. Any medical enterprise has two ends like this. At one end are the treatments of the disease after it has occurred. At the other end is the research and the development and the application of treatments that prevent that disease from occurring in the first place.

Why do parents who have children with small jaws and big overbites persist with a belief that orthodontics alone fixes everything? If someone asks me what the true cost is of treating someone with a small jaw, then that total cost must include tonsillectomies, dentistry, oral surgery, orthodontics, TMJ therapy, rhinoplasties, chin implants, sleep studies, CPAP (continuous positive airway pressure) therapy, and finally remedial jaw surgery. But I can only collate these costs if I tie all those things together as one linked or total series. So this question of whether adolescent dental crowding, or bad bites, or even small jaws has any other consequence apart from braces is obviously a very pertinent one. Is there really a link to adult obstructive sleep apnea (OSA)? Will the adult eventually insist on cosmetic intervention? Are impacted third molars inevitable or can they be prevented? Is there any way of correcting a bad bite before it starts? Is there any way to prevent snoring or OSA from ever developing?

There were a number of events that occurred in my life that set me on the intellectual and professional pathway that I now lead. At some point it occurred to me that a narrow dental arch was more a case of a narrow nasal airway. At some point it occurred to me that a small jaw and an obstructing tongue were part of the same condition. At some point it occurred to me that dental crowding and impacted teeth in adolescents presaged the development of OSA in late adulthood. At some point it occurred to me that everything that I was taught in becoming a dentist was not the sum of everything I could know and that it could be built upon.

This book is in effect a chronicle of those ideas and their assimilation into a complex philosophy and then a practical set of new operations and new treatments. My six ways to design a face include IMDO, GenioPaully, custom BIMAX, SuperBIMAX, custom PEEK, and SARME. I am not the inventor of any of these things. The appearance of their originality is a silk screen, behind which lies an indescribably complex history and the serial and compounded efforts and stories of millions of people.

It is unimaginable to me that any person would willingly submit themselves to any of these operations, however simple or complex. Although I have always acted gently and hopefully painlessly, and with compassion and with precision, it is another level completely to trust themselves to be the first to an operation never before performed, let alone believed. So I'd like to thank the patients whose stories illustrate this book. If there is an inventor, it was the individual child who would suggest to me that their condition was curable.

If only I would become as imaginative as their own mind in describing their own condition, and a match to their inspirational hope.

1
REIMAGINING ORTHODONTICS AND ORAL SURGERY

History should never be ignored, but it always is. In every clinical discipline, fundamental premises or truths exist to drive the culture, practice, and scientific enterprise of that specific clinical group. History establishes how one thought or practice began and of course leads to another and the next. Through history we see why we do things a certain way today. It is in history that we see how our forebears interpreted the same observations we still see, and how their older philosophies of care underpin our modern clinical practices and wider community expectation.

Not all clinical disciplines are necessarily in agreement with each other. Chiropractors, osteopaths, and naturopaths undoubtedly disagree with physicians over many things. But no matter their underpinnings (respective of philosophical or scientific premise), almost all clinical groups were initially founded by a single person (or guru or saint). And yet we pretend that because we live in today, that it specifically equates to modernness or betterness, and what was in the past—which is by default old or ancient—has no part to play in how we think or practice today.

Our modern disciplines have evolved to be rooted only in new science, eternal debate, and collective polite argument. We can only accuse the other distant craft group of quackery. As proper scientific doctors we simply cannot believe that deception and magic and nonscience and esotericism can exist in ourselves. But is there really any true separation of modern practice from older practice? Are our modern treatments really so different to our founding fathers' so many centuries or decades or years ago? Are we really doing so much better? Consider Fig 1-1.

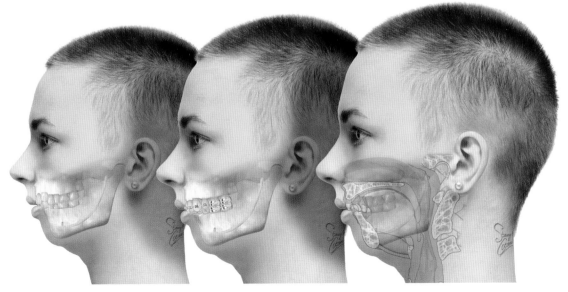

FIG 1-1 Traditional orthodontics alone with dental extractions and removal of impacted third molars will result in straight anterior teeth, but this century-old, well-established, and universally accepted treatment ignores the why and how of tooth crowding, as well as how the airways, face, tongue, jaws, and teeth are all indivisibly interrelated.

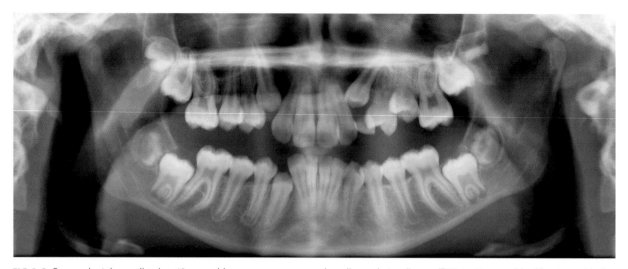

FIG 1-2 Severe dental crowding in a 12-year-old as seen on a panoramic radiograph. In a "normal" 12- to 13-year-old, without considering the third molars, the 28 permanent teeth should all erupt into a Class I occlusion, and there should be no retained primary teeth. Multiple impacted canines and second molars and impending impacted third molars can be orthodontically seen as a dental state of "late eruptive development" or of "premolar or third molar redundancy" or simply as "too many teeth." By contrast, the maxillofacial surgeon's view is to see that there is a normal developing complement of 32 adult teeth, there is a primary smallness of the jaws, there are codeveloping facial and airway problems, and all of it can only formally be evaluated by total-head 3D head analysis, or via volumetric medical CT imaging.

ORTHODONTIC DIAGNOSIS

Orthodontics was largely introduced by Edward Angle in 1895. He described the classification of "malocclusion"—a Latinization he invented to describe a "bad bite"—as Class I, Class II (division 1 or 2), or Class III. Orthodontists today still use the Angle classification of malocclusion to "diagnose" orthodontic cases, adding words such as "mild" or "severe" to further describe these classes followed by other descriptors such as "redundant" or "impacted" teeth or incisor relationship or jaw-profile association.

In the context of a purely dental clinical examination, a 12-year-old child with prominent maxillary anterior teeth may be described as a "severe Class II bilateral molar malocclusion, with significant incisor overjet, deep incisor overbite, and moderate mandibular incisor crowding, with impacted maxillary canines and impending third molar impactions" (see Fig 1-2).

Further dental analysis can be given with lateral cephalometry (Fig 1-3). The measurements of angles and proportions of certain points and positions of the facial bones and skull base began in the late 19th century, alongside the science of anthropometry, which eventually incorporated radiographic imaging in the early 20th century. The language of modern cephalometry is orthodontically oriented. It has its own culture bred from a hundred different voices with racially separated data sets identifying what

is "normal" and "abnormal." It exists only for orthodontists and today is rarely used by jaw correction surgeons.

Dental orthopantomogram (OPG; Fig 1-2) analysis, also known as *panoramic radiography*, allows a better assessment of the teeth and mandible, but it is a highly distorted view. Even used together, panoramic radiography and lateral cephalometry are still poor descriptors of jaw and facial volumes and proportionality, and they are completely inadequate in assessing both airways and faces (Fig 1-4).

Yet the extrapolation from dental radiographic analysis to dental clinical pathway persists because it is formalized. Parents believe it to be true, and of course dental professionals believe it to be true. We all collectively and repeatably participate. The orthodontic waiting room is full of kids with braces and elastics. Our society is convinced that braces and dental extractions and orthodontics are all noninvasive and essentially benign and normal processes. But what we potentially ignore is the obvious fact that the 12-year-old sitting in front of us now will be an adult later on (Fig 1-5). And all of the dental analysis that is geared toward directing an adolescent orthodontic process, a process centered only on the negative esthetic of big anterior teeth, intrinsically ignores the biggest issue of them all—the ongoing lifetime effects, which started at birth and will end in old age, of what caused the bad bites and dental crowding and permanent tooth impactions to occur in the first place: the small mandible.

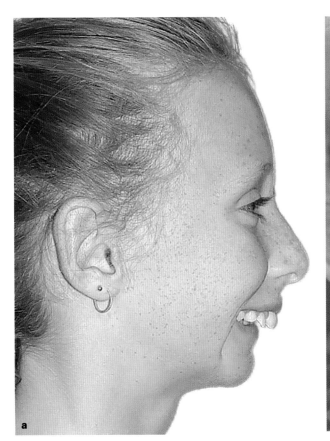
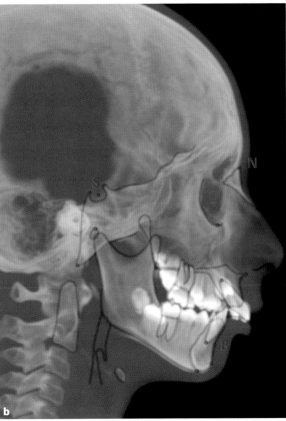

FIG 1-3 *(a and b)* An assessment of the profile of the same 12-year-old child with prominent maxillary anterior teeth may now include an orthodontic description of the jaw base. The cephalometric analysis evolves the orthodontic diagnosis as "severe Class II bilateral molar malocclusion, with significant incisor overjet, deep incisor overbite, and moderate mandibular incisor crowding, with impacted maxillary canines and impending second and third molar impactions, on a platform of anterior maxillary excess shown by excessive SNA angle and mild SNB angle deficiency." While the airway can be imagined on a lateral cephalogram, it is often poorly seen. Inherent postures such as neck uprightness and unnatural head position coupled with the awake state as well as transient states such as breath holding, swallowing, jaw posturing, general movement, and lip pursing, not to mention the general anxiety of the child entering the x-ray machine, all affect how the soft tissues tense and move as well as how reliably they can be interpreted or referenced. In my view, which is supported by meta-analysis,[1] the best measurement to determine whether a mandible truly lengthens due to an interventional orthodontic or surgical mandibular treatment is to compare the SNB angle on serial lateral cephalometry. Measuring changes in the SNB angle is relatively free of the confounder of growth and is not affected by genioplasty or GenioPaully. An accurate SNB measurement requires that the child does not posture the jaw forward—a notoriously difficult thing, as natural jaw joint position on lateral cephalometry is extremely difficult to confirm. The full treatment for this case is presented in chapter 9, along with our method of validating her surgical outcomes.

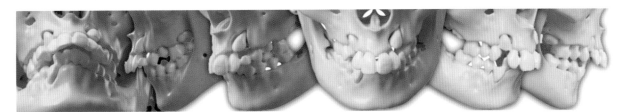

FIG 1-4 A better way than lateral cephalometry is to assess the interplay of teeth and bone as volumes in three dimensions. But this hard tissue 3D view does not see the soft tissues, and it does not visualize the airway or those anatomical structures that influence it. The competition of the dental perspective, which sees excessive and crowded teeth that together form a malocclusion, versus the medical perspective, which sees small jaw volumes and compromised airways and altered facial form, catches the parent between complex philosophical arguments. The crystal clear alternatives are divided as *(1)* traditional camouflage orthodontics based on dental extractions (including third molars) and *(2)* early interventional surgery through the intermolar mandibular distraction osteogenesis (IMDO) protocol. The winner or loser of that choice can only ever be the child and future adult.

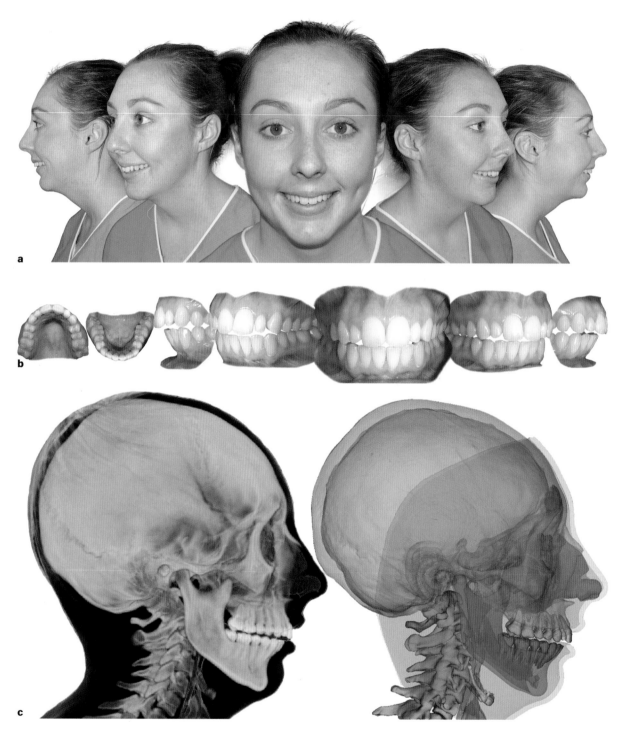

FIG 1-5 This patient had been treated with orthodontic bite splints and expert nonextraction camouflage orthodontics since the age of 12 years for a significant dental overjet and severe dental crowding. *(a)* At age 20 years, after having her third molars removed, she presented with complaints of significant breathing issues, general exercise intolerance, and a chronic forward head posture that she found impossible to correct by "standing up straight." While she had not yet developed full obstructive sleep apnea (OSA), she knew she snored, and she knew her small mandible had a big part to play in the history of her issues. For this patient, remedial jaw surgery coupled with repeat orthodontics offered a significant chance of permanent cure for her airway, bite, and posture problems. *(b)* With her jaw seated anatomically in its natural joint positions, her teeth only met at the back of her mouth, with a significant anterior open bite. The forward head posture and poor chin-neck contour are significant esthetic concerns. *(c)* Digitally derived lateral cephalometry with medical computed tomography (CT) or dental CBCT has significantly evolved from the traditional plain x-ray machine. Segmentation of color rendering allows for clear visualization of teeth, jaws, airway, and cervical posture. Such rendering not only improves diagnostic performance for the dentist but also helps the patient understand the complex interlinks of airway, bite, skeleton, and face. In this case, even with extreme forward head positioning, forward collapse of the cervical spine is still pushing into the back of the tongue, significantly reducing airway lumen and causing pronounced airway obstruction during sleep and during erect exercise.

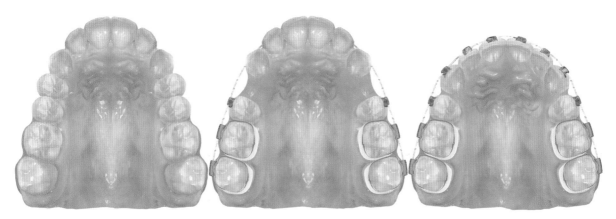

FIG 1-6 Extracting premolars to create dental space for orthodontic decrowding, or retraction of prominent anterior teeth, is the basis for all camouflage orthodontics used for the treatment of Class II, division 1 malocculsion.

DENTAL EXTRACTIONS AND TRADITIONAL ORTHODONTICS

Almost all humans have the genetic potential to develop and keep 32 adult teeth. But almost all adolescents have dental crowding as their adult dentition erupts, giving the visual illusion that there are an excessive number of adult teeth. And almost all adolescents with dental crowding will develop impactions of the third molars; this near-universal impaction in people with crowded teeth gives an illusion that third molars are redundant or evolutionarily unnecessary to modern human existence. Because we have people in modern society whose craft it is to treat this human commonality of dental crowding, if a child with crowded teeth has a mother wanting to treat that crowding or crookedness with classical orthodontics, then braces combined with dental extractions of any of those 32 adult teeth through oral surgery is inevitable.

Crowded or overly prominent anterior teeth, or any bad bite (whether Class I, II, or III) for that matter, usually results in premolar extractions (Fig 1-6). While this is considered "minor oral surgery" because it is performed in-office by the dentist, it is by no means "minor" to the individual losing these teeth. Combine this with third molar removal, and a given orthodontic patient is losing a minimum of six to eight permanent teeth. Even if "nonextraction" treatment is selected in clinical orthodontics (Fig 1-7), third molar removal is still almost universally required. So if an adolescent has dental crowding, or a malocclusion, or dental impactions, or all of these together, then dental extractions carry an almost 100% certainty in late adolescence or early adulthood.

From a total of 32 teeth, and following classical orthodontic treatment for dental crowding, the end result will almost never be 32 teeth. The end result will be 28, 26, or 24 teeth. If you lose four premolars and four third molars, these lost eight "back" teeth represent a certain loss of occlusal table and dental volume, not to mention upward of ~33% loss in total dental mass (Fig 1-8). These lost teeth will also not develop associated alveolar bone or gingiva to support them, and they will not support the face that surrounds them.

Non-jaw surgeons may empiricize that corrective jaw surgery is invasive. But what equal professional rationalism exists to explain or accept that permanently removing one-third of a child's dental mass through a combination of classical orthodontics and traditional oral surgery is not considered invasive? In my view, traditional orthodontics inherently relies upon invasiveness and is quite the opposite of conservative.

Nevertheless, this competition between ideas of conservatism, easiness, or invasiveness only considers the teeth. Are there other things we are ignoring by insisting on focusing and diminishing our diagnosis or treatments to the teeth alone? In demonizing the other professional, it's easy to ignore what we do not know or see or talk about, or worse, what we refuse to acknowledge.

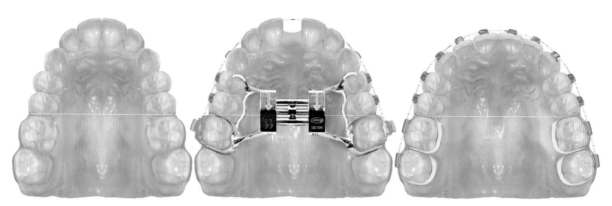

FIG 1-7A For Class II, division 1 malocculusion, not extracting premolars requires expansion and then orthodontic retraction of prominent anterior teeth as the created midline gap is closed. This backward retraction further potentiates the chance of maxillary third molar impactions. How this combination or pattern of orthodontics ultimately leads to other facial and airway effects is described in chapter 12.

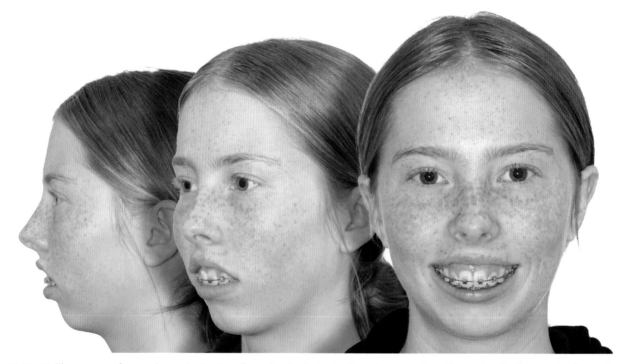

FIG 1-7B The process of expansion and retraction of prominent anterior teeth produces an elongation and vertically excessive "gumminess" to the anterior teeth and accentuates the original lip incompetence associated with the small mandible. This pattern of camouflage orthodontics is a leading cosmetic drive and preamble to later remedial BIMAX surgery. This patient's treatment is explained in Fig 15-14.

NONDENTAL CONSEQUENCES OF TRADITIONAL LEAD-ORTHODONTICS

Lead-orthodontics is what I call treatment where orthodontics comes first. The orthodontist is the first to assess the bad bite and the dental crowding. Everything that follows is as a consequence of the orthodontic event that preceded it, or of the orthodontic assessment, or of the orthodontic diagnosis. The entire conversation revolves around the orthodontic management of teeth (Figs 1-9 and 1-10).

As a maxillofacial surgeon, I clinically see three broad age groups of people. The first group are adolescents (10–21 years old) with a full complement of crowded adult teeth and a bad bite looking to keep everything and in a perfect face, forever. The second group are adults (22–49 years old) unhappy with the gummy smiles and cosmetic facial disproportions they attribute to camouflage orthodontics. And finally there is the middle-aged group (50+ years) with a history of orthodontics and dental extractions who now snore and have thick necks and uncontrollable

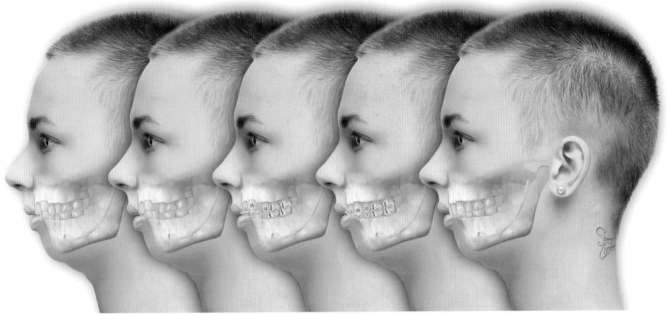

FIG 1-8 Extraction-based orthodontics of Class I dental crowding in adolescence. Four premolar extractions are a staple of almost all orthodontic practice. The third molar impactions that almost inevitably co-arise will eventually lead to a consideration of their extraction, premised on an idea of them being redundant or unnecessary. But removing eight teeth leads to a ~33% reduction in dental mass. In assessing only the bite, there is no assessment of the face or future adult airway. Forward planning toward how the adult face will look—after the orthodontics is completed—is entirely ignored.

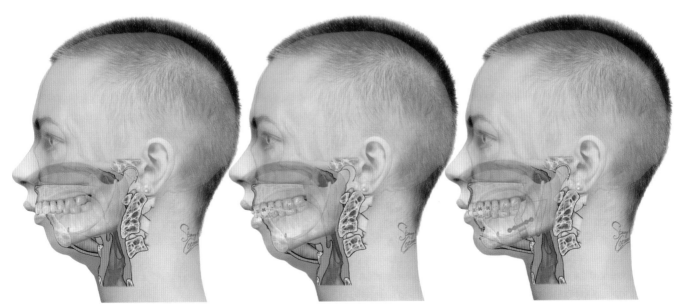

FIG 1-9 In treating without orthodontic extractions, traditional lead-orthodontics for Class II, division 1 malocclusion aims to attempt some retraction of the maxillary anterior teeth. A vertical gumminess results, with parted lips, accentuated by the lack of chin often associated with anterior mandibular hypoplasia (AMHypo). Orthodontic retraction (Class II) elastics also train the patient to hold the mandible forward while awake. After the impacted third molars are removed, the lip incompetence and chronic forward jaw posturing can be relieved with a small advancement bilateral sagittal split osteotomy (BSSO) into a Class I bite, with upward sliding genioplasty to improve lip seal. This basic form of jaw correction surgery is always and only done under the primary direction and recommendation of the treating orthodontist, and almost always with current orthodontics in place in order to help "settle the bite." Because the geniohyoid is not greatly stretched or advanced by either the sliding genioplasty or the small BSSO, there is only a small advancement of the airway—certainly not to a degree that would permanently overcome the total effect of glossoptosis or future risk of developing OSA.

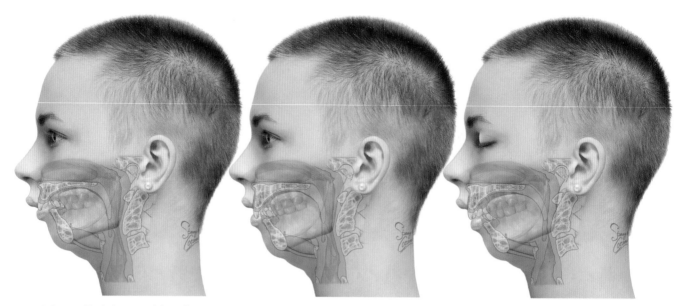

FIG 1-10 By their constraining effect and pull-back on the maxilla, all jaw splints, including MyoBrace, TwinBlock, Herbst, and Frankel, will partially "correct" the maxillary anterior tooth prominence of Class II malocclusion, but this effect is entirely by restricting growth of the maxilla, by pulling the maxillary anterior teeth backward and downward, and by positioning the mandible forward during waking hours. As a Cochrane review demonstrates,[1] there is no proof that jaw splints will grow a child's small mandible or act any differently to any other form of camouflage orthodontics. MyoBrace offers no scientific support for their marketing and therapeutic claims that they "grow the small mandible." At night, the supine child, adolescent, or adult will fall asleep, and as conscious tone is lost, the tongue and jaw will completely relax backward to obstruct the airway, thus reversing any daytime influence of such presumed tongue training and awake forward jaw posturing. The eventual effect of all camouflage nonextraction orthodontic therapies for Class II is therefore the same—to shrink the maxilla, produce a gummy smile, and help train the adolescent to hold the mandible forward, but only when awake.

> For every person with a bad bite,
> there are three combined, interwoven,
> inseparable treatment considerations:
> occlusion, airway, face.

weight gain. In reality these three groups are really the same people, with the same anatomical conditions, just at different stages of their lives.

This book explains how each of these groups can be managed with one overlying simple clinical philosophy, and that is to include a surgical treatment from the start. The jaw surgeon has never *not* been part of the equation of the treatment of bad bites. Likewise, it is not possible to ignore or delete orthodontics from that equation either. But the relationship between the two sides must be reinterpreted to correctly solve it. As I will come to elaborate in this book, orthodontics and oral surgery go hand in hand. They developed together from the start. Whether I operate on jaws to remove third molars or operate on jaws to fundamentally fix jaw size, the operations are fundamentally the same, and

they are performed almost the same way, and with a similar collaborative orthodontic effort. All that changes is primacy.

Maxillofacial surgeons are the absolute and only experts in facial disease and of facial abnormality and skeletal facial issues, all of which are associated with bad bites, crowded teeth, airways, and of course the face. The maxillofacial surgeon still needs orthodontics, but the relationship has changed. The roles have swapped.

For every person with a bad bite, there are three combined, interwoven, inseparable treatment considerations: occlusion, airway, face.

OUR ILLUSTRATIONS

In order to properly compare all the treatment types and ideas of anatomical derangement that lead to malocclusion, and in order to make meaningful assessments of the effects of treatments on facial proportions and airways and across ages, this book uses a single model—an imaginary female as she transitions through life. In the 7th century Pythagoras described six ages of man: infancy (0–6 years),

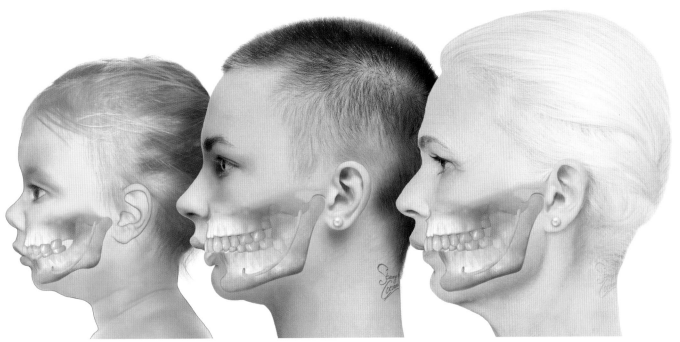

FIG 1-11 Seeing a person through the ages. In this case at 24 months, 17 years, and 65 years, respectively. Proportionally, the small mandible is eternal. Understanding why small mandibles are so common, and their link to dental crowding, bad bites, and airway obstruction, is a primary subject of this book.

adolescence (7–21 years), adulthood (22–49 years), middle age (50–62 years), old age (63–79 years), and advanced age (80+ years). This book illustrates the model at three of these ages (Fig 1-11): infancy (around age 2 years), adolescence (around age 17 years), and old age (around age 65 years). Throughout the book you will see only her relaxed facial profile with teeth together, both awake and asleep.

This model was built by merging data from real CT scans, precise anatomical segmentations of hard and soft tissues, and a lifetime of study involving many thousands of people to determine the interlinks between facial profile, airway, jaws, and occlusion. Peppered among these illustrations are real examples of actual patients and procedures that best illustrate my concepts that underlie both facial surgical and orthodontic diagnosis, as well as the comparative therapeutic and cosmetic benefits of this treatment or that.

For instance, the illustrations explaining the mechanism of thumb sucking were directly derived from the volumetric scans of a real infant who had developed anterior open bite. The images were donated by a Sydney-based radiology house who had examined an intubated child in a Sydney-based pediatric-care ICU. He had developed life-threatening suppurant pansinusitis following advice to his mother to actively cease his thumb sucking habit.

CT scans of infants are profoundly rare. But with this single image set came our first proof of the importance of nasal breathing to developing a normal healthy state of the nasal sinuses. With it too came an understanding of the developmental compromise committed upon the maxilla and sinuses by the small mandible and glossoptosis, as well as the contribution that normal nasal breathing gave to normal midfacial development. It also pointed out to us that dental advice that demonizes thumb sucking in order to prevent the development of anterior open bite was harmful in that it deleted the "why" the child was thumb sucking in the first place.

Another illustration base focused on a single midadolescent female and the effect that IMDO had upon correcting her Class II malocclusion and in normalizing her small mandible. It was through this patient that we precisely studied the effects of tongue muscle pull, particularly the geniohyoid muscle, and its relief upon glossoptosis. These CT scans were painstakingly rendered in 3D to accurately demonstrate the multiple dental, facial, and airway issues associated with anterior mandibular hypoplasia (AMHypo).

There is very little that differentiates one human from another. The tiny genetic differences that distinguish a Finn from a native Peruvian would account for less than 0.0001% of the entire human genome. Yet it is in the expression

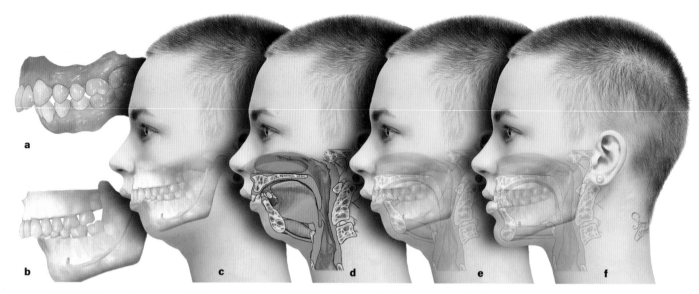

FIG 1-12 How various anatomical layers are interpreted. *(a)* View of how a dentist, parent, or orthodontist may see the relationship of maxillary and mandibular teeth in the mouth, or within an intraoral photograph. The patient may hold the mandible forward, altering the true bite relationship, but this visual oral examination is blind to jaw joint position. *(b)* A radiograph such as an OPG or even a lateral cephalogram gives little obvious further elaboration upon the visual beyond an examination of tooth roots, or at best the mandibular outline. There is no true elaboration on jaw joints, neutral jaw joint seating, or the overlying face itself. *(c)* The skeletal, dental, and facial relationships can be married, but this view still ignores the internal. *(d)* Cross-sectional views help understand toned (awake) tongue muscle contraction and airway patency. *(e)* Fusion of all pretreatment elements allows us to see the combined awake and erect relationships of the tongue, jaws, teeth, occlusion, airway, jaw joints, and facial effects that combine as a result of the small mandible. *(f)* The directed surgical treatment of part *c* to fundamentally correct the mandibular volume demonstrates a comparative means of seeing how dental impactions, malocclusion, airway collapse, tongue contraction, and facial profile may change toward an ideal anatomical state.

of this tiny genetic difference that we examine all that is different between ourselves, or groups of ourselves. In studying faces and jaws and bites, what we are looking for is a common fundamental link that gives the human commonality for all the various patterns of dental crowding and the connected link to inner airways and overlying facial form. And it is through these same illustrations that we can examine the effects of bespoke facial design that augments the therapeutic facial surgical intervention—six ways.

ORTHODONTIC CLASSIFICATIONS OF MALOCCLUSION

Malocclusion is a dental term, and it relates to the teeth alone. The Angle classification was invented before we had radiographs or CT scans or even a modern understanding of functional facial anatomy. As such, the Angle classification of malocclusion is outdated and, frankly, not useful to a description of orthognathics. More importantly, this classification is exclusionary in that it does not define why the condition of malocclusion exists. By only looking at teeth, the Angle classification inherently excludes any understanding

of the volume effects of jaws, particularly their effect on facial profiles, the postural effects on the tongue, and the overall lifetime effects of the compromised inner airway.

In my worldview, there are six methods for looking at malocclusion in profile (Fig 1-12). First, you can look at the teeth and gingiva and their intra-arch relationship. Second, you can look at how the malocclusion state relates to the underlying local dental skeleton. Third, you can look at how the dental skeleton and bite relate to the profile of the face. Fourth, you can look at how the whole facial skeleton relates to the inner airway. Fifth, you can look at the way the occlusion, skeleton, face, and airway combine simultaneously. And finally, you can look at the way that a given therapy affects all four anatomical states in terms of dynamic posture (asleep vs awake, smiling vs relaxed, supine vs erect).

Considering the different orthodontic classifications for malocclusion, this chapter presents 1:1 illustrations (see Figs 1-13 to 1-16) to demonstrate that all forms of common malocclusion are derived from the same basic common smallness of the mandible, or what I call *anterior mandibular hypoplasia* (AMHypo). Illustrations are made with a chin button (normogenia) or without a chin button (agenia), but note that almost all people with AMHypo also have some form of agenia. You will notice that those who have a chin button have a subtly greater pull on the geniohyoid muscle, with slightly greater patency of the airway behind the epiglottis (the so-called C3ERPO point, or 3rd **C**ervical, upper **E**piglottic, **R**etropharyngeal **O**bstruction point), and slightly more defined chin-neck contour. This may indicate a view that the natural chin button has an evolutionary function in stretching the geniohyoid to help overcome glossoptosis, but this is not my opinion. I honestly do not know why some humans have chin buttons, except that they look good. My therapeutic opinion is that the surgical GenioPaully, which creates a chin button, does have these therapeutic airway effects, as well as a primary effect on the lower lip posture, lip competency, and general esthetic lines that are drawn.

> Which profile the patient displays, and which treatment philosophy you choose, will define everything that will follow. The only fundamental differences are whether there is agenia or not, AMHypo or not, and maxillary hypoplasia or not.

All illustrations have a full complement of 32 teeth—in various patterns of eruption or crowding or alignment or development or impaction. In each series of this set of four, part *a* shows a normal mandible, with or without a chin button. Parts *b* to *f* show AMHypo with and without agenia, respectively. In *b* to *f*, the small mandible proportions are exactly the same between each illustration, and only the pattern of dental crowding is different. All have impacted third molar development as well.

Parts *c* to *f* show AMHypo as well as relative small-ness of the maxilla, known as *maxillary hypoplasia*, which is always associated with additional nasal airway issues further complicated by the small mandible.

Which profile the patient displays, and which treatment philosophy you choose, will define everything that will follow. The only fundamental differences are whether there is agenia or not, AMHypo or not, and maxillary hypoplasia or not. The decision to treat the malocclusion class is not based on numbers contrived through lateral cephalometry. It is based on rationalizing that 32 teeth are normal and

that we must volumetrically assess the ideal positioning of these 32 teeth, a normally spaced airway, and a normally proportioned profile, all within patient-specific facial volumetric needs to accommodate all internal anatomy.

The questions then become: How do I fit everything in? How do I keep everything? What do I need to make bigger? What steps do I need to take to move from small to normal? How do I make this specific individual with all her myriad issues "normal"? And how do I reclassify everything to see the pattern of it all and at once?

A NEW ORTHOGNATHIC CLASSIFICATION

In order to merge all the different themes of treatment, I propose that there is a need for a different way to orthognathically classify the average profile of a face. By *average*, I mean 98% of us, excluding the 2% that fall into a battle of an infinite variety of subtle or imagined abnormality. This classification therefore is of facially normal variance based on the almost absolute commonality of AMHypo. Ours is not a discussion on the pathologic variances of a thousand other vague and rare conditions. Of course not every single person in every single instance will fall easily into this subclass of this or that, but the overwhelming majority will.

In my assessment, the current means of orthodontic malocclusion classification ignores everything outside of the bite anyway, including the "why" of how a particular and common malocclusion occurs. And if we don't know the common "why," then we will never know how to fix almost everything.

> AMHypo is so ubiquitous, and so common, that we see it as normal; and because it is normal, we don't see it at all.

In my classification (Figs 1-13 to 1-16), I still use the principles of Class I, II (including divisions 1 and 2), and III malocclusions that Angle first defined, but I also give an added viewpoint of how anterior open bite develops. In my mind, these abnormal states of facial profile and bad bite fall on a spectrum (*b* through *f*), but they all have exactly the same small mandible. The base condition is always AMHypo. In my mind, AMHypo is so ubiquitous, and so common, that we see it as normal; and because it is normal, we don't see it at all.

FIG 1-13 Orthognathic malocclusion series 1: Agenia, with and without AMHypo, with and without maxillary hypoplasia, looking only at the teeth and facial profile and jaw size. *(a)* Normally proportioned mandible and maxilla without a chin button (agenia). There is a full complement of 32 teeth in full natural occlusion. Without a natural chin button, the lips are slightly parted, and the molar and incisor occlusion is an Angle Class I without dental crowding. With the lips slightly parted, the anterior teeth are prominently seen, and the appearance is of anterior dental fullness. Orthodontically, this would be called maxillomandibular protrusion with Class I occlusion without crowding. *(b)* AMHypo with agenia with the maxillary arch drawn normally. The appearance is of prominent upper lip protrusion and prominent maxillary tooth display. There is significant dental overjet and deep incisor overbite. The mandibular teeth are not crowded, and the first molars are in a Class II relationship. Orthodontically this is classified as Angle Class II, division 1 malocclusion. Division 1 implies that the maxillary incisors are well forward of the mandibular incisors. *(c)* AMHypo with agenia with the collapse of the maxillary anterior teeth, creating crowding or retrusion of the maxillary incisors, which deepens the dental overbite but reduces the dental overjet. There is less mandibular dental crowding, but there are impacting third molars. The molar relationship is Class II. The orthodontic classification here is Angle Class II, division 2 malocclusion. *(d)* AMHypo with agenia leading to mandibular crowding. There is also maxillary crowding and impacted maxillary canines due to a secondary small maxilla. The molars are in a Class I relationship. This would be called Angle Class I malocclusion with severe dental crowding. *(e)* Severely small maxilla with extreme dental crowding. This is caused by a lack of pneumatization of the maxillary sinuses and is an extension of the state shown in *d*. Both are caused by open mouth breathing due to the inherent AMHypo. The extreme smallness of the maxilla means the maxillary anterior teeth lie in line with or behind the mandibular anterior teeth, and there is a negative Class III molar relationship. This "malocclusion" gives the illusion that the mandible is too big. The orthodontic classification is Class III malocclusion with severe dental crowding. *(f)* Here the smallness of the maxilla and the dental crowding are associated with the anterior teeth not meeting at all. This is called *anterior open bite*, and its genesis pathophysiologically is related to the inherent smallness of the mandible—AMHypo—and is almost always associated with an infantile habit of airway-compensating thumb sucking (see Fig 1-17).

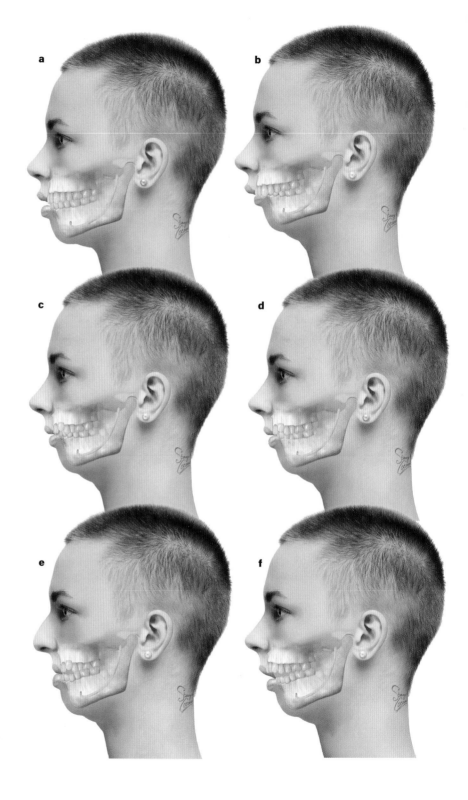

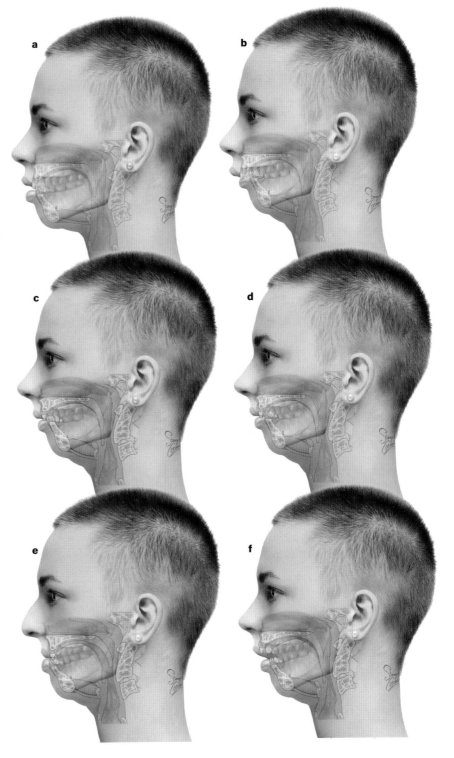

FIG 1-14 Orthognathic malocclusion series 2: Agenia, with and without AMHypo, with and without maxillary hypoplasia, looking at the teeth, tongue, airway, facial profile, and jaw size. By saying that 98% of all malocclusion is caused by AMHypo, our new orthognathic classification can rationalize simultaneously the airway and facial profile effects, in addition to malocclusion of dental crowding patterns. The only additional considerations are therefore *(1)* Is there a chin? *(2)* Is there an effect on maxillary development? *(3)* Is the condylar anatomy normal? *(a)* Normally proportioned mandible and maxilla without a chin button (agenia). *(b)* AMHypo with agenia with the maxillary arch drawn normally. *(c)* AMHypo with agenia with the collapse of the maxillary anterior teeth. *(d)* AMHypo with agenia leading to mandibular crowding, in addition to a secondary small maxilla leading to maxillary crowding and impacted maxillary canines. *(e)* Severely small maxilla with extreme dental crowding. Because there is chronic nasal blockage, innate glossoptosis, and agenia (short geniohyoid distance), this state poses the greatest lifetime anatomical risk of OSA. *(f)* Here the smallness of the anterior maxilla and the dental crowding on a primary base of AMHypo and agenia are associated with the anterior teeth not meeting at all.

FIG 1-15 Orthognathic malocclusion series 3: Normogenia looking only at the teeth and facial profile and jaw size. *(a)* Normally proportioned mandible and maxilla with a chin button (normogenia). With a chin button, the lips are closed at rest, and a proportion of the maxillary front teeth are esthetically seen below the line of the relaxed upper lip. The appearance is of a full and complete smile. Orthodontically this would be called Class I normal occlusion without crowding. With a more defined jawline, this is still a very feminine profile but less neotenic (young looking). The geniohyoid is at full stretch, and there is good chin-neck contour. I call this "the California look." *(b)* AMHypo with normogenia with the maxillary arch drawn normally. The outward curl of the lips and the slight prominence of the maxillary anterior teeth normalizes nasal projection and nasal-lip balance, and the slight retrusion of the normal chin button is considered in combination very feminine and neotenic. I call this "the soft French look." *(c)* AMHypo with normogenia with the collapse of the maxillary anterior teeth. There is relative collapse of the upper lip relative to the base of the nose, giving a sense of overforward nasal size or projection (a common cause to seek cosmetic nasal tip reduction). *(d)* AMHypo with normogenia leading to mandibular crowding, in addition to maxillary crowding and impacted maxillary canines. There is a prominent lower lip curl because of the collapse of the upper lip. *(e)* AMHypo with normogenia with a severely small maxilla with extreme dental crowding, leading to buccal crossbite and a high arched palate. The illusion is that the mandible is too big, which is further accentuated by what is essentially still a normal chin button. I call this the "wicked witch of the west" look. *(f)* Here the smallness of the anterior maxilla and the dental crowding are associated with the anterior teeth not meeting at all. All anterior open bite is associated with infantile glossoptosis, which remains present throughout the lifetime of the individual and is pathologically expressed as OSA in adulthood.

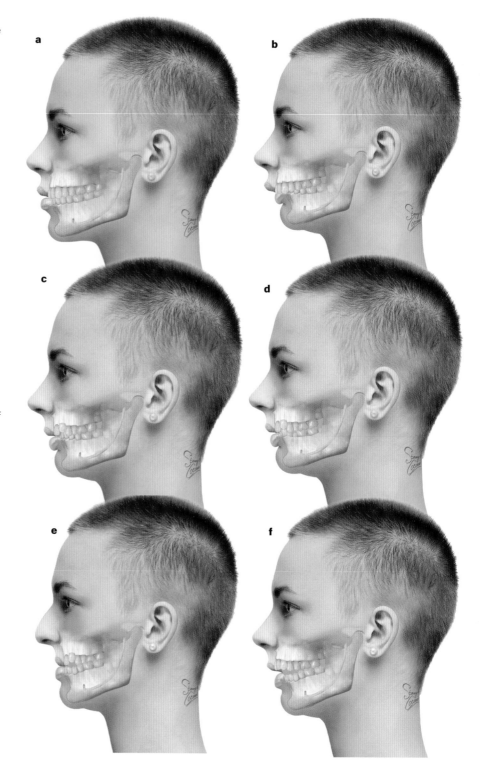

FIG 1-16 Orthognathic malocclusion series 4: Normogenia looking at the teeth, tongue, airway, facial profile, and jaw size. *(a)* Normally proportioned mandible and maxilla with a chin button (normogenia). This person is at least anatomical risk of lifetime development of OSA. *(b)* AMHypo with normogenia with the maxillary arch drawn normally. *(c)* AMHypo with normogenia with the collapse of the maxillary anterior teeth. *(d)* AMHypo with normogenia leading to mandibular crowding, in addition to maxillary crowding and impacted maxillary canines. *(e)* AMHypo with normogenia with a severely small maxilla and extreme dental crowding. *(f)* Here the smallness of the maxilla and the dental crowding are associated with the anterior teeth not meeting at all in anterior open bite. In all these cases *(b to f)*, the degree of glossoptosis and OSA risk is the same. Assessment of airway state in an erect, toned, and relaxed posture is a different assessment to being supine, relaxed, and in deep sleep, as will be explained in later chapters.

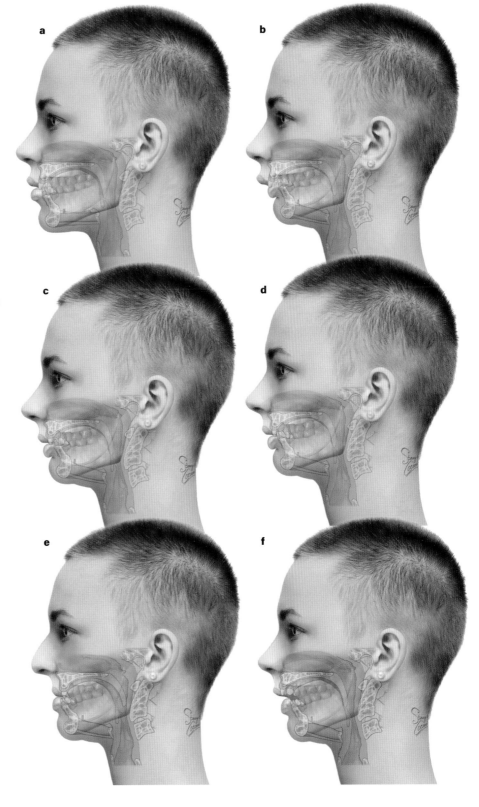

But to say AMHypo is abnormal, my first classification type is to describe the ideal. Thus I define the first state—Class I normal occlusion with 32 uncrowded teeth in a normal adult face. This is the anatomical and treatment ideal toward which we convert the AMHypo state, and from it relieve the patterns of airway, facial, and dental issues AMHypo causes. To accept this state is to believe that all of us should functionally develop 32 teeth—our teeth—as a normality of being our individual versions of human.

If you cannot accept this premise of my view of the ideal universal Class I occlusion founded on 32 teeth, then the rest of this book will be nonsense to you.

Pretreatment profile classification

My baseline dental assumption is that if there is nondevelopment of individual permanent teeth, it is because the teeth did not bud and therefore develop crowding or impaction. In my view, the lack of an individual random tooth is due to lack of local volume and not the result of specific genetic predetermination. A normal human complement of teeth is 32.

CLASS A

Class A describes a normal complement of 32 teeth without crowding in Class I orthodontic occlusion, with or without a chin button. There is no AMHypo. This may be called "Class I occlusion with no dental crowding and full dentition." This state is the gold-standard ideal outcome for all treatments that we apply to a face, jaws, and occlusion. There is no glossoptosis.

CLASS B

Class B describes the presence of AMHypo, with or without a chin button, with normal development of 32 teeth but with at least the mandibular third molars impacted. There is little remaining dental crowding, and the prominent anterior teeth are in an Angle Class II, division 1 pattern. There is normal maxillary development, though it is usually narrow posteriorly. This may be called "Class II malocclusion with prominent anterior teeth" or "Class II, division 1 malocclusion." There is inherent glossoptosis.

CLASS C

Class C also describes the presence of AMHypo, with or without a chin button, with normal development of 32 teeth but with all third molars impacted. There is significant dental crowding in the maxilla, such that the anterior teeth lean inward, reducing the natural dental overjet. The maxilla is not typically narrow, but it may be slightly shorter anteroposteriorly. There is relatively little mandibular dental crowding. This may be called "Class II malocclusion with collapsed maxillary anterior teeth" or "Class II, division 2 malocclusion." There is glossoptosis.

CLASS D

Class D describes the presence of AMHypo, with or without a chin button, with normal development of 32 teeth. There is severe dental and incisor crowding in both jaws, but a Class I molar relationship is preserved. This may be called "Class I malocclusion with dental crowding." The third molars are usually all impacted. The maxilla is developmentally small, and there is glossoptosis.

CLASS E

Class E describes the presence of AMHypo with normal development of 32 teeth but with almost universal impaction of the third molars, particularly in the maxilla. The teeth are severely crowded, and the very small relative size of the maxilla brings the incisor relationship into a reverse overjet (the maxillary anterior teeth lie behind the mandibular anterior teeth). The overwhelming etiologic cause is the primary AMHypo, leading to chronic open mouth breathing and severe pneumatic underdevelopment of the maxilla and the midfacial sinuses. The chronic nasal obstruction associated with the deformed and reduced upper nasal airways is often seen as secondary to the open mouth breathing. In my view, AMHypo has led to supine open mouth breathing, which has lead to chronic nasal obstruction. Chronic nasal obstruction does not primarily lead to open mouth breathing. Because the mandible appears larger than the maxilla, a visual association is made between the large mandible and the severe dental malocclusion state. The presence of a hooked or aquiline or proportionally large nose, or dropped Caucasian nasal tip, is always because of developmental hypoplasia or smallness of the underlying piriform, nasal spine, and maxilla and is primarily caused by the primary smallness of the mandible and inherent glossoptosis. Overall, this pattern may be called "Class III malocclusion," and it is linked to the orthodontic description of "adenoid facies" and is the entire pathophysiologic pathway leading to the "Hapsburg jaw." The glossoptosis is chronic, with profound nasal obstruction.

CLASS F

Class F describes the presence of AMHypo, with or without a chin button, with normal development of 32 teeth. The third molars may or may not be impacted. Dental crowding is present in the maxilla, but the maxillary anterior teeth only partially overlap, or they openly overlap the line of the

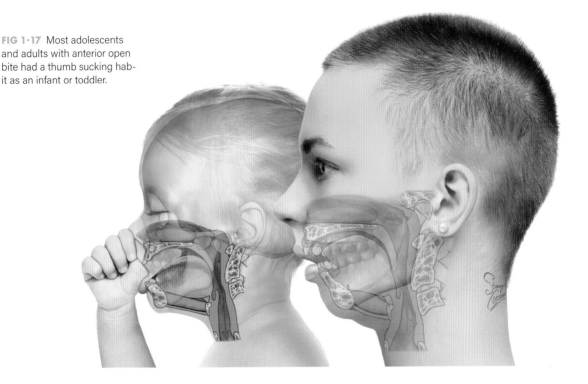

FIG 1-17 Most adolescents and adults with anterior open bite had a thumb sucking habit as an infant or toddler.

mandibular anterior teeth. This condition occurs because of chronic open mouth breathing, where there is over-eruption of the molars, which further props open the front of the mouth, leading to severe lip incompetency. Where the open mouth breathing has been closed because of adaptive thumb sucking in order to drive nasal breathing, there is worsening of the anterior dentoalveolar deformity in the maxilla. Overall the condition may be called "anterior open bite" and is often associated with tongue thrusting (see Fig 1-19), which helps close the oral lip seal and thus enables for normal nasal breathing while awake. Tongue thrusting does not cause the anterior open bite. Anterior open bite is overwhelmingly present only with AMHypo. The association of anterior open bite and glossoptosis is pathognomonic.

ANTERIOR OPEN BITE AND THUMB SUCKING

The adolescent presentation of prominent anterior teeth, a small mandible, tongue thrusting, and anterior open bite malocclusion is seen to be associated with an infant or child-hood habit of thumb sucking (Fig 1-17). How infantile thumb sucking transitions into anterior open bite in the adolescent, and why the infant sucks their thumb in the first place, has been an eternally confused area of clinical philosophy and

conjecture involving many craft and interest groups, and thumb sucking is an almost universally demonized child-hood habit. In my view, thumb sucking is actually an adaptive response to glossoptosis and a life-saving habit for babies with abnormally small jaws (see Fig 1-19).

To understand anterior open bite is to also understand the interrelationship between concepts of obligate nasal breathing, tongue thrusting, glossoptosis, AMHypo, anterior oral seal, and thumb sucking. Neonates are naturally obligate nasal breathers, and to nasally breathe, the mouth and jaws must be closed and sealed. But in a neonate with a small mandible, and with innate glossoptosis, the baby may find it desperately difficult to nasally breathe while asleep and lying on their back (Fig 1-18).

Pierre Robin was the first person to describe the reasons behind the phenomenon of the "blue baby." He taught mothers and doctors how to nurse and lay these small-mandible babies prone and on their stomachs to help with breathing. Unfortunately, his insight and knowledge on the dangers of glossoptosis are barely remembered. After all, mothers today are taught to always place their babies on their back to sleep—"back is best" —to reduce the risk of sudden infant death syndrome. But for babies with a small mandible and glossoptosis, there is inherent tongue collapse that blocks normal breathing during supine sleep. Cue the thumb.

A distressed newborn, lying on their back and unable to nasally breathe with a closed mouth, will be reactively

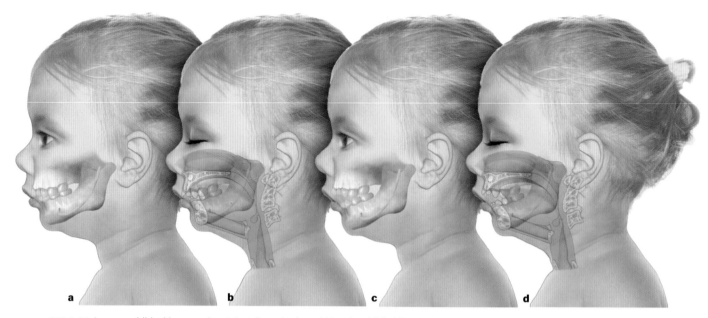

a   b   c   d

FIG 1-18 A young child with a prominent dental overjet *(a and b)* and a child with anterior open bite *(c and d)* have the same inherited small mandible (AMHypo). All that differs between them are the different postural habits that enable them to overcome glossoptosis and nighttime airway collapse. The child with the prominent overjet learns to sleep with their mouth open, lying on their front or side. The child with anterior open bite, on the other hand, learns to suck their thumb to help hold the mandible forward when they sleep in any position. Which way the child randomly selects will lead eventually to an adolescent orthodontic and orthognathic classification.

unsettled. They will thrash and cry, and the thumb waving in front of them becomes the soother. Not just for comfort like many believe, but because the simple act of sucking the thumb naturally closes the mouth, seals the lips, and holds the tongue and small mandible forward, thereby relieving the glossoptosis and permitting nasal breathing again (Fig 1-19).

Seen this way, then, thumb sucking is a functional and life-saving adaptation to a fundamentally abnormal anatomical condition. Eventually this thumb sucking becomes a functionally dependent behavior whereby normal nasal breathing, even during supine sleep, becomes possible and dependable and necessary (and terribly hard to break as an unconscious habit later in childhood).

Many dentists and speech pathologists recognize the association between thumb sucking and anterior open bite and small jaws and erroneously assume that the thumb sucking causes the small jaws. But it is actually the other way around. Adolescents and adults with anterior open bite and small jaws have always had an inherently small mandible, and the resulting glossoptosis made it difficult for them to breathe during sleep, hence the natural neonatal survival mechanism of thumb sucking. While almost all people who have anterior open bite sucked their thumbs as children, thumb sucking did not cause their small jaws.

REFERENCE

1. Batista KB, Thiruvenkatachari B, Harrison JE, O'Brien KD. Orthodontic treatment for prominent upper front teeth (Class II malocclusion) in children and adolescents. Cochrane Database Syst Rev 2018;3:CD003452.

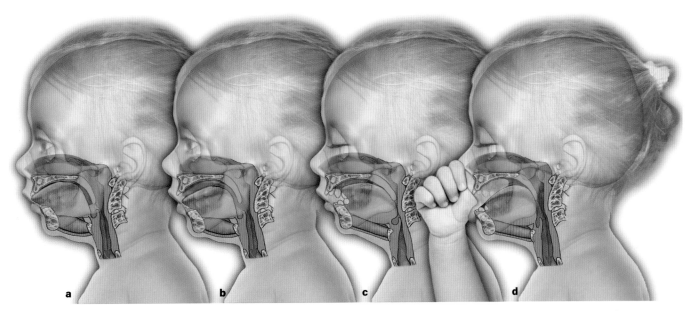

FIG 1-19 A common complaint of orthodontists treating anterior open bite in adolescents is persistent tongue thrusting that they say complicates successful orthodontic therapy. Tongue thrusting *(a)* as an adaptive position of the tongue has its origin in the infantile period and is only present during the awake state. By closing the hole between the anterior open bite and parted lips, it simultaneously brings the back of the tongue forward and restitutes normal nasal breathing. Tongue thrusting, as with general tongue tone, can only occur during fully awake or light sleep states. Without tongue thrusting, there is no innate oral seal, and obligate open mouth breathing occurs *(b)*. During deep sleep, with loss of tongue tone and under the influence of gravity with supine sleeping, the relaxed tongue collapses the retroglossal airway completely, which is called glossoptosis *(c)*. Lying on the side, along with the natural discovery of the thumb, enables the mandible to translate forward and thus opens the retroglossal airway. The second metatarsal joint of the thumb locks behind the incisor teeth, and the lips form a natural seal. The combination enables natural nasal breathing, and a simultaneous natural relief of both oral seal and of glossoptosis *(d)*. There is nothing unnatural about thumb sucking. Thumb sucking is a naturally adaptive measure to the primary state of AMHypo in order to overcome glossoptosis—and thus survive the neonatal and infantile period. It leads to normal midfacial development and normal sinus health. But it is demonized for the deformation of the anterior maxilla and is blamed as a cause for the development of the small jaw.

2

WHY OBSTRUCTIVE
SLEEP APNEA OCCURS

The baby with Pierre Robin syndrome born with a small jaw. The Class II adolescent with braces and impacted third molars (Fig 2-1). The middle-aged overweight person with sleep-disordered breathing (SDB) and a new diagnosis of obstructive sleep apnea (OSA) supported by a high apnea-hypopnea index (AHI) score. These are all the same person but at different stages of life.

I am 52 years old as I write this, and behind me lies a professional lifetime of treating small jaws, treating the effects of small jaws, and avoiding the effects of small jaws. As a maxillofacial surgeon, I offer a perspective that is not as a sleep dentist offering a mandibular advancement device (MAD), a throat surgeon offering uvulopalatopharyngoplasty (UPPP), an otolaryngologist prescribing tonsillectomy, a craniofacial surgeon treating a neonate with jaw distraction, an orthodontist offering braces, an oral surgeon recommending tooth extraction, a psychiatrist prescribing amphetamines to a sleepy schoolchild, or a respiratory physician offering a sleep study and a continuous positive airway pressure (CPAP) device.

As a maxillofacial surgeon, my training is as a dentist, an oral surgeon, a bite specialist, a general medical doctor, and as a primary medical-surgical specialist in corrective jaw surgery.

I can stretch a small jaw, and with it I stretch out the tongue behind it, the face in front of it, and the spaces between the crowded teeth as well. I have particular insight into these issues because I suffer from the same diseases that I treat. But how do my surgical therapies also medically treat my patients? What are my overall therapeutic aims?

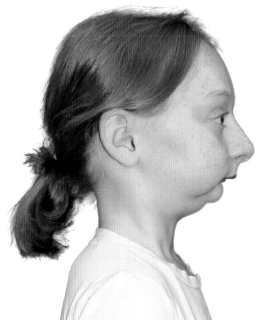

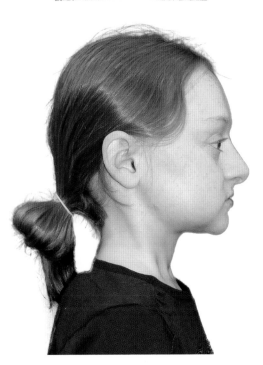

FIG 2-1 Before and after photographs (taken 6 weeks apart) of a 12-year-old adolescent girl with severe mandibular hypoplasia (caused by Melnick-Needles syndrome; see Fig 8-1) associated with snoring and sleep-disordered breathing (SDB). Weighing only 51 pounds, this patient's small size reflects the scientific evidence that SDB has significant negative effects on growth hormone (GH) assay and associated growth retardation. Early adolescent treatment by modern jaw surgery correction methods such as intermolar mandibular distraction osteogenesis (IMDO) have clear benefit.

MY JOURNEY WITH OSA

I was innately skinny as a young adult and adolescent. Until I was 28 years old I weighed only 150 pounds and had a body mass index (BMI) of 21, with only about 5% body fat. I always had mildly small jaws (see Introduction), but I never snored. I was just a mouth breather drooling silently into my pillow.

As my active young adult life increasingly became settled, my children were born, and work started to dominate my life, I sat more, exercised less, socialized with more dinners, traveled in planes, and lived in more hotels. So I started putting on weight. My new external environment eventually gained a new equilibrium, and internally my equilibrium changed to suit. I put on more muscle. I was physically stronger. But I was also putting on much more fat too.

By the time I was 34 years old, I was up to 174 pounds with a BMI of 25. When I hit 42, I weighed 209 pounds and my BMI was 30. By 51, I was almost 245 pounds, and my BMI was a shocking 35. My fasting blood glucose, which should have been below 5.5, was now 6.0. My fasting insulin, which should have been 8.0 at most, was now 11. My knees and ankles hurt when I walked. I was grumpy. After plane trips my ankles swelled. My wardrobe was a museum of thin to fat.

In the 8 years previous, I had successfully tried four diets, each of which lasted a year and brought me down to 165 pounds, but something always stopped the momentum, and my weight would return to a newer and bigger number. And if I plotted these new weights (y) on an age (x) scale, they fell on the one straight line.

What was happening was that I could not change my environment, and I could not permanently keep a low weight to suit that environment. I still worked at the same job. I still had the same social world, the same town that surrounded me. The same kids, the same food, the same supermarket, the same kitchen, the same subtle pressures. So when you combined everything into one big ball of different-colored strings, it all really meant I just lived in the same inflexible universe of modern human life.

My weight was essentially an end-point expression of my internal balance point. My internal equilibrium was always reverting back to the same point that was defined by the static equilibrium that surrounded me. And I was aging. And everything was getting unnoticeably and slowly worse. It was all so subtle. But what really woke me up was when I started snoring. Literally.

It's a horrible feeling. The choking. And it would force me to suddenly sit up, trying to catch my breath. And I'd stay propped up with pillows scared to fall asleep again. I put on a home monitor, and it gave me an AHI score around 5. Not much. My phone had an app that recorded how well I slept. It wasn't good. Another app recorded my snoring sounds. It sounded like a freight train. More frightening was when I fully obstructed, and I wasn't breathing at all.

I woke up tired. My thoughts were muddled. I spontaneously fell asleep. Everywhere. In movies. Watching TV. Lying in the grass under a tree. My mood changed too. I was less patient. Maybe I was more curmudgeonly. So I had bariatric surgery, and had almost 90% of a very large stomach permanently removed. It is called a "gastric sleeve." The weight loss was dramatic and relentless and permanent. By 212 pounds my snoring had stopped, and my old shirts started fitting around my neck. At 198 pounds my blood glucose and fasting insulin levels were completely normal. My blood pressure returned to 120/70. By 165 pounds I was completely healthy again. I wasn't hungry at all, and I easily maintained small meals. My ankles were normal. My knees worked normally. And of course I was sleeping fully, my dreams returned, my emotional balance was regained, and my thinking restored.

I couldn't change the equilibrium of my external world, so I forced permanent change on my own internal equilibrium. Even as surgeons, we are all dependent consumers on our own craft and colleagues.

SNORING AND DENTISTRY

Snoring has an enormous impact on people and society. Sleeping partners are the first affected, and eventually our bodies too start telling us that something's wrong (Fig 2-2). The health effects of poor sleep, including poor rapid eye movement (REM) cycles, chronic hypoxia, hypocognition, cardiovascular hypertension, and of course obesity, bleed into our personal lives, and this has become a real problem for society at large. When seen across a lifetime, the individual and economic effects of SDB make snoring a major health crisis that has real effects across the world economy.

Snoring causes lethargy. Poor sleep translates into reduced cognition and reduced physical activity. Snoring has a direct effect on every facet of the way each of us performs, lives, and remains healthy. While we can see the direct day-to-day effects of a poor night's sleep, in the long term, snoring's effects are cumulative—and relentless.

In 1923, Pierre Robin was the first person in the world to relate dentistry to snoring. While we associate Pierre Robin syndrome (and the micromandible) to his name, what he actually described were three things. First, Robin

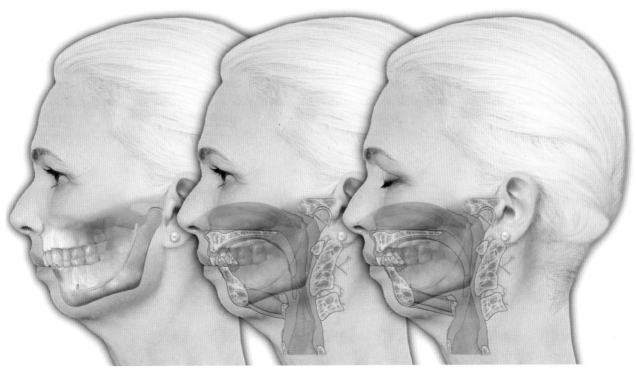

FIG 2-2 The symptom of snoring coupled with an AHI score from a sleep study ignores completely the anatomical reasons underlying why the patient has recurrent apnea episodes during sleep. Our faces are so much a part of the consideration of personal identity that we forget that faces are functional objects. A person born with a small mandible relative to the rest of their body will always have that disproportion as their body ages. Overbites, camouflage orthodontics, big tonsils, and eventually OSA are all part of the same life journey that many of us travel.

recognized that at least 40% of all Europeans (he was a Parisian dentist) had small mandibles. He called this condition mandibular hypoplasia. Second, Robin observed that all people with a small mandible snored. He saw the effect of a collapsed tongue on the back of the throat and gave the condition a name—glossoptosis. Third, Robin developed a jaw splint to hold the mandible forward, and with it the back of the tongue. The use of the device was life-changing for patients who suffered from breathing difficulty at night. Pierre Robin called this invention the Monobloc. It lives on today, with little recognition of his profound ideas, in the form of modern orthodontic MADs.

Today, the management of SDB represents an enormous worldwide medical economy. We know that snoring, upper airway resistance syndrome (UARS), and its end-expression of OSA is a major contributor to the development of obesity, diabetes, and cardiovascular disease in the forms of hypertension, stroke, and heart attack risk. We also know that OSA, UARS, and SDB have primary effects related to childhood cognitive performance and physical growth (see Fig 2-1) and adult-related risk of traffic accidents or workplace injury.

The Australian government, along with the Royal Australasian College of General Practitioners, has dedicated enormous economic and medical resources to the endeavor of surveillance, diagnosis, and management of SDB. Australia has led the way with developing treatments for snoring. Both the CPAP machine and at least one major dental (MAD) device company, SomnoMed, began their lives in backyard Australian garages. For almost 100 years, the dentist has been front and center of the war against snoring, and Australian dentists have helped lead the way for the past 20 years.

Most of us really don't know what causes UARS. And people may not know the small mandible is a major primary cause of snoring. Physicians find this difficult to see, because a fat neck and obesity and aging often mask the small chin. In older kids, dentists recognize the Class II malocclusion associated with the small mandible relatively easily. But in adults, this dental sign of the small mandible can be obscured by the camouflage orthodontics the patient had during adolescence.

By identifying the small mandible and recognizing glossoptosis, the dental practitioner is the primary means of identifying the risk of snoring. Whether it is in the child presenting with a big dental overbite or in the adult presenting in the late stages of full-blown OSA,

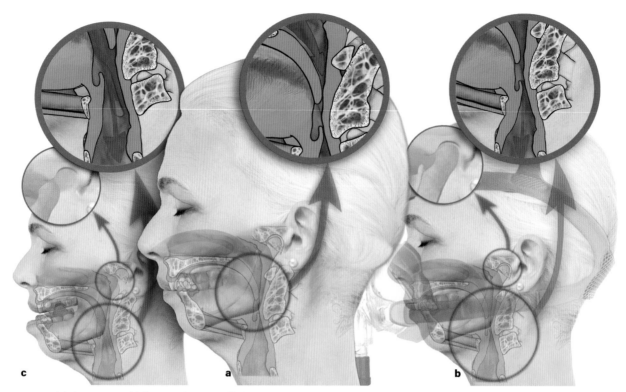

FIG 2-3 *(a)* The person with increased UARS will obstruct their upper airway between their soft palate and upper epiglottis at approximately the level of the 2nd and 3rd cervical vertebrae (inset). This is called a *closed torus* or *horn torus*. The author anatomically calls this C3ERPO, or 3rd cervical, upper epiglottic, retropharyngeal obstruction. *(b)* Using increased air pressure will drive air via the nose and push open the collapsed airway (torus) through the collapsed C3ERPO column (large inset). Increasing nasal air pressure through the CPAP can be titrated against the upper airway resistance, pneumatically opening the collapsed torus, until airway passage occurs through the C3ERPO region. The temporomandibular joint (TMJ) remains in its normal position (small inset). *(c)* Pulling the mandible forward through use of a MAD will directly pull the lower part of the C3ERPO column forward and hold the mouth partially open, allowing mouth breathing to occur (large inset). The forward position of the mandible moves the TMJ out of its fossa (small inset), which can lead to the development of TMJ pathology. The splint itself can orthodontically retrude the maxillary teeth and procline the mandibular teeth, eventually leading to development of a chronic malocclusion.

the dentist is front and center in the ability to offer definitive help.

By working with the orthodontic practitioner, sleep physician, or maxillofacial surgeon, the dentist becomes much more than someone giving fillings, extracting teeth, or applying splints. They become a frontline oral physician, applying their expertise of head and neck anatomy and clinical diagnosis for the cure of a first-world medical disease.

OBSTRUCTIVE SLEEP APNEA

The stories that many older people offer when discussing why they are on a CPAP machine often start with the terrifying discovery of their unconscious apneic states (Fig 2-3). What started as innocent weight gain, or complaints of daytime tiredness or general mental fogginess, or a sleeping partner's complaint of relentless snoring, eventually becomes a cry of an unbearable, life-dependent, and desperate need for medical help.

Diagnosing OSA

The general medical practitioner's referral to a sleep specialist can be a frustrating one for their patient. Linked up to machines and monitors through wires and stickers—and in a hospital bed with technicians and soft lights, strange sheets, and different pillows—is not a true replication of your own bedroom and your own natural state. In this anxious environment, many people find it hard to fall asleep. Or they wake up early and often.

And the test, unless it is repeated regularly and averaged, is not truly a reflection of how well or poorly a patient naturally sleeps at home and over many months. For many people who snore and who take part in a sleep study, they may still come away without a positive test outcome to

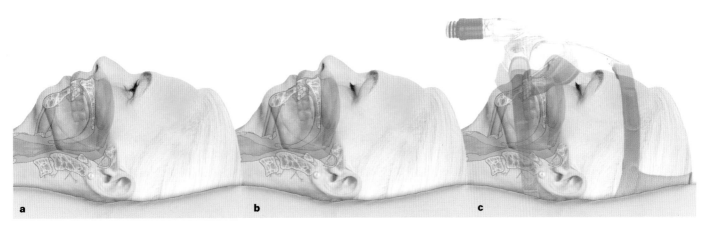

a   b   c

FIG 2-4 *(a)* Lying awake, the tongue has enough tone to resist gravity, and the retroglossal airway is patent. *(b)* With deepening sleep, there is a loss of tongue tone, and under gravity the retroglossal airway collapses—producing airway obstruction—and apnea occurs. *(c)* A positive increase in airway pressure using CPAP can partially overcome retroglossal airway collapse for most (but not all) people. Mathematically, CPAP works best up to the horn torus, but not past the horn torus.

confirm that they have OSA. Without a critical AHI score barrier (> 5 apnea or hypopnea episodes an hour), the offer of relief through CPAP may be frustratingly denied; or, at best, a repeat sleep study, with all the attendant inconveniences of that, is all that may be offered.

AHI SCORE

Usually, an admission to the hospital provides a sleep technician who will monitor a range of physiologic activities during sleep. Restlessness, blood-oxygen saturation, brain wave activity, nasal air movement, blood pressure, heart rate, and breathing effort are all measured. In the morning, the sleep physician will then analyze the data in a way that will give a number. This number is called the apnea-hypopnea index or AHI. It is a reflection of the number of sleep-wake cycles and low oxygen periods—or choking attacks—a person may or may not have per hour and averaged over the sleeping period. It is scored as mild (5–14), moderate (15–29), or severe OSA (30+).

While snoring, poor sleep, or daytime tiredness is often part and parcel of why people attend a sleep study, for the sleep physician the important medical question is to confirm whether a person is suffocating in their sleep or not. Having apnea literally means you are not breathing. And without breathing your blood-oxygen levels can fall low enough that you may simply not wake up. Ever.

Having a high AHI number (> 5 in adults), along with other measurement parameters, will help confirm a diagnosis of OSA. Being diagnosed with OSA is important to know, because the condition is linked to developing high blood pressure as well as myriad irreversible problems such as arterial wall thickening, stroke risk, heart disease, kidney

disease, and diabetes. Most importantly, OSA is associated with a real association of reduced life span, which is a product of developing diseases that directly arise from having chronically low blood-oxygen levels.

Even though it may be the reason why a person first went for a sleep study, a complaint of snoring fundamentally does not primarily support a diagnosis for OSA, and there are no physical signs, other than the AHI score, that a doctor can search for that will positively support a diagnosis of OSA. Some patients who snore are not actually measurably choking in the night. Hospital-based studies exist to assess whether the patient has a critical number of apnea or hypopnea episodes; they are not designed to determine whether that patient has the risk factors that may or may not meet the criteria for OSA in the future. Nevertheless, the diagnosis of OSA is one that belongs to the sleep physician. For an AHI score above 5, CPAP is the remedial treatment of choice by the sleep physician to reduce the AHI score.

Treating OSA

Unfortunately, the medical profession is less interested in "why" or "how" a patient is obstructing their airway than whether or not they are actually suffocating in their sleep. We know that medically treating airway collapse during sleep, regardless of the reason, is relatively accessible. And as long as you haven't reached a physical end-point, for most people there is at least a limited promise of potential relief.

All a person needs is two things. The first is a mask and a machine that can deliver continuous positive airway

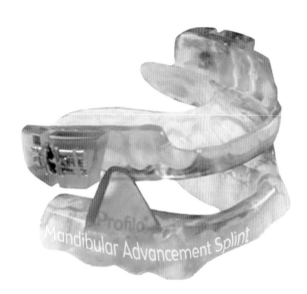

FIG 2-5 For some patients, the CPAP can be intolerable. Also, with extensive obstruction, CPAP pressures may not be enough to overcome airway collapse. The only other device that has been shown to provide a known and objective (nonsurgical) improvement to the AHI score, and possibly also to other symptoms, is the MAD. These dental splints are given a range of different proprietary names and are marketed on a broad range of therapeutic claims or comfort levels. But all of them are variations of Pierre Robin's original Monobloc invention. The one main advantage of the MAD is that by activating the wedge and screw in the top appliance, it can incrementally extend the mandible forward. In achieving symptomatic relief, and a reduction of AHI score, it is possible to ascertain the distance that jaw surgery may need to permanently overcome to open the collapsed nighttime airway.

pressure via the nose and mouth (Fig 2-4). This is called a CPAP device.

The second thing is personal tolerance. Without tolerance, a person with OSA will not be able to use a CPAP machine for 8 hours a night, every night, for the rest of their life.

CPAP THERAPY

The effectiveness of CPAP therapy is measured by the AHI score through repeat sleep studies. The practical effective goal of CPAP is to reduce the AHI score by reducing the average number of apnea or hypopnea episodes per hour a person suffers while they are asleep.

However, CPAP does NOT reverse hypertension, diabetes, obesity, heart disease, or stroke risk. And, more importantly, CPAP does not cure a person of OSA. CPAP will never give anyone a permanent AHI of 0 because, fundamentally, a sleep study does not acknowledge or eliminate the reasons why OSA is happening in the first place.

CPAP does NOT reverse hypertension, diabetes, obesity, heart disease, or stroke risk. And, more importantly, CPAP does not cure a person of OSA.

SYMPTOMS AND COMPLAINTS OF OSA

Ironically, the very same complaints that often bring the patient to the clinic for testing are not measurable or primary goals of CPAP therapy—things like getting a better night's sleep or feeling better during the day.

A person's set of symptoms and complaints may be wide, and they may even seem oddly disconnected to OSA or to each other. They can include insomnia in bed—they may be having an arousal as they fall asleep lying on their back—while somehow easily falling asleep at their desk with their head forward over a book. General anxiety and depression is commonly reported, as is poor concentration or poor work or scholastic performance. There may be specific complaints, seemingly unrelated to each other, such as muscle soreness, neck problems, recurrent headaches, or teeth grinding or jaw clenching or TMJ problems. People can complain of general fatigue, poor sports participation, general unfitness, and maybe even more general problems such as vague stomachache, irritable bowels, general muscle pain, restless legs, or chronic tiredness. And they may complain of ongoing weight gain that is almost impossible to control, slow down, or reverse.

All of these personal concerns are not measured or reported in a sleep study. And these complaints are not reflected in an AHI score either. Even though they may be considered effects or associations of OSA, whether they go away or not using CPAP is unpredictable and unmeasurable.

MAD THERAPY

Another treatment option for OSA offered by sleep dentists is the MAD, or mandibular advancement device (Fig 2-5). The MAD helps to hold the mandible and back of the tongue forward and may help with breathing at night (Fig 2-6). Like CPAP, the effect of the MAD can be measured by an AHI score, and the sleep physician may suggest a MAD if CPAP does not seem to be tolerable for their patient.

Just like CPAP, the MAD is also not a permanent cure for OSA, and it may or may not assist in addressing daytime symptoms and complaints. Unlike CPAP, however, a MAD can only enable oral breathing, not nasal breathing. And, unlike CPAP use, which really does not have any secondary

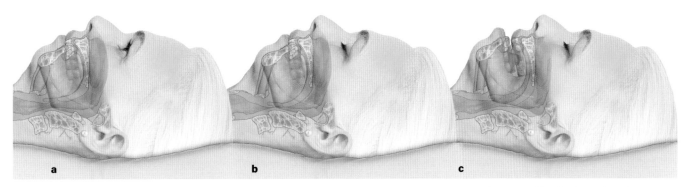

FIG 2-6 *(a)* Lying awake, the tongue has enough tone to resist gravity, and the retroglossal airway is patent. *(b)* With deepening sleep, there is a loss of tongue tone, and under gravity the retroglossal airway collapses—producing airway obstruction—and apnea occurs. *(c)* Opening the mouth and advancing the mandible pulls the hyoid and epiglottis forward (the lower part of the C3ERPO column), but only allows for oral breathing to occur. The MAD is far more effective at opening the closed torus surrounding the obstructed airway than the CPAP device. Unlike CPAP, the MAD does not allow for nasal airflow to occur. Successful use of a MAD to relieve someone of OSA absolutely confirms the presence of glossoptosis.

side effects apart from intolerance, the MAD can lead to significant TMJ issues such as pain, joint clicking, and jaw muscle discomfort. Because the MAD holds the whole bite and mandible forward, chronically it can also lead to permanent negative effects on a person's bite and normal chewing patterns.

How body fat aggravates OSA

Obesity is seen so often with snoring and OSA that it is casually seen as causative. We also see OSA occurring in people who have thick muscular necks, such as weight lifters. This common association of obesity, thick necks, increased intra-abdominal fat, and older age—and the simple fact that we see OSA so rarely in people who have thin necks and who are generally skinny—means we assume that being fat is the cause of snoring and OSA.

However, these co-observations of obesity and OSA reflect more of an association, or at best an aggravation. The association between the two is not true causation. There are many people who are fundamentally skinny, and young, and who still have upper airway collapse. What really causes OSA is far more fundamental and detailed than a simple blame upon obesity. That being said, it is absolutely true that weight reduction can eliminate OSA, but only where weight gain caused and fueled and aggravated the full end-point expression of OSA to finally occur.

When considering how obesity aggravates OSA, it is helpful to imagine the neck as essentially a donut (Fig 2-7). As fat is deposited under the skin and around the intestines, so too does fat thicken the neck and constrict the soft flabby tissues that surround the upper airway. As

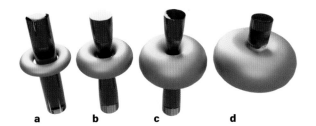

FIG 2-7 A radial neck and inner airway can be teratologically represented and topologically considered as a simple toroid (T). *(a)* A thin neck has a wide hole and allows for normal laminar noiseless airflow (T > 1). *(b)* A thickening neck, induced by increasing muscle mass or inner fat, makes the hole smaller (T → 1). The passage of air thins and increasingly becomes turbulent and noisy. Air resistance increases. The venturi of increased inner airflow, particularly with aerobic exercise, induces further collapse. *(c)* Eventually the neck can be so wide, and the inner airway so small, that we approach a horn torus (T = 1). Increasing airflow pressure through CPAP can overcome this near-complete toroidal collapse, but barely. *(d)* Once the toroid has collapsed, only increasing air pressure can reliably recreate an already closed airway (0 < T < 1). The greater the toroidal collapse, the more the torus approaches the shape of a sphere (T = 0), where air pressures to regain an airway approaches infinity. Therapeutically creating an incollapsible airway occurs only by making the toroid thinner—through weight loss—or by coring the inner walls through ablative ear, nose, and throat (ENT) surgery; physically stretching the toroid through a MAD; or permanently by advancing the jaw surgically. The toroid provides a physical mathematic model to explain why people become intolerant of CPAP, or are CPAP resistant, where AHI scores do not adequately reduce with CPAP therapy.

the donut gets bigger, the hole in the middle gets smaller. If the hole was already small to begin with, the donut doesn't need to get much bigger before the inside hole doesn't exist anymore. When the hole just pinches, this is called a *horn torus*. As neck thickening advances, the inner hole closes more and more, until the donut achieves the shape of a sphere. A patent torus can be given a value > 1, meaning airway passage is absolute. A horn torus, where the inner hourglass airway has just pinched, has a value of 1. A perfect sphere has a value of 0. Between 1 and 0 is the mathematic chance that a CPAP or MAD has the ability to regain the inner hole and regain nighttime airflow.

Weight control is a huge part of controlling OSA. Fat scans such as dual-energy x-ray absorptiometry (DEXA) can accurately see and monitor fat store loss through diet-selective high-protein, low-carbohydrate ketogenesis. Very low–calorie or food volume–restrictive diets (portion control) can be enhanced by use of intragastric balloons inserted by a gastroenterologist. Weight loss can be more permanently obtained through surgery such as gastric sleeve or gastric bypass procedures performed by an upper GI surgeon.

Surgical treatment of OSA

ENT SURGERY

The common surgical referral given for a person who is unable to control their OSA or snoring—either with CPAP or with a MAD—is ear, nose, and throat (ENT) surgery. ENT surgery traditionally looks at the nasal septum, nasal turbinates, nasal valves, adenoids, tonsils, soft palate, and back of the tongue.

For the nasal septum, the ENT surgeon will resect, carve, and straighten it. This is called a functional septoplasty. ENT surgeons can also open the doorways and remove the walls between the sinuses. This is called fine endoscopic sinus surgery or FESS.

For the turbinates, the ENT surgeon can reduce them. This is called a turbinectomy. For the nasal valves (nostrils), grafts can be placed to widen them. These are called nasal alae, nasal tip lifts, or nostril battens or overall may be called a functional rhinoplasty.

For enlarged or encroaching adenoids behind the soft palate, the ENT surgeon can scrape them away. This is called an adenoidectomy. For enlarged tonsils that seem to fill the back of the mouth behind the tongue, the ENT surgeon can remove them. This is called a tonsillectomy.

For a vibrating soft palate, the ENT surgeon can tighten and scar it using radiofrequencies or surgery and also remove your uvula, especially if it is long. This is called a uvulopalatopharyngoplasty or UPPP. If the back of the tongue is considered too large for the throat, the ENT surgeon can surgically partially remove it. This is called a partial posterior wedge glossectomy.

> I place corrective jaw surgery at the top because fundamentally it should correct the absolute "why" behind choking in your sleep in the first place.

The aim of all of these procedures is to reduce the encroachments of the walls and sides and roof and passages of the sinuses, nose, and back of the throat into the airway. In the small rooms and corridors of the upper airways, the ENT surgeon is removing the furniture and inner walls, scouring the paint, and opening the doorways. If, after all this surgery, the patient is still snoring, the ultimate ENT option is to bypass the whole house and create a direct and permanent breathing tube in your trachea. This is called a tracheostomy.

CORRECTIVE JAW SURGERY

At the bottom of the OSA treatment list is corrective jaw surgery, or maxillomandibular advancement (MMA) as ENT surgeons call it. It runs dead last, and it is the only surgical procedure that is not performed by an ENT surgeon. It is also the least understood operation of them all.

For me, and for the reasons I explain in this book, an assessment toward corrective jaw surgery should be at the top of the medical pile. I place it at the top of the list not because it is the best at treating an AHI score. I place it at the top because it is the best at treating everything else that isn't an AHI score. I place corrective jaw surgery at the top because fundamentally it should correct the absolute "why" behind choking in your sleep in the first place.

THE TRUE CAUSE OF SNORING AND OSA

The fundamental premise of this book is that upper airway obstruction, which leads eventually to apneic episodes during sleep, is caused by a collapsing tongue. This tongue obstruction is called *glossoptosis*, and it has been a known phenomenon since at least 1923 when it was first described by Pierre Robin in Paris. This tongue collapse occurs more easily when you lie on your back—and during a state of deep sleep—when the body and the tongue lose all tone.

The second fundamental premise of my book is that glossoptosis is inherently associated with people who have small jaws. Small jaws are very common in Western society. Small jaws lead to bad bites and crowded teeth in adolescents,

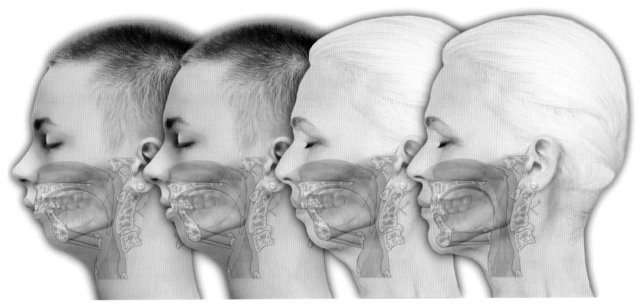

FIG 2-8 Treating the older patient who had camouflage orthodontics as an adolescent through the process of remedial BIMAX is curative for the glossoptosis that is intrinsically linked to the small mandible. Corrective jaw surgery permanently holds the upper airway open (the C3ERPO column) and effectively resists the development of OSA. How that surgical process occurs, and the links that tie all the bits that make up a face together, is explained in the remainder of this book.

The fundamental premise of this book is that upper airway obstruction, which leads eventually to apneic episodes during sleep, is caused by a collapsing tongue.

which itself leads to adolescent orthodontic interventions. In older adults, especially as weight is naturally gained, this same small jaw, and the same glossoptosis, inherently leads to a reduced airway lumen, which, promoted by weight gain and the laxity of aging, evolves into the development of snoring and then OSA during deep sleep (Fig 2-8).

The third and most important premise I make is that there is a surgical remedy that can reverse the associated glossoptosis of the small jaw in adolescents as well as correct for the orthodontic consequences of the small jaw. The evolution of this philosophy is to recognize that variants of the same surgical jaw procedures can be used in older people who already have developed OSA in order to cure them of their glossoptosis and therefore reverse their tongue obstruction that is actually causing their OSA.

Remedial corrective jaw surgery

For me, the common reports of adolescent dental crowding, dental extractions, impacted teeth, and orthodontic problems such as a bad bite or prominent anterior teeth in younger years are just as indicative of the reasons underlying why a person has glossoptosis than a standalone

consideration of AHI score, CPAP history, diet trials, BMI measure, or medical background. Orthodontics, oral surgery (by way of dental extractions), and ENT procedures (tonsil removal and nasal surgery) are common stories of childhood, and they are also common to many older people who snore or who have OSA.

A lot of what follows in this book is an explanation of how crowded teeth, bad bites, and big tonsils occur as a result of the general and common smallness of our jaws. Permanently making small jaws a normal size is a well-documented and scientifically supported fundamental and permanent cure for OSA. Corrective jaw surgery is designed to work whether you are in deep supine sleep or wide awake, breathing heavily and running on a treadmill. By curing people of breathing difficulties, such as snoring, or of the risk or presence of OSA, the jaw correction surgeon is also helping to prevent a range of other diseases that are very commonly associated with OSA.

Very fundamentally, maxillofacial surgeons are not sleep physicians. We are jaw correction surgeons. We are not here to treat an AHI score or to compete against CPAP or snoring splints or ENT surgeons wanting to remove tonsils. As jaw surgeons, we are not treating what the

As surgeons, we are not treating what the obstructions are causing.
Instead we are treating what causes the obstructions.

obstructions are causing. Instead we are treating what causes the obstructions. We want to change the collective story. The summation of the airway anatomy, apneic episodes, snoring, daytime tiredness, and all the other potentialities of the problem.

Unlike sleep physicians, we do not have Band-Aid cures. And unlike ENT surgeons, we are not wanting to take bits and pieces away. We are not here to remove the furniture from the room. Everything we do is about making the room bigger to help patients keep all their anatomical furniture. And to keep patients living better and more healthily, and hopefully for a much longer period of time—free of the common diseases we usually associate with abnormal aging.

3

DECIDING ON JAW SURGERY

The responsibility of the facial orthognathic surgeon is to provide a scaffold to support the soft tissue and dental structures of the face (Fig 3-1). While the appearance of the smile may be enhanced as a result of orthodontics alone, the core objectives of orthognathic jaw surgery are to correct for a combination of esthetic-facial, functional-dental, and medical health issues. We want our patients to be able to chew pain free, to taste, and to enjoy food. We also want our patients to be able to breathe, to sleep, to run, and to be socially normal.

Our jaw surgery is still typically planned with an orthodontist and performed by a medical surgical specialist in a specialist medical facility, using sophisticated titanium biomaterials. Imaging involves use of specialist radiologic and 3D optical-scanning technologies. While a specialist orthognathic surgeon is usually medically trained, they will also usually have qualifications in dentistry. However, the orthodontic practitioner or general dental practitioner has primary responsibility for their patient's dental health care. As a team, everyone will be working together, from family dentist and medical physician to orthodontist and surgeon. Global care means everyone understanding the overall plans and goals and coordinating with each other.

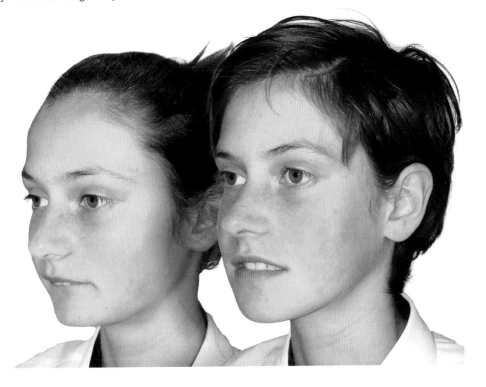

FIG 3-1 Adolescent girl with severe anterior mandibular hypoplasia (AMHypo), secondary small maxilla, and mild snoring. Photographs show an 8-month facial difference following pre-IMDO (intermolar mandibular distraction osteogenesis) palatal widening using a tooth-borne HYRAX appliance by her orthodontist, 14-mm IMDO, 6-mm custom titanium maxillary advancement via LeFort 1 osteotomy, and a second IMDO with 8 mm of distraction. The patient achieved Class I orthodontic occlusion following completion of the surgical series. Photographs show the patient at 13 and 14 years, respectively.

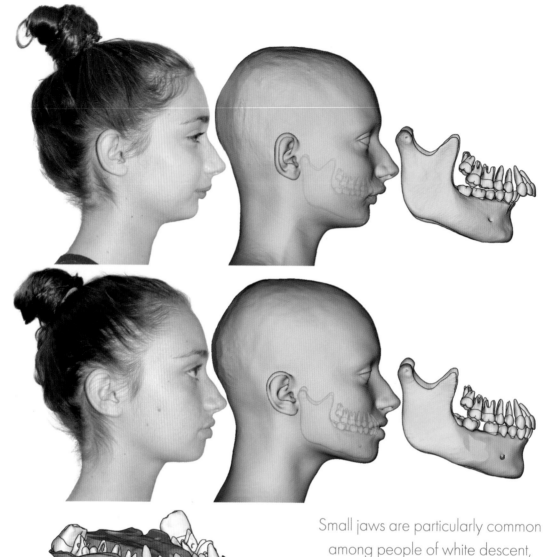

FIG 3-2 There is a clear link between having a small mandible and an underdeveloped or bad bite. Correcting jaw size discrepancy through surgery not only corrects for associated malocclusion but also gives opportunity for retaining a maximum number of teeth as well as correcting facial proportion, neck posture, and airway patency.

> Small jaws are particularly common among people of white descent, and the bad bites they cause are nothing new.

THE SMALL JAW

In the previous chapters I have explained that almost all bad bites have their origin in a small mandible (Fig 3-2). But small mandibles are hard to recognize in children with only baby teeth. We really only know a jaw is small when we see crowding, nondevelopment, or impactions of the permanent teeth.

Small jaws are particularly common among people of white descent, and the bad bites they cause are nothing new. Sepsis from infected, crowded, and decayed teeth was the leading cause of death and morbidity in London during the 1700s and 1800s. While the development of Western dentistry essentially eliminated dental mortality, it did not address the underlying problem that caused them.

Now, 200 years later, the most prevalent diseases of Western civilization are linked to snoring and obesity (see chapter 2). Some of the worst aspects of living in the modern world are the easy access to calories and the constant time pressures to deplete our lives of real physical activity. In some countries, and in those aged over 50 years, obesity is as high as 60% of urban populations, which severely aggravates snoring, breathing difficulties, and by extension, tiredness, which only encourages the medical supercycle to spin and spin.

CHOOSING BETWEEN ORTHODONTICS AND ORTHOGNATHIC JAW SURGERY

For most people, the aim of orthodontic treatment is simple: To achieve straight teeth and an even bite. But this treatment does not address the real problem for why the teeth were crooked in the first place—the disproportion in the size and shape of the maxilla and mandible. Having proportional jaws matched to the natural number of human teeth (32) will create a natural alignment of all teeth in a natural bite, as nature originally intended.

Traditional orthodontics, almost always combined with dental extractions, camouflages the underlying cause of dental crowding. This is in fact the genesis for the term *camouflage orthodontics*. Not only does traditional orthodontic treatment NOT address the root cause of the crooked teeth, dental crowding, and bad bite, but prolonged use of appliances combined with extractions is more likely to make jaws smaller. Despite many false claims, nothing belonging to orthodontics allows jaws to be grown or made bigger.

As orthodontics cannot treat the underlying jaw size discrepancy, it also cannot treat any medical conditions associated with a jaw size discrepancy, including airway and breathing disorders, temporomandibular joint (TMJ) disorder, headaches, and the lifetime ability to normally masticate and eat with all teeth. If left ignored, these basic medical conditions can lead to jaw arthritis, dental disease, and tooth loss later in life as well as the medical effects of advancing sleep apnea such as hypertension, obesity, diabetes, heart disease, and stroke risk in old age.

The cornerstone of orthognathic jaw surgery is in realigning or altering the size and shape of the jaws and co-arranging a maximum number of teeth in order to improve the way the teeth and bite work. Jaw surgery, usually in combination with traditional orthodontic treatment, is in

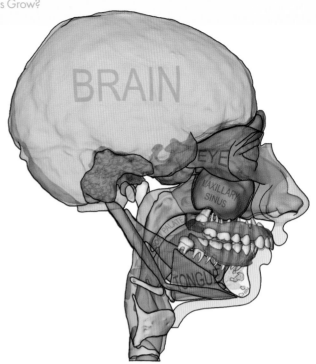

FIG 3-3 Faces and facial bones are reactive tissues; they expand rather than actually grow. There are underlying expansion forces that help faces develop. Broadly, these expanding influences on our "growing" facial bones are the brain, nasal airflow, and the muscular development of the anterior tongue. Breathing problems and abnormal tongue size inevitably go hand-in-hand and almost always lead to dental crowding and bad bite problems that are first noticed as the permanent teeth start erupting.

> The cornerstone of orthognathic jaw surgery is in realigning or altering the size and shape of the jaws and coarranging a maximum number of teeth in order to improve the way the teeth and bite work.

my view the only solution for adolescents and adults in treating their underlying jaw discrepancy. Jaw surgery is not just about correcting a bite. It's also about freeing the airway to make breathing easier—to prevent wider medical disease—and enhancing and normalizing the patient's facial proportions and profile.

HOW DO FACES GROW?

Despite what most people believe, the bones of the face do not really grow so much but rather expand as a surrounding crust or strut (Fig 3-3). Understanding how faces develop will help you understand why dental crowding and bad bites occur and what wider problems can also arise. There are three major regions of the face, and we can roughly divide them into thirds.

The forehead

The upper third of the face is dominated by the forehead. It is expanded by the brain. A small component around the eyebrows is expanded by healthy frontal air sinuses.

The middle face

The middle third of the face develops as a combination of enlarging eyes and expanding air sacs called the nasal sinuses. The most prominent of these expanding sacs is the maxillary sinus (one on each side). Acting as a pair, the maxillary sinuses help develop the bony shell of the maxilla that will eventually surround and support the maxillary arch of permanent teeth.

> There is a clear and well-established primary link between small jaws, dental crowding, bad bites, and breathing problems.

Natural nasal breathing occurs as a back-and-forward airflow: 14 times a minute, 60 minutes an hour, 24 hours a day. If nasal breathing is constant and throughout the developing period of an individual, the positive airflow maintains a low yet constant pneumatic stimulus to help inflate the nasal air sacs. Regular bilateral nasal airflow also maintains healthy mucosa and optimal nasal health.

As the maxillary sinuses expand and the inner nasal passages develop, the thin crust of bone that surrounds the air sacs contributes to a stable supporting structure to the middle face. This expanding bone also helps to hold and align developing and erupting permanent teeth as they replace smaller primary teeth.

The maxillary arch of teeth is connected by the palate. The palate is also the floor of the nose. The palate and maxillary dental arch is formed by the molding influence of the dome, or upper surface of the tongue. With a closed mouth and sealed lips, the tongue dome seals itself against the palate to enable normal nasal breathing to occur.

If the maxilla is small, dental crowding occurs. Childhood difficulties with nasal breathing are a prominent cause. In order to breathe through your nose, especially when you sleep at night, the mouth must be passively closed and the lips naturally sealed. Passive, natural, and constant nasal breathing with the mouth closed and the tongue dome seated in the palate is extremely important for normal midfacial and dental arch development.

The lower face

The size of the anterior muscular tongue determines the size of the lower third of the face. The anterior tongue and anterior mandible development go hand in hand (a first arch derivative). If the tongue is small, the supporting mandible is also small, and dental crowding and a recessive dental bite occur. A small tongue is also associated with glossoptosis, where the normally sized backside of the tongue (a second to fifth arch derivative) falls backward to block the upper airway and cause snoring.

When you are awake, the tongue muscles that connect the posterior side of the chin to the back of the tongue (hyoid) are contracted. This helps hold the airway behind the posterior tongue open, so that you can easily breathe. With especially small jaws, the tongue muscles cannot contract enough to open this airway, forcing the person to either hold their head and neck forward or to open their mouth in order to breathe.

For most people with small jaws, tongue muscles contract to allow for normal awake breathing; but when they fall asleep, these muscles relax and block off the airway behind the tongue. This can lead to a condition called *noisy breathing* or *primary snoring* or *sleep-disordered breathing* (SDB). In adults, these basic airway conditions can evolve into obstructive sleep apnea (OSA). There is a clear and well-established primary link between small jaws, dental crowding, bad bites, and breathing problems.

WHY ORTHOGNATHIC JAW SURGERY?

For 98% of people who have malocclusion, the mandible has not grown into a correct size with the maxilla. How this discrepancy impacts one's overall health and well-being depends on the individual, the extent of the discrepancy, and the age of the person. Nonetheless, jaw surgery should be a part of the informed consent when discussing options for treating *any* condition that is the result of a discrepancy in the size or shape of the jaws. Only a jaw correction surgeon can give definitive and specialist medical advice concerning the role of orthognathic jaw surgery, but the family dentist should also be involved to aid in that discussion.

While there is still clearly a role for traditional orthodontics and minor dental compensations with minimal long-term health impact, malocclusion cases should still require initial assessment by a trained specialist surgeon to predict whether surgery will be of benefit or not.

Where there is a larger discrepancy between the jaws, the relationship to the effects of glossoptosis becomes more apparent, and there is likely to be a history of one or more of the following:

- Tiredness
- Lack of concentration
- Breathlessness on exertion
- TMJ problems
- Headaches
- Difficulty chewing
- Affected speech
- Open mouth breathing
- Chronic nasal congestion
- Snoring
- Neck posture issues

Where there are already comedical problems, traditional orthodontic treatments will not address these concerns. Of greater issue is that independent dental treatments may actually risk potentiating some serious medical conditions into older age. These wider medical risks, as with the underlying jaw discrepancies, will still be present after the teeth are orthodontically camouflaged and straightened. In some cases, frank medical conditions such as OSA may arise from small jaws, and formal surgical treatment to correct jaw size may be complicated by previous camouflage orthodontic treatments. More importantly, the extraction of teeth so commonly associated with camouflage orthodontics is irreversible.

People who have large jaw discrepancies may also express unhappiness with their profile or facial proportions. Common complaints include that the patient feels they have no chin or that they have a big nose or big ears. While traditional orthodontics may straighten the teeth, when used alone it cannot enhance the shape or profile of the face. If, after orthodontic treatment, the patient is still unhappy with their overall facial esthetics, or the bad bite persists, the orthodontist may offer a suggestion to seek remedial corrective jaw surgery. Remedial corrective jaw surgery following camouflage orthodontics is complicated and expensive. Final treatment results are rarely ever as good as corrective surgery that is planned from the very

beginning. Most importantly, nothing can replace already extracted teeth.

For many reasons, it is vitally important to be informed about the prospect of orthognathic jaw surgery before an adult or child starts orthodontics. Advice as to the appropriateness of corrective jaw surgery can only be given by a specialist orthognathic jaw surgeon. And it is important that the family dentist, and of course the patient, be made aware of all treatment options available, their costs, and the expected benefits of care. This information should ALWAYS be given prior to embarking on any form of irreversible treatment, particularly those that lead to orthodontic extractions.

QUESTIONS TO AID DECISION-MAKING

Many questions can help determine whether jaw surgery is appropriate and indicated for a given individual:

1. Will the individual keep 24, 28, or 32 teeth?
2. Will they gain an open airway titrated against normal exercise tolerance?
3. Will they gain an open airway titrated against a full night sleep free of snoring?
4. Can there be an expected normalization of cervical postural control, or at least improvement?
5. Is speech lisp improvement a possibility (sibilant and fricative control)?
6. Will the patient achieve a wide smile, without buccal corridors, and full upper lip projection, or will the bite be narrow and set back or long?
7. Will treatment achieve a fully functional Class I occlusion in full dentition, with TMJs in a normal anatomical position, free of asymmetry or risk of joint disease?
8. Will the treatment achieve eventual centric occlusion–centric relation synchronicity?
9. How stable is the treatment result, and what is the chance for teeth to move away from their treatment positions?
10. Will there be esthetic improvement to overall frontal facial balance, symmetry, and proportion?
11. Will the individual achieve idealized facial profile balance?
12. Will the individual achieve symmetry of their face or jaw, or chin point or dental midline?
13. Will treatment eliminate a poor chin-neck contour (dewlap)?
14. Will treatment gain vertical facial height proportionality?

15. Will treatment achieve normal lip competence?

16. Is there a chance that treatment will cause a dorsal hump in the nose, or will treatment improve a dorsal hump or sense of nasal size or projection?

17. How will treatment affect nasal tip projection?

18. Will treatment improve nasal alar base widening?

19. Will treatment improve nasal airflow?

20. Will treatment achieve jaw widening?

21. Will treatment achieve cheekbone widening?

22. Will treatment eliminate the dark circles beneath the individual's eyes (venous pooling)?

23. Will treatment improve a sense of tiredness or alertness or energy or sense of inattention during the day?

24. Will treatment eliminate dental crowding without the need for dental extractions?

25. How is this treatment or that treatment compared in terms of overall treatment time?

26. Will treatment extend an individual's life span through reduction of risk factors associated with development of obstructive sleep apnea (OSA)?

27. Will there be general growth normalization through growth hormone assay normalization if the child is already "small for their age"?

28. Is there any possibility for reduction of lifetime cardiovascular and cerebrovascular risk associated with OSA?

29. Will treatment improve or worsen socialization?

30. Will treatment improve or worsen self-esteem?

31. Is there a chance for improved developmental and functional eruptive potential for third molars?

32. Is there any potential that treatment may spontaneously achieve natural decrowding of crowded teeth?

33. Will there be correction of lip projection and fullness, with better dental support in a passive (nonsmile) state?

34. Will the individual achieve normal esthetic chin point projection with this treatment?

35. Will the eventual jawline be feminine or masculine, and can the appearance of either be accentuated or diminished?

36. Will there be smile leveling and dental midline centralization?

37. Will treatment prevent the need for tonsillectomy or adenoidectomy or palatopharyngouvuloplasty as treatments for OSA, SDB, primary snoring, or upper airway resistance syndrome (UARS)?

38. Will treatment avoid dental extractions or impacted third molar removal?

39. Is the treatment chosen avoiding or eliminating or accentuating a risk of periodontal or root resorptive effects?

40. Will the treatment chosen produce a "gummy" smile, or will it produce a "normal" smile line?

41. Is there a potential that the treatment chosen will aggravate or cause TMJ disease, TMJ dysfunction, or tension headaches, or will the individual be trained to adopt an abnormal jaw joint posture or position?

42. Does surgery have real or common surgical side effects like persisting numbness to skin, lips, or tongue?

43. What are the costs of treatment?

44. Which treatments offer a minimum or maximum of treatment time?

45. Are there risks of not having a certain treatment versus risks of having a certain treatment?

IT'S ALWAYS A JOURNEY

When we travel, we have a specific destination in mind and a specific time frame for traveling there. We know where we want to go and when and for what reasons. There are often multiple routes or modes of transportation we could take, and some are faster, more convenient, and most costly, while others are slower, less convenient, and less costly. All of these factors are considered before we book the flight, hop in the car for the road trip, or jump onboard the cruise ship. The journey is planned from the start.

Much like traveling, where we have many options and narrow down our choices based on our wish list and travel needs, there are also many options available to patients walking through our doors. Making a choice to include jaw surgery away from traditional orthodontics is always going to be hard, and patients must have a list of ideals, wishes, wants, and expectations if they are truly going to make a rational choice. They must know what they want at journey's end.

The job of the clinician, then, is to define the patient's origin (the problem) and the methods available to get them to their destination (the solution). The predictive success of this care then becomes dependent on how many boxes of the wish list are checked.

I am a facial orthognathic surgeon, and as such I can be criticized for only offering treatments that are surgical. That same argument can be applied to orthodontists, who

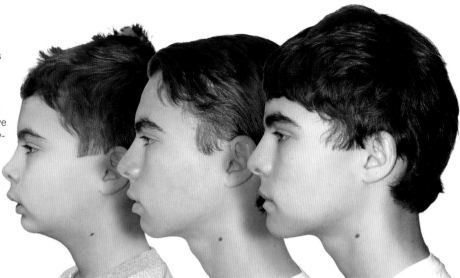

FIG 3-4 The child of a medical general practitioner. IMDO was performed first at 11 years, 10 months with natural dental settling, followed by Class I orthodontics at age 14 years for a short 12/12 period. At 16 years, he returned for GenioPaully to also advance the chin and fully relieve what was a Class B AMHypo with hypogenia and profound glossoptosis.

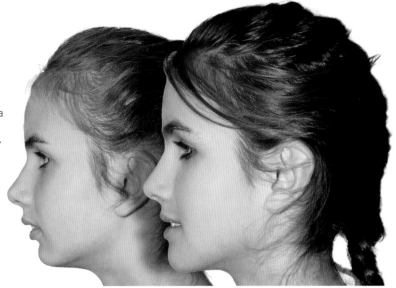

FIG 3-5 The child of a veterinary surgeon. IMDO and GenioPaully were performed together at age 12 years, 11 months to relieve a Class B AMHypo with hypogenia and childhood effects of glossoptosis. Post IMDO was a short 12-month period of orthodontics, with a full Class A 32-tooth dentition by age 16 years.

may only offer an orthodontic solution to a person's given problem. But much like travel, there is often more than one way to reach a destination, and the journey depends on how fast, how convenient, and how costly the patient wants it to be. Each journey will be different.

Indeed there are treatment regimens in dentistry that take an unnecessarily long journey, and there are treatment regimens used in dentistry that try to achieve an outcome that will have the same degree of success as catching a train from Sydney to New York (that is, none). Ultimately, however, it is up to the clinician to offer appropriate options, ask questions, and give sound answers to patients. Fundamentally it is up to the patient to decide whether the treatment (the journey) will match the condition (the origin) and the desired treatment outcome (the destination).

CASE EXAMPLES

Figures 3-4 to 3-13 demonstrate the individual treatment journeys of patients from my practice. For each, a brief description of the original condition, the treatment employed, and the time frames involved are described. Each patient had a set of functional issues that were related to either a current set of symptoms and signs or a perceived risk of future symptoms or medical disease. Before treatment, each had a list of questions given to them, all of which they wanted individually explained. It was only after a long consideration that each patient was allowed to make a rational choice from among the range of care options. None were rushed or forced into treatment, and each individual was treated with an appropriate surgical option for their unique set of circumstances and goals for treatment.

FIG 3-6 The child of a dental surgeon. At 21 years old, the agenia, oligodontia combined with dental extractions, bite splint trials, and an adolescence dominated by camouflage orthodontics has left a 22-tooth dentition and profound mandibular retrusion and glossoptosis. Treatment was initially IMDO-LeFort surgery, then Super-BIMAX and eventually custom PEEK implants for jaw angles and cheekbones as well as dental implants.

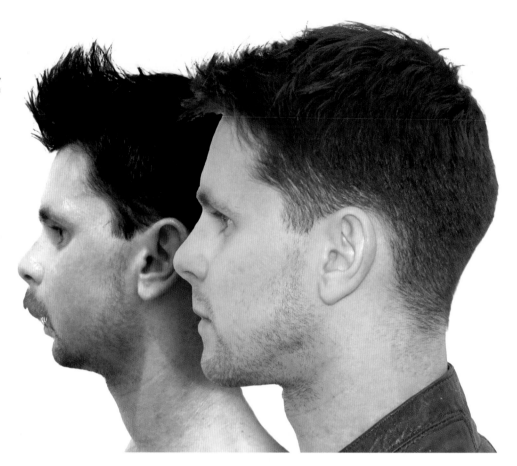

FIG 3-7 From early childhood there are myriad features of glossoptosis with ENT intervention such as tonsillectomy and adenoidectomy. In this case, treatment of the classic Class C orthognathic AMHypo began with pre-IMDO orthodontic widening of the maxilla with dental HYRAX, then proclination orthodontics beginning at age 12 years, 11 months and progressing for about 4 months. This was followed by IMDO-GenioPaully, which led to further natural dental settling and Class I orthodontic mechanics for about 12 months. Overall treatment was completed by age 14, with third molars continuing to develop normally toward 32 teeth.

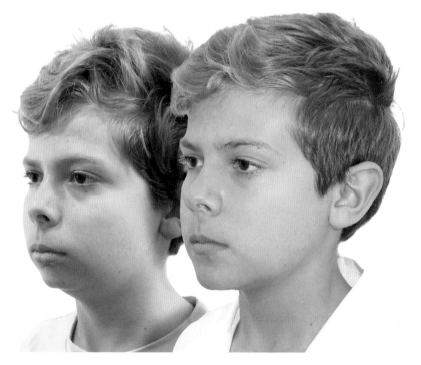

FIG 3-8 A 41-year-old man with severe maxillomandibular retrusion and prominent dewlap based on an original primary AMHypo. Unable to tolerate sustained aerobic exercise, and a prominent snorer, he underwent a sleep study that did not confirm a formal diagnosis of OSA. He was intolerant of CPAP and MADs. He was originally treated with 8-mm LeFort 1 posterior surgically assisted rapid maxillary expansion (SARME), followed by 14-mm IMDO, 6-mm maxillomandibular advancement surgery, and 8-mm GenioPaully using custom titanium to achieve normal full Class I occlusion and full relief from snoring and exercise intolerance issues.

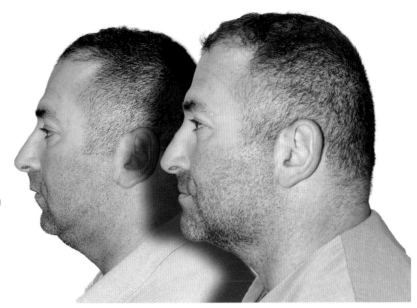

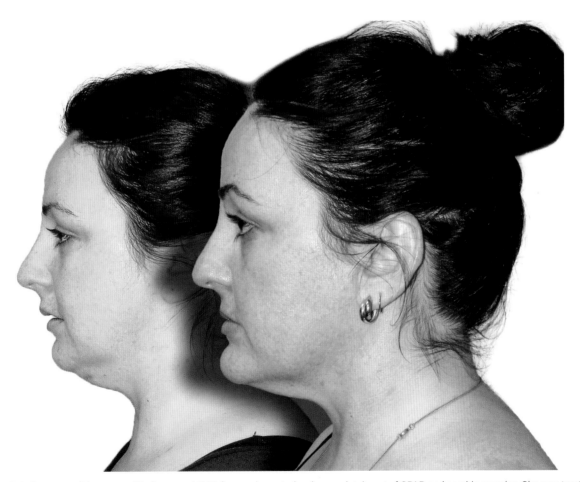

FIG 3-9 A 41-year-old woman with diagnosed OSA from a sleep study who was intolerant of CPAP and aerobic exercise. She was treated as a child with premolar and third molar extractions as camouflage orthodontics for primary AMHypo presenting as Class II, division 1 malocclusion, and consequently she had only 24 teeth remaining. She was surgically managed with an 8-mm LeFort 1 posterior SARME, 14-mm IMDO and BIMAX advancement (net LeFort advancement of 10 mm), and 8-mm GenioPaully. She is now in complete OSA remission. Overprominence of the chin button can be feminized later with contouring and reduction, or "softening." Functionally overcoming the OSA should be the primary goal of orthognathic surgery; cosmetics is secondary.

FIG 3-10 This 27-year-old woman was treated as an adolescent with camouflage orthodontics for her orthodontic Class III malocclusion. As an adult she sought skeletal remediation (see Fig 15-15) in co-ordination with her cosmetic dentist. Initial SARME with a Mommaerts device was followed by complex custom BIMAX. Her cosmetic dentist was able to use Invisalign therapy to maximize and improve smile alignment, which ultimately was augmented by custom lithium disilicate veneers to produce a perfect smile-facial coordination as well as complete medical reversal of her OSA state.

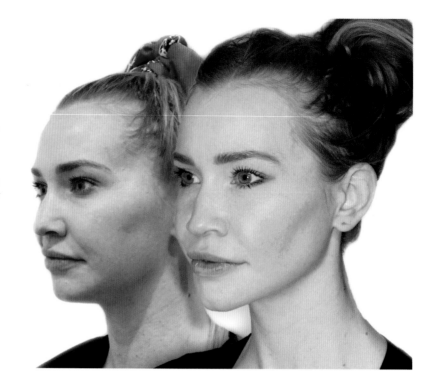

FIG 3-11 A 15-year-old adolescent boy with severe AMHypo, hypo-genia, and moderate maxillary hypoplasia. He was originally treated orthodontically and with 8-mm IMDO to overcome mild dental overjet and conversion of Class II, division 2 to Class I occlusion. He later had advancement genioplasty (10 mm) and full advancement BIMAX (12-mm BSSO and 10-mm LeFort 1) as coun-terclockwise rotation for a full pogonion change of 28 mm. Photographs show the patient at 15 and 18 years, respectively.

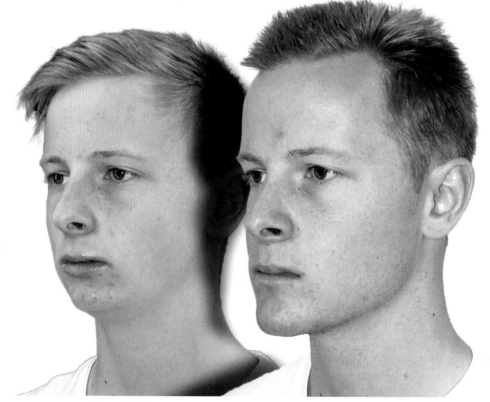

FIG 3-12 Following a few years of camouflage orthodontics, the vertically long face, open lips, and gummy narrow smile compete with the esthetic of the originally small jaw to produce a distinct face. Remediation could only be achieved by careful planning and eventual remedial BIMAX surgery, not only to lengthen and shape the jawline but also to widen and normalize the maxilla and dental arch position (see Fig 12-13). The airway is, however, always the dominant medical theme.

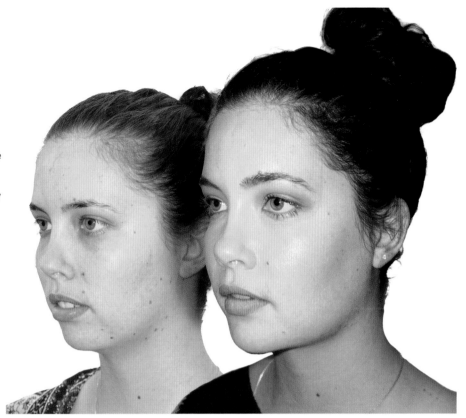

FIG 3-13 The sense of a large nose and diminutive chin and jawline can lead to an esthetic drive that includes patient demands for nasal reduction and chin augmentation by silastic implant. A more medically oriented examination identifies the primary smallness of the jaws and the inherent lifetime risks of OSA and of medical disease from this. Custom titanium solutions and forward diagnostic and surgical planning should always be toward the remedial BIMAX, with a view to managing airway, bite, and overall facial esthetics.

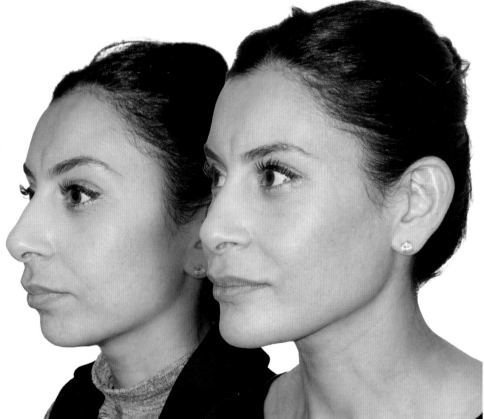

4
THE DIGITAL DIAGNOSTIC PROCESS

This chapter explains the steps involved in diagnosing and planning toward jaw surgery treatment.

Establishing medical and dental primary support is very important for successful future surgical care.

STEP 1: THE FIRST VISIT

A referral is always needed for orthognathic surgery. The first meeting between the surgeon and the patient is about getting to know each other. It is vitally important that the surgeon understands the personal circumstances of their future patient. It is also important that a patient is given complete information about the vast range of treatment options available to them by a broad range of practitioners. You want the patient to be able to make an objective assessment of all available options (not just the surgical ones) and to compare the potential of those treatments against their own expectations and general understanding about their condition.

Most patients find an orthognathic surgeon through their dentist, orthodontist, or physician. Increasingly, however, still many find a surgeon directly via the Internet and hence may not have an appropriate referral in place. Establishing medical and dental primary support is very important for successful future surgical care.

To help patients understand this complex area of surgery, any surgeon should have a wide selection and series of printed 3D models of real people that have undergone actual surgical and orthodontic treatments by the practice. An experienced surgeon will more than likely have close

examples of the patient's condition. Models can help show the steps necessary to achieve the treatment goals that all agree to expect.

Orthognathic jaw surgery procedures almost universally require the involvement of an orthodontic practitioner to optimize treatment goals. It is important that whoever provides the orthodontics (either the dentist or the orthodontist) is demonstrably experienced in working with patients undergoing orthognathic jaw surgery and is happy in providing ongoing orthodontic support as required. The orthodontic practitioner must be happy to become a working member of the surgical team and be willing to provide and accept feedback from the surgeon.

The first surgical appointment is a discussion of ideas and how treatments may or may not benefit the patient (Fig 4-1). It typically lasts 30 to 60 minutes. At this first appointment, the surgeon may provide a sleep-monitoring device or refer to a sleep disorder specialist if there is a concern about obstructive sleep apnea (OSA) or snoring. The surgeon's acceptance of seeing the patient for a first appointment is not an automatic agreement to treat by either party. If the patient and surgeon both agree to the prospect of jaw surgery, then they may progress to Step 2.

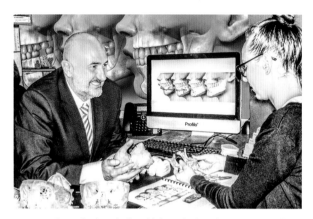

FIG 4-1 Consultations help with introducing the surgeon and patient to each other. For surgical operations, patients need a valid referral from their orthodontist, medical practitioner, or family dentist as well as full medical insurance before they can be accepted for treatment.

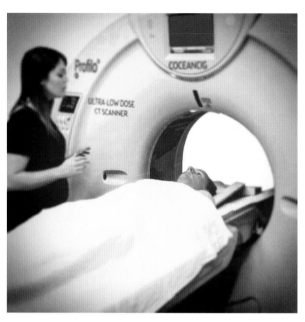

FIG 4-2 Data obtained from medical-grade CT, using ultralow-dose scanners, enable the surgeon and orthodontist to see how teeth and bites relate to wider airway and total facial structures.

It is impossible for any software to replicate precisely the dreams, desires, or projected surgical outcomes with respect to facial esthetics.

STEP 2: DATA ACQUISITION AND PLANNING

Once the patient and the surgeon have decided to advance the doctor-patient relationship, both will work together toward developing a definitive diagnosis of the condition and constructing a treatment plan idealized to the patient's wants and needs. The first diagnostic step is to arrange an ultralow-dose medical computed tomography (CT) scan, which is obtained with a strict imaging protocol and using specialist medical radiology partners (Fig 4-2). Prior to the CT, a patient-specific oral device may be made and worn to help natural jaw position during the scan.

For many reasons, medical CT scans offer superior diagnostics in comparison to "dental" CBCT devices. CBCT data, while appropriate for dental assessments, is not appropriate for medical-diagnostic purposes that assess for total soft tissue, cervical, and airway purposes in orthognathic settings.

The raw CT data obtained is used to digitally "segment" the jaws, airway, facial soft tissues, and of course teeth using specialized orthodontic and orthognathic (O&O) software. This software is used both to diagnose the overall condition and to "digitally operate" to see what series of surgical and orthodontic treatment steps are needed to provide a surgical "cure."

CT scans are combined with the optical scans of the teeth and bite. Later, the fused CT and optical data sets can be used to "print" facial bones and to create patient-specific surgical guides, surgical bite splints, and bespoke titanium bone plates. These devices are the new gold standard for most corrective jaw procedures, except for adolescent intermolar mandibular distraction osteogenesis (IMDO). In adolescent patients seeking IMDO correction for anterior mandibular hypoplasia (AMHypo), a presurgical planning CT is optional, unless directly asked for by the treating surgeon.

There is a lot of preparatory work performed by the surgeon and ancillary staff before seeing the patient for the planning appointment. There is a cost for such planning, and prepayment may be required before the planning appointment.

During the diagnostic appointment, which takes between 45 and 75 minutes, the surgeon uses the segmented images to demonstrate the baseline condition and airway, the occlusal and facial esthetic effects of that, and then a range of surgical treatment options to correct each identified anomaly.

The overall surgical movements can be combined with a soft tissue facial simulation to showcase the possible facial esthetic effects of this or that surgical option. It is important to remember that all esthetic/facial simulations are not real. It is impossible for any software to replicate precisely the dreams, desires, or projected surgical outcomes with respect to facial esthetics. The best way for a patient to assess what is esthetically possible or achievable is by comparing their own pretreatment portrait photography against examples given by other treated patients.

Regardless of all best intentions, the vast range of perceptions of what is ideal beauty and the beauty one sees in themselves is all extremely subjective. For this reason, the surgeon is limited to offer only medically relevant and objectively measurable medical/clinical outcomes. To this end, orthognathic jaw surgery is designed to be a functional, balanced, and proportional means to realign and objectively correct facial bones, occlusion, and airway. Whether that also offers an additional benefit of positive esthetic change is entirely a secondary consideration.

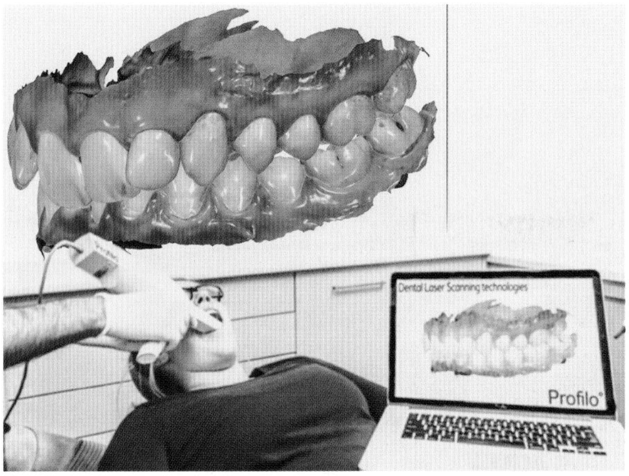

FIG 4-3 Dental impressions have been replaced with digital optical scans of teeth and bites. These will later be "fused" to CT scans to provide accurate representations of the total face, which is important for diagnosis, treatment planning, and later for bespoke titanium engineering manufacture. The process of obtaining optical and CT scans (the data) and the subsequent digital segmentation of bone, teeth, and soft tissue is an expensive and time-consuming exercise. It is only undertaken if there is an agreement to undergo further diagnosis, planning, and treatment.

STEP 3: THE CONSENT PROCESS

At the diagnosis and planning appointment, it isn't always immediately possible to provide estimates of treatment costs. This may be for a range of reasons, including a lack of agreement as to what surgical treatment plan is ideal for the condition the surgeon is seeing or the need for more time for the patient to consider their treatment options.

If both the surgeon and the patient agree (and formally consent) to a formalized surgical operation (or series of operations), the surgeon will endeavor to provide formalized estimates of surgical costs along with the item numbers used by insurers for rebate purposes. Financial estimates usually only occur where the patient has full and current private hospital (medical) insurance approval, and where the specific surgical step is likely to proceed within the next 3 months. We call these forms of understanding "formal treatment consent" and "formal financial consent." The surgeon can proceed with surgery only when both are given.

Any costs for co-orthodontic procedures, anesthetist costs, or hospital copayments (dependent on the level of private medical insurance) are given separately by these third parties and usually not by the surgeon. Private hospital and operating room expenses and the surgical assistants that are used during surgery are costs usually entirely borne by the medical insurer (as long as the patient has

the right level of coverage). IMDO distractors, titanium medical devices, and planning biomodels are also usually paid for by medical insurance coverage, but only if the patient proceeds with surgery.

STEP 4: BESPOKE TITANIUM MANUFACTURING AND ENGINEERING

The patient should be given time to think about their proposed treatment before they can be allowed to book any surgical appointment. Their "informed treatment consent" and "informed financial consent" is usually valid for 3 months from the time of signing.

For people requiring LeFort, bilateral sagittal split osteotomy (BSSO), genioplasty, GenioPaully, or BIMAX procedures, surgical planning files require upload and coordination with a titanium design-team engineer (Fig 4-3). The team I work with is located in Europe, so the surgical booking date can only be made at a minimum of 6 weeks into the future (due to manufacturing and delivery timetables).

Bespoke titanium plates and guides are "printed" using state-of-the-art titanium sintering technology (Fig 4-4). Titanium is the most biologically compatible material available for corrective jaw surgery procedures. Titanium is

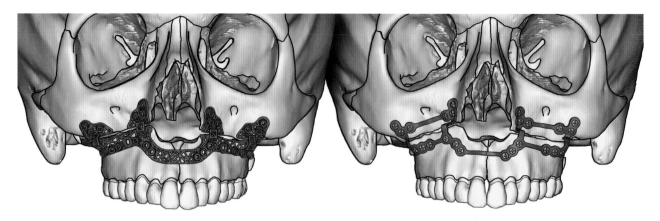

FIG 4-4 Creating "virtual" biomodels enables surgical planning as well as the engineering design and manufacture of bespoke drill guides and repositioning plates. These are first designed by bioengineers and surgeons, then printed in 3D in titanium using laser sintering technology based in Europe. The entire process, from design to delivery, is usually covered under private medical insurance as a custom medical prosthesis.

> Bespoke titanium and specialized jaw distraction techniques
> have greatly increased the predictability and successful outcome
> of jaw surgery procedures.

also used in the manufacture of specialized jaw distraction devices. Titanium printing is an extremely expensive process, but costs are essentially covered by the medical insurance policy as custom-made medical devices.

While "normal" orthognathic plates and distractors may be "off the shelf," patient-specific plates are designed to fit only the patient they are designed for, and only in the position that has been planned. They cannot be used for other patients. Bespoke titanium and specialized jaw distraction techniques have greatly increased the predictability and successful outcome of jaw surgery procedures. Both have replaced traditional jaw surgery plating systems as the gold standard for corrective jaw surgery.

STEP 5: SURGERY IN A HOSPITAL

Procedures requiring only limited distractor or localized plate removal can be outpatient hospital procedures. Surgically assisted rapid maxillary expansion (SARME), LeFort, BSSO, and IMDO patients (requiring insertion of distractors), require an overnight or weekend stay in the hospital. The surgeons will normally arrange reviews the next working day in the surgeon's office to initiate instructions on IMDO and SARME distractor usage.

SARME, LeFort, and BIMAX patients will require removal of nasal sponges 24 hours after surgery in the hospital bed or clinic. GenioPaully and genioplasty patients usually require one overnight stay only. BIMAX patients will usually have a 1- to 3-night stay in the hospital. The surgeon may normally visit the hospital daily during their stay to check on the patient's progress.

There may be multiple stepped operations involved in a patient's care. Not all surgical procedures are 100% predictable, and remedial "tweaking" operations are a distinct reality of all surgery.

STEP 6: ONGOING MONITORING

There is normally a timetable of regular monitoring of the patient in the surgeon's office. The recall schedule is determined by the procedure. Review appointments often require the taking of in-house, low-radiation digital panoramic radiographs. The surgeon may also offer review by email, Skype, Zoom, specialized dental or snoring monitoring apps, or by third-party review such as by their orthodontic practitioner. These reviews do not replace in-person reviews. A surgeon will manage each patient on an individual basis and take into account whether they are a local resident or primarily living interstate or overseas.

For IMDO, SARME, GenioPaully, and genioplasty patients, there is never a requirement for intermaxillary fixation (IMF). For LeFort, BSSO, and BIMAX patients, IMF is becoming increasingly rare but is not entirely eliminated.

If there is a requirement for IMF, then there is a requirement to visit the surgeon on a daily basis for elastics changes.

A soft or puréed diet is essential for several weeks following any form of jaw surgery. No dairy products can be consumed until all sutures are removed on day 10 to 14. The surgeon will also provide detailed instructions on oral hygiene protocols.

Jaw surgery often (but not always) involves more than one surgical procedure and is not 100% predictable in 100% of patients. If surgery has not exactly achieved an anticipated outcome, remedial or "tweaking" surgery may be required. The costs of remediation are usually minimal, but never zero. Agreement to any form of surgery accompanies an agreement to undergo any remedial surgery if it is required or deemed necessary by the surgeon.

Only once the surgeon has agreed that surgery has been successful will the patient be directed to reengage the orthodontic copractitioner, unless there is an agreement in the presurgical planning to involve the orthodontist at an earlier stage.

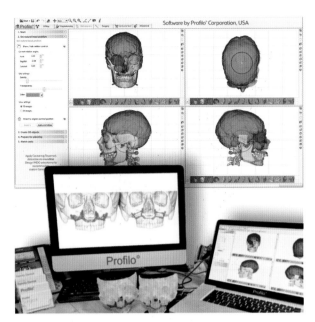

FIG 4-5 Virtual 3D diagnosis and treatment planning involves a range of specialized diagnostic and planning software and access to multiple medical manufacturers and approved medical devices. Most medical appliances used are covered under private insurance when performed by an accredited maxillofacial surgeon in an accredited surgical facility.

DIAGNOSING AND PLANNING TOWARD JAW SURGERY

ORTHODONTIC AND ORTHOGNATHIC ASSESSMENT

There are many types of jaw growth problems, and some people can have a combination of conditions. Often the person's primary jaw growth problem will have secondary distortion or expansion effects on other parts of the face.

Diagnosing what kind of bad bite a patient has can focus all clinical attention on the teeth. A total facial assessment, given by facial growth specialists, will link the dental bite pattern to the broader facial condition as well as help assess for any potential medical co-conditions. Facial development and dental development go hand in hand. A doctor cannot assess one without the other. Bad bites and crowded teeth are an end-point expression of how a face has properly or improperly grown.

Faces and mouths don't just hold teeth. They give attractiveness; they express emotions; they allow one to eat, to taste, to swallow, to speak, and to breathe. Looking at how everything comes together can help coordinate complicated modalities of care and help maximize opportunity for treatment of many associated conditions, as well as prevent some very common adult medical and dental diseases.

> Among all the things that a face or jaw correction specialist can assess for, airway function is probably the single most important one.

A range of sophisticated software is available to assess the combination of teeth, jawbones, airway, and facial profile (Fig 4-5). We call this process an orthodontic and orthognathic (or O&O) assessment. The O&O assessment has three purposes: *(1)* Define the origin (the diagnosis), *(2)* define the destination (the desired face and bite), and *(3)* define the journey (the series of orthodontic and orthognathic steps) required to reach our agreed outcome or set of objectives.

WHY IS AIRWAY ASSESSMENT SO IMPORTANT?

Among all the things that a face or jaw correction specialist can assess for, airway function is probably the single most important one. Airway compromise and dental crowding are parallel conditions that only a specialist trained in both dentistry and medicine, in combination with a team of

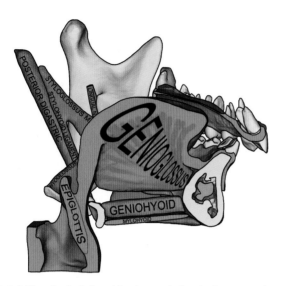

FIG 4-6 The physical size of the tongue is the single greatest influence on mandibular development. The connection of muscles that link the back surface of the chin to the back of the tongue and epiglottis means that there is a primary association between a short bite and breathing difficulties.

The combination of custom titanium printing and minimalist surgery means we can predict the ideal position of facial bones and accurately move them to idealized positions to create new occlusions and new faces.

people dedicated to fixing airway and orthodontic problems, is truly capable of assessing for the patient.

Jaw and tongue size go hand in hand (Fig 4-6). A small "anterior" jaw is intrinsically linked to a small "anterior" tongue. Having a bad bite and the presence of impacted or crowded teeth can be a real indicator for small tongue size, "bad" tongue position, and a compromised airway.

SEEING THE UNSEEN

Facial development in the child is a relentless progression and interplay of many natural factors. The brain grows. Primary teeth are replaced with permanent teeth. Normal nasal breathing slowly but surely inflates a healthy midface. The developing occlusion and relative sizes of the maxilla and mandible each influence the other. In combination, these processes and a hundred others all superimpose themselves. There is a constant interweaving and dynamic

and almost infinite expression of how the final face will develop.

In almost 20 years of specialist surgical practice, my experience is that of all the forms of jaw growth problems that present in otherwise normal adolescents and adults, almost all of them have an origin in an innately small mandible. Almost everyone has impacted third molars. Almost everyone has crooked teeth. Almost everyone has an imperfect bite. Almost everyone snores. True beauty, true symmetry, and true facial proportionality are actually very rare.

Advances in technology allow us to virtually recreate our anatomy and separate and reassemble the component parts. As facial surgeons, we can see how crowded teeth, small jaws, the tongue, and airways can interplay and create the final face. More importantly, we can see which domino fell first, and the series of dominos that subsequently fell in the development of the not-so-perfect adult face. Almost always, that first domino was intrinsically the small mandible.

Our technologies also allow us to print faces. We can now design what the skeleton of our faces should look like. As a maxillofacial surgeon, I can see how muscles and skin and cartilage and teeth and bone can be pushed and pulled in certain directions to give an overall precision to how the face should be (Fig 4-7). I can see how an initial smallness can be made normal. I can see how an airway can be made incollapsible during sleep (Fig 4-8). I can see how I can prevent a child's future third molars from impacting.

I am really privileged to be able to work with an international team of manufacturers, engineers, hospitals, like-minded surgeons and orthodontists, and of course our patients. Together we are able to practically and predictably apply these new technologies, sourced from different countries, to benefit everyone. New distractor designs are allowing us to predictably and three-dimensionally grow small jaws, expand the face, and superstretch airways (Fig 4-9). In orthodontics, we can design and print wires and brackets and splints to predictably move and coordinate teeth into precise patterns to match our distractor treatments. The combination of custom titanium printing and minimalist surgery means we can predict the ideal position of facial bones and accurately move them to idealized positions to create new occlusions and new faces.

When we combine everything together—diagnosis, planning, digital design, minimalist surgery, and intelligent orthodontics—we are truly entering a realm where everyone has the potential to be perfectly functional, and the chance to be naturally and maximally beautiful. It is truly a magical time for us all.

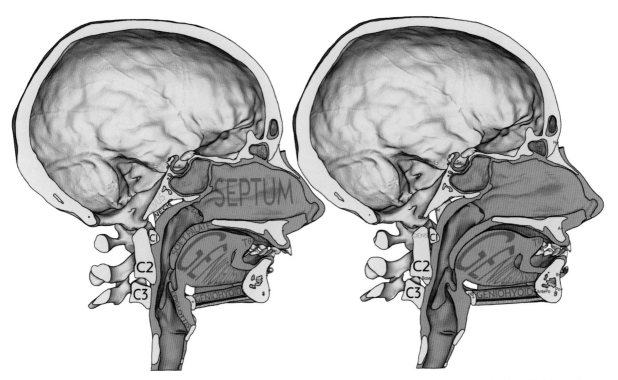

FIG 4-7 Distracting the mandible to help correct a bad bite and crowded teeth can give a dramatic change to facial profile. These changes can be measured by lateral cephalometry and can be actively measured by the cotreating orthodontic practitioner.

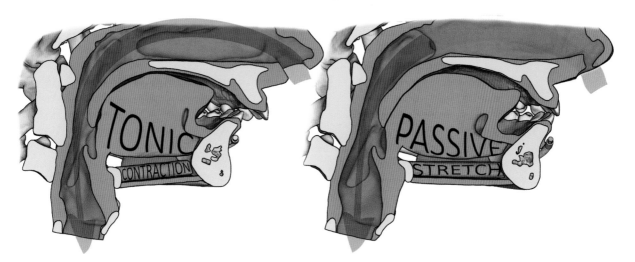

FIG 4-8 Jaw correction surgery stretches tongue muscles that connect the backside of the chin to the back of the tongue. Surgery to lengthen the mandible can prevent tongue collapse during sleep. "Growing" the small mandible like this in young children who do not yet have symptoms of airway problems can help prevent postural, dental, and airway problems arising later in life. Our surgical claims to "grow the mandible" should not be confused by nonsurgical claims that dental splints can also cause small jaws to be "grown" or "stimulated" as an alternative to jaw distraction surgery. The conceptualization of "growth" is explained later in this book.

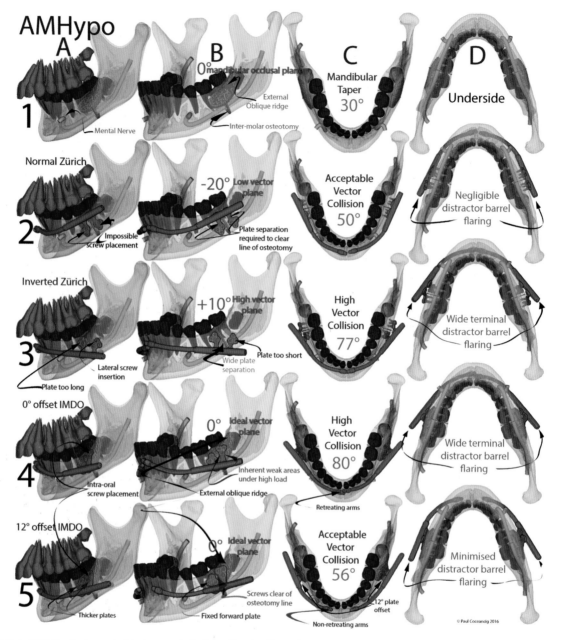

AMHypo

A | **B** | **C** | **D**

1 — Normal Zürich | 2 — Inverted Zürich | 3 — 0° offset IMDO | 4 — 12° offset IMDO | 5

A column:
- Mental Nerve
- Impossible screw placement
- Lateral screw insertion
- Plate too long
- Intra-oral screw placement
- Thicker plates

B column:
- 0° mandibular occlusal plane
- External Oblique ridge
- Inter-molar osteotomy
- -20° Low vector plane
- Plate separation required to clear line of osteotomy
- +10° High vector plane
- Plate too short
- Wide plate separation
- 0° Ideal vector plane
- Inherent weak areas under high load
- External oblique ridge
- 0° Ideal vector plane
- Screws clear of osteotomy line
- Fixed forward plate

C column:
- Mandibular Taper 30°
- Acceptable Vector Collision 50°
- High Vector Collision 77°
- High Vector Collision 80°
- Retreating arms
- Acceptable Vector Collision 56°
- 12° plate offset
- Non-retreating arms

D column:
- Underside
- Negligible distractor barrel flaring
- Wide terminal distractor barrel flaring
- Wide terminal distractor barrel flaring
- Minimised distractor barrel flaring
- © Paul Coceancig 2016

FIG 4-9 In 2015, the final round of design was to further refine the distraction vectors that were intrinsic to a universal IMDO distractor. The first cognitive step was recognizing the vast majority of adolescent and adult small jaws as equally and proportionally small. By calling it AMHypo, it was possible to apply a universal distractor design that applied equally to treating all AMHypo cases. This involved analyzing literally hundreds of AMHypo mandibles and averaging out the angles, lines, and distances that were able to predictably convert "small" to "normal" volumetrically. Because these principles are fundamentally four-dimensional, I call the distractors "tesseract" appliances due to the way they force volume changes in the mandible.

PROFILO° SURGICAL

Profilo° Surgical is an international interdisciplinary group comprising oral surgeons, orthodontists, and maxillofacial surgeons with higher levels of information technology and software tools that enable precise 3D assessments of facial structures as well as access to international manufacturers for both implantable devices and surgical instrumentation. With these software programs, we are able to coordinate separate clinical disciplines to maximally enhance facial esthetics as well as facial functions such as mastication and airway patency.

The initiating role of the medical radiographer is critical to the success of Profilo° Surgical procedures being

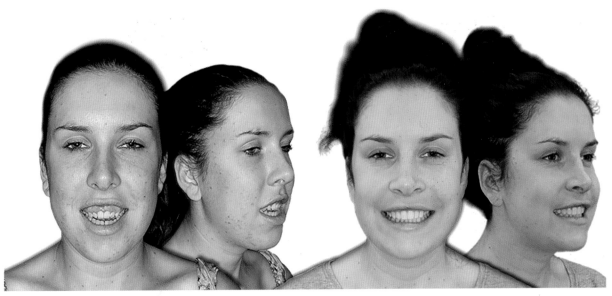

FIG 4-10 Proper surgical planning of combined facial, occlusal, dental, and airway structures enables maximum coordination of interdiscplinary treatments.

performed correctly and to maximize patient "opportunity of benefit" (Fig 4-10). This section explains the critical element of CT data, its interplay with 3D facial surgical science and diagnosis, and the dependence of surgical success upon it.

CT PROTOCOL

Profilo° Surgical uses CT scans for detailed surgical-facial, orthodontic, and orthognathic surgical treatment planning. The CT scans are further processed using 3D modeling software to enable analysis and surgical treatment planning, and potentially also for 3D printing purposes.

The use of scan data is very dependent on the cooperation of the radiographer to do the following:

- Maximally minimize radiation to the patient (despite all current claims, modern medical CT is superior to dental CBCT in all aspects and is usually much lower in radiation risk or exposure)
- Simulate patients in their most natural (erect) cervical posture and neutral jaw (occlusal) and facial positions, while lying supine
- Present data to enable ease of data handling as well as input into third-party interpretive software by Profilo° Surgical technicians or other third-party services

The best way to minimize radiation dosage to patients is to ensure that the first scan taken is performed perfectly. This includes the following parameters being met:

- The supine patient posture should replicate the natural erect head, neck, and jaw posture.
- The scanning field must be set to include the whole face (the ears, vertex, forehead, and nasal tip), the back of the head, and the entire jaw and neck (Fig 4-11).
- There can be no additional materials, straps, buttons, headrests, or hair accessories in the scan (see Fig 4-16) to minimize or eliminate the presence of metal.

1. Patient positioning

Before the patient is positioned, all metallic dentures, jewelry, hair pins, and metal objects must be removed from the scan field. The patient's hair should be placed in a high ponytail on top of the head to ensure that no hair falls beside or on the ears.

Before the patient assumes the supine position, the radiographer should observe the natural profile and posture of the patient while erect in order to replicate it while the patient is supine. Any head support should be small and rest only on the occiput, and there should be nothing behind the neck itself. No straps should be used to prevent distortion of the soft tissues.

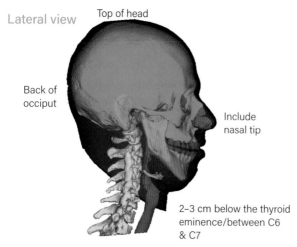

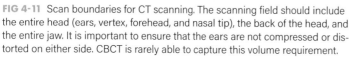

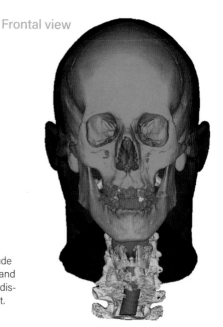

FIG 4-11 Scan boundaries for CT scanning. The scanning field should include the entire head (ears, vertex, forehead, and nasal tip), the back of the head, and the entire jaw. It is important to ensure that the ears are not compressed or distorted on either side. CBCT is rarely able to capture this volume requirement.

The patient should be instructed to bring their teeth together into a normal and naturally comfortable bite with only a slight separation of the posterior teeth, which should only just be touching (see Fig 4-12). The mandible must be positioned back with the mandibular condyles naturally and comfortably high in the mandibular fossa. Note that most patients with short jaws will position their jaw forward (see Fig 4-12b). It is important that this does not happen during the scan. The patient should be advised to keep their jaw in their "comfortable" position. Occasionally the surgeon will provide a bite splint to help stabilize this position.

The lip posture must be relaxed, and the ears should not be folded or compressed. The patient should be instructed not to swallow during scanning or purse their lips closed.

2. Image acquisition

The field of view and scan range must include the entire skull and surrounding soft tissues as well as the neck. CT scanners should have no less than 128-slice scan capacity to minimize radiation dose and maximize data quality. Images acquired must use helical fine overlapping slices of ≤ 0.5-mm slice thickness, with ≤ 0.4-mm spacing and no gantry tilt. Erect CBCT is not recommended as data manipulation will take more time and cost the patient more, and the volume of 3D quality will never be as good or as complete as with medical-grade CT imaging.

3. Image presentation

All CT scan and radiograph files should be saved in the DICOM format. All files should contain the patient name, date of birth, and sex; date of the scan; referring doctor; radiology practice name and location; and CT scanner model and software used. Only the fine slice image data should be archived, and both bone and soft tissue data sets should be included.

CONSIDERATIONS FOR POSITIONING

Getting the natural occlusion correct

Getting patients to position their teeth together can be a difficult and frustrating task. Most people with facial growth abnormalities have bad bites that lead to abnormal jaw postures or displaced temporomandibular joints (TMJs). Asking patients to simply "put your teeth together" can be confusing and lead to improper 3D assessment of their facial proportions or TMJ positions.

The best scans have both TMJs sitting in neutral or "comfort" positions in their respective fossae, with the posterior teeth lightly touching (Fig 4-12a). This position ensures that an abnormal occlusion is not abnormally influencing the balanced TMJ position. However, it can take

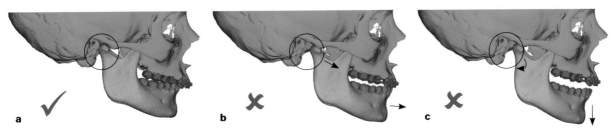

FIG 4-12 Proper and improper positioning of the teeth and jaws for CT scanning. *(a)* Proper positioning with the condyles in the fossae and the posterior teeth lightly touching. *(b)* Improper positioning with the anterior teeth touching but the jaw positioned forward. *(c)* Improper positioning with no teeth touching and the jaw positioned forward.

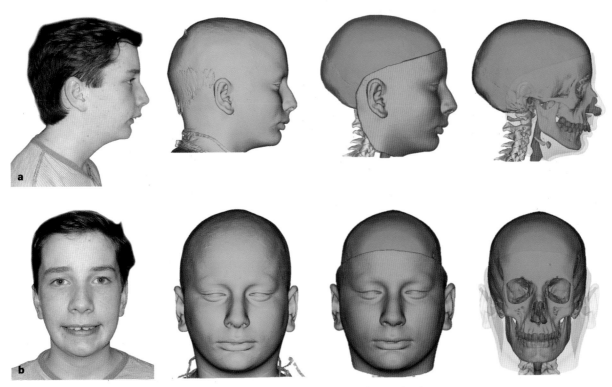

FIG 4-13 Natural cervical posture of a patient with a small jaw. *(a)* Lateral view. *(b)* Anterior view.

considerable practice in giving appropriate directions to achieve this positioning.

The "forward bite" is typical for patients with a naturally small mandible to compensate for a cosmetic discrepancy, and some may not have a naturally comfortable bite at all (Fig 4-12b). An abnormal position will likely occur if the radiographer asks the patient to "put the front teeth together."

An open bite appears when the patient simply does not follow the radiographer's instructions (Fig 4-12c). The condyles are positioned too anteriorly when the bite is open like this. A scan taken with the teeth and jaws in this position will affect the assessment of TMJ position, occlusion, airway, and soft tissue facial structures, and accurate surgical planning is impossible.

Replicating natural (erect) cervical posture

Most people with small mandibles will have an airway issue that forces them to hold their head forward (cervical hyperlordosis) in order to maintain a patent retroglossal airway (Fig 4-13). When lying supine, the cervical hyperlordosis is naturally lost and is a cause for airway obstruction when asleep. When positioning patients onto the supine CT scan bed, the occiput may need to be supported with a silicone ring in order to replicate this cervical hyperlordosis in the scan.

When assessing asymmetric facial growth, it is common for patients to have cervical torticollis as well. It is vitally important to make sure that the entire axial skeleton is

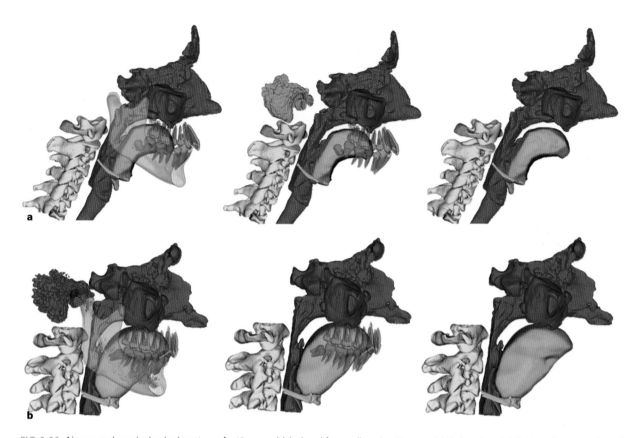

FIG 4-14 Airway and cervical spinal posture of a 12-year-old (a; head forward) and a 28-year-old (b; head upright). Note the narrowing of the airway in the 28-year-old due to the small mandible and the compression of the airway from behind by the cervical spine in the "stand up straight" neck posture. It is important to remember that an ideal field of view for a CT scan includes the whole upper airway down to the vocal cords (mid thyroid cartilage, or no lower than above C7). Imaging the soft tissue of the anterior neck also allows for visualization of the dewlap and the thickness of subdermal fat contributing to it.

straight and aligned on the CT scan bed and that the neck is not unnaturally or abnormally bent or kinked away from its natural erect posture.

Airway analysis

Airway patency is dramatically affected by patient positioning. For airway analysis to be objective between patients, between scans, and between radiographers, a consistent and repeatable patient positioning protocol must be obtained.

EFFECT OF VERTEBRAL AND JAW POSTURE ON TONGUE POSITION AND AIRWAY WIDTH

Airway volume is closely related to the vertebral column posteriorly and the tongue anteriorly. Figure 4-14 illustrates the airway of a 12-year-old compared to a 28-year-old. Note the size and positioning of the airway in relation to the vertebral column and the tongue. In the 28-year-old, the airway appears constricted and narrow (see Fig 4-14b). The

narrow-caliber airway is due to both the small mandible and the uprightness of the neck.

If the patient swallows during the scan, or if their neck or jaw is poorly positioned, there can be an artificial compression and distortion of the retroglossal airway.

EFFECT OF HEAD TILT ON AIRWAY AND VERTEBRAL POSTURE ASSESSMENT

Torticollis and neck tilt can impact vertebral posture and thereby affect assessment of the airway. Figure 4-15 illustrates three possibilities of head tilt resulting from torticollis and poor supine axial alignment.

Peripheral head devices and hair braids

Avoid using additional head straps or head guards because they will appear in the scan. Head straps distort skin and can affect facial image quality and assessments of facial proportionality or balance (Fig 4-16a). Use of surrounding head guards can distort the ears and can

FIG 4-15 Effect of head tilt on airway and vertebral posture assessment. *(a)* Torticollis from cervical scoliosis (strong association with facial asymmetry). The associated head tilt is chronic and difficult to correct for by postural manipulation. *(b)* Torticollis from hemifacial microsomia and cervical malformation. The associated head tilt is chronic and difficult to correct for by postural manipulation. *(c)* Neck tilt acquired by poor supine axial alignment. The radiographic vertebral axial misalignment causes offset or kink in the axial upper airway.

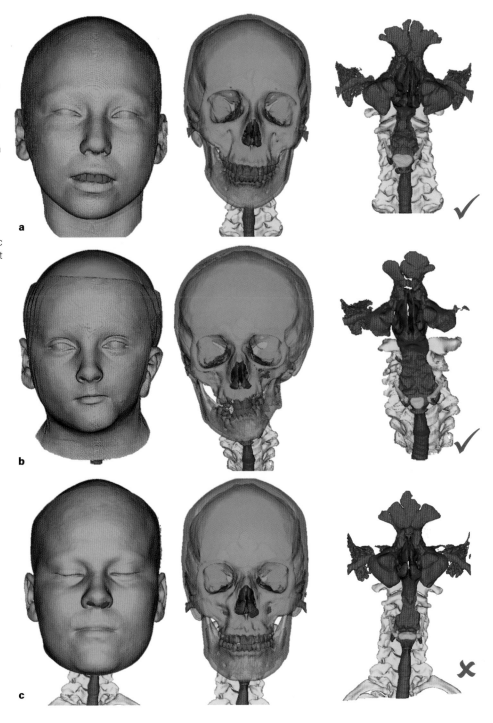

a

b

c

abnormally affect radiographer positioning and later assessment of facial proportions (Fig 4-16b). Peripheral devices lying on the skin are difficult to digitally remove from 3D assessments.

Hair bands and braids can interfere with facial assessment and distort soft tissues (especially ears) by their bulk and radiodensity (Fig 4-16c).

Effect of CT MPR and CBCT imaging

CT scans should not be reformatted into MPR (multiplanar reformation) data. Images saved in this format appear distorted with reduced image quality (Fig 4-17a) and abnormal voxelization. Likewise, CBCT should not be used because voxel size is usually coarse, unless the radiation energy is massively increased. For maxillofacial surgery,

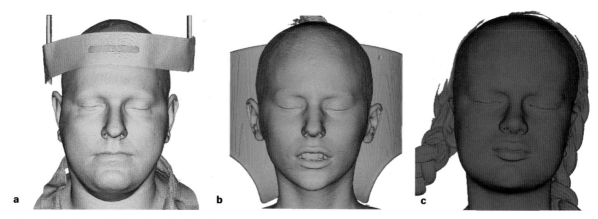

FIG 4-16 Head straps *(a)*, head guards *(b)*, and hair bands or braids *(c)* should be avoided to prevent distortion in the scan.

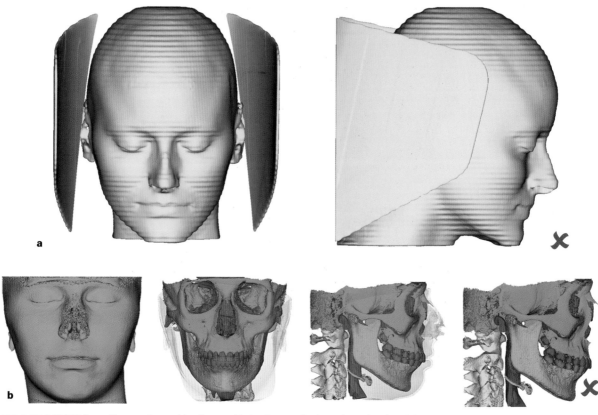

FIG 4-17 *(a)* MPR formatting produces ridge lines and is inadequate for formal 3D planning. *(b)* In CBCT imaging, the field of view is often restricted, there is soft tissue burnout, particularly at the nasal tip and cranial vertex and ears, and the overall dosage will be greater than high-slice medical CT imaging.

this modality is poor for imaging soft tissues and the airway, and in particular causes soft tissue burnout artifact of the nasal tip, and is naturally restrictive of volume, often eliminating the neck (Fig 4-17b).

Abnormal jaw positioning

Abnormal jaw positioning negatively impacts assessment of the scans. An unnaturally open jaw distorts lip posture and soft tissue proportions of the face (Fig 4-18a). This affects skeletal, soft tissue, airway, postural, and occlusal surgical correction planning. Correct posture facilitates undistorted assessments of all facial structures (Fig 4-18b).

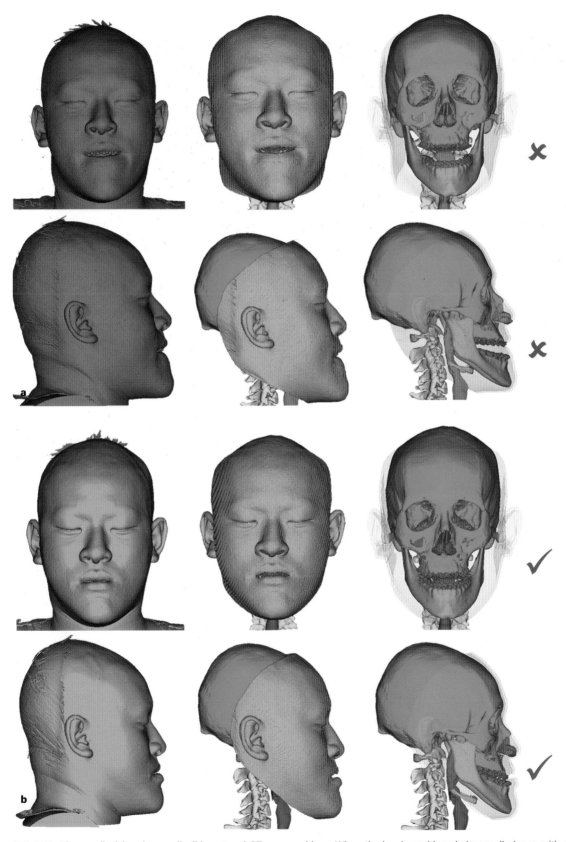

FIG 4-18 Abnormally *(a)* and normally *(b)* postured CT scan positions. When the jaw is positioned abnormally (open with a sucked-in lower lip), the shape and position of the vertebral column and airway can be affected, as well as the profile of the face. When the jaw is positioned normally, there is no distortion.

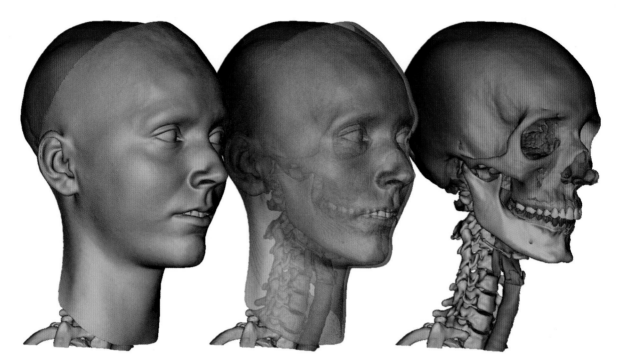

FIG 4-19 Diagnostic segmentation is performed with the patient in natural posture, with the teeth lightly and normally touching, and includes the creation of a calvarium, mandible, vertebrae, hyoid, maxillary and mandibular teeth, the occlusion (including gingiva and hard palate), airway column, facial skin shell, and finally the nasal and sinus mucosa. There can be nothing in the taking of the image data that distorts or deletes any of the entirety of the whole head and neck. A combination of ideal posture, ideal centrality, ideal volume, ideal imaging machine, ideal intraoral scanning, and ideal computer segmentation allows for a baseline digital presentation that establishes the diagnosis of everything that forms a face—with component parts seen both digitally together and separately. The next step is to define the ideal proportion of all the mechanics and internal machinery and the imagined journey through a combination of digital surgery first, then orthodontics, and finally dentistry—and then in the real world, the add-on surgical cosmetic and medical bits and pieces—that will guide us in arriving at a mutually agreed therapeutic-airway, occlusal dental, and esthetic-facial destination.

Obtaining correct bite position and relaxed lip postures enables predictive software algorithms to correctly interpret potential surgical treatments.

DATA COLLECTION AND SEGMENTATION

The CT scan data together with the digital dental scan forms a composite volume, and segmentation should be learned by the surgeon. While instructions are normally a part of any given segmentation software, it does require a mathematic understanding of Booleans, morphology operation, and Hounsfield ranges.

Ultimately eight structures should be visualized for ideal patient planning processes: *(1)* teeth and roots, *(2)* teeth and gingiva, *(3)* mucosal hard palate, *(4)* mandible, *(5)* calvarium, *(6)* hyoid bone and vertebrae, *(7)* facial skin, and *(8)* airway—from nose through larynx, including the sinus and nasal/sinus mucosa (Fig 4-19).

A critical step, however, is in the creation of the fused calvarium (Fig 4-20). This single entity contains four elements: the bony calvarium, the nasal and sinus mucosa, the maxillary teeth, and the palatal and gingival mucosa. It is this single combined image that allows the jaw correction surgeon to simultaneously manage the nasal airway as well as 3D orientation of the maxilla—particularly where maxillary impaction is required.

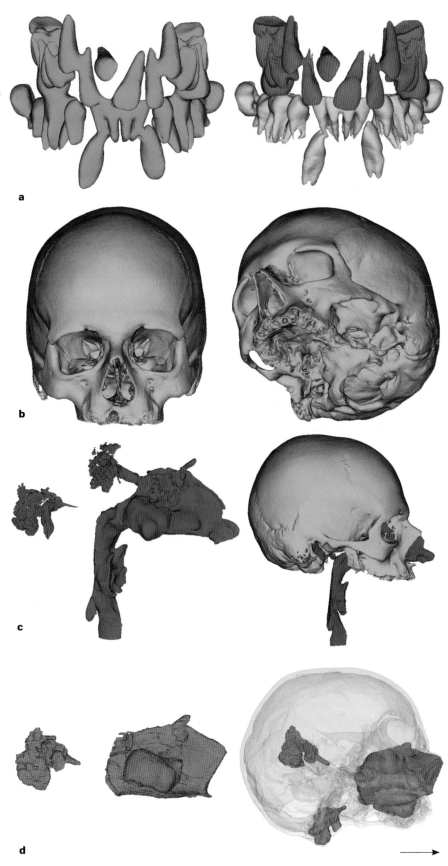

FIG 4-20 Imaging sequence for creating a normal calvarium. *(a)* Step 1: Create two sets of teeth. *(b)* Step 2: Create the calvarium. *(c)* Step 3: Create the airway. *(d)* Step 4: Create the intracranial sinus mucosa, including from the piriform to the choanae, as well as mastoid air cells.

FIG 4-20 (CONT) *(e and f)* Step 5: Create the nasal and sinus mucosa. This involves a complex series of mathematic steps, not easily sequenced or autoformatted by software protocols. An experienced segmentation engineer can dissect the midfacial nasal mucosa and merge that with a morphologically dilated intracranial airway. Using "smoothing" and Boolean subtractions, a simulated nasal and sinus mucosa can be recreated and later added to the calvarium to produce a true digital re-creation of the patient's real-time midface *(g)*. This in turn is used for final airway diagnostics and jaw surgery corrective planning decisions.

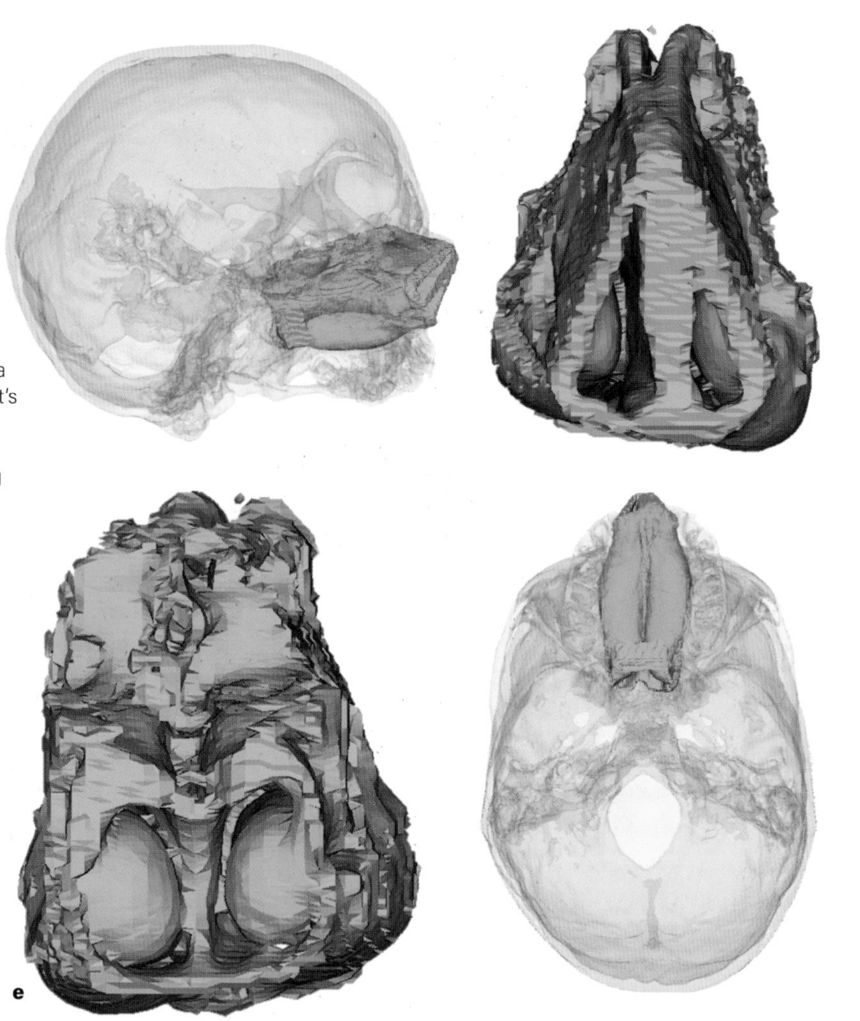

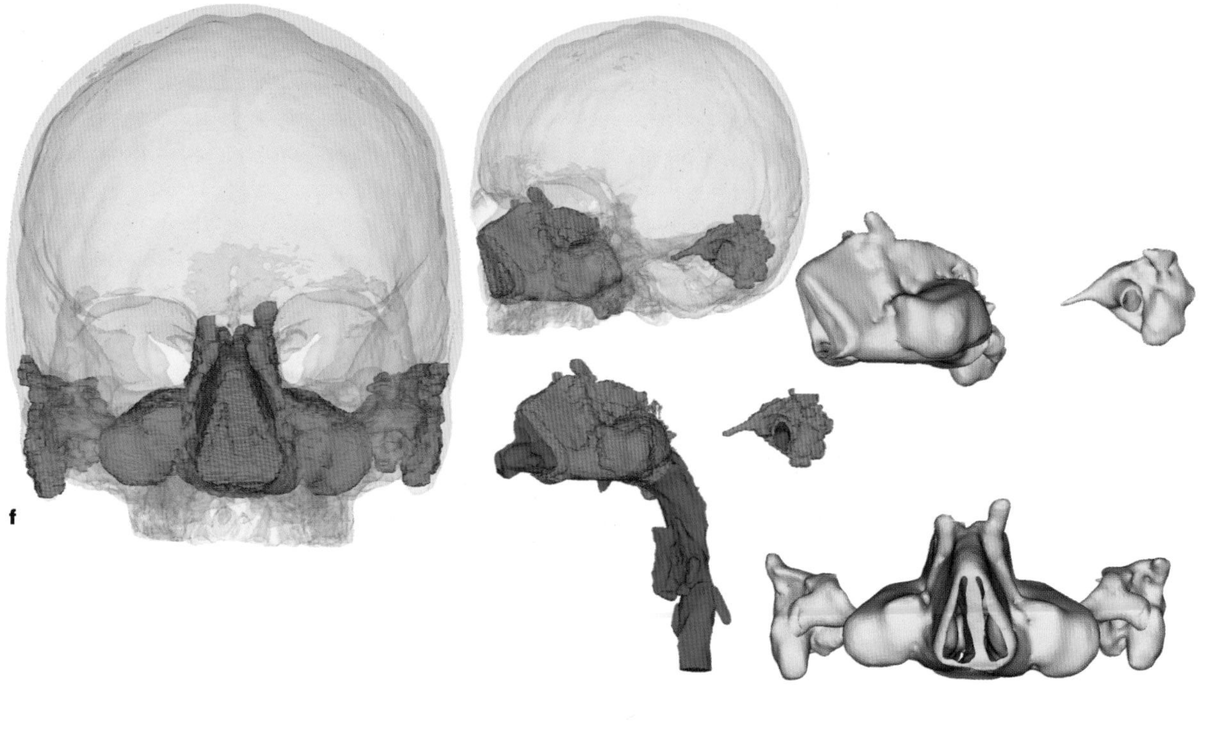

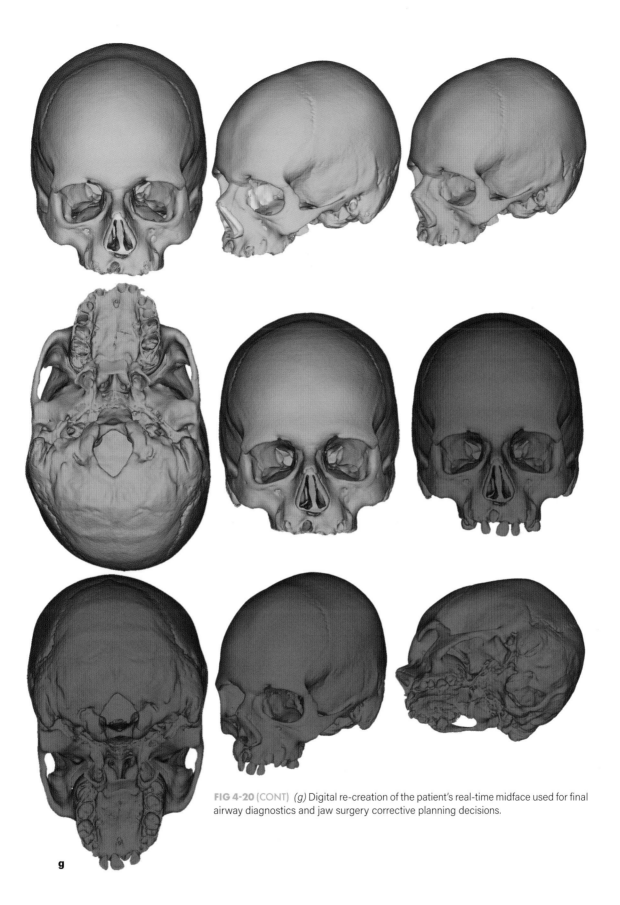

FIG 4-20 (CONT) *(g)* Digital re-creation of the patient's real-time midface used for final airway diagnostics and jaw surgery corrective planning decisions.

g

5

WHAT IS AMHYPO AND WHY SHOULD CLINICIANS UNDERSTAND IT?

Anterior mandibular hypoplasia, or AMHypo, is the most common form of the small mandible in people of Caucasian descent. AMHypo arises because of a small anterior tongue (with normal jaw joints), and it leads to dewlap (poor chin-neck contour), dental crowding, impacted third molars, a range of dental malocclusions (see Figs 1-13 to 1-16), and retroglossal tongue displacement into the upper airway (with associated neck posture issues). But why do so many people have AMHypo in the first place? And what are the barriers to it being treated effectively? To answer this question, we must first consider the ways humans have evolved over time (and commonlly held misconceptions about this process) as well as the forces that have defined Western culture and modern dentistry in particular.

There are speculative socioanthropologic causes for malocclusion that have entered into the culture of dentistry as assumed fact.[1,2] *Mandibular hypoplasia* as a descriptive term encompasses a dental view that the mandible has developed or "grown" in a relatively small though proportional way and, as a growth diminution, involves the entire mandible, inclusive of vertical rami and condyles. This paradigm assumes that the small jaw and its associated dental crowding is the endpoint diagnosis rather than a dental expression of an underlying anatomical condition. In Western orthodontic literature, population incidence studies of Class II malocclusion is widely reported as ~25% to 38%. If we invert the orthodontic paradigm and instead assume that simple symmetric Class II malocclusion is not the disease but rather the dominant effect of a common anatomical trait, then almost all cases of symmetric Class II malocclusion, additionally extending to almost all forms of dental crowding and malocculsion class, would be due to a fundamentally

AMHypo is really not about having a small jaw at all—it's about having a small anterior tongue—and it is very much about all the secondary anatomical problems that an embryologically small anterior tongue also brings.

uniform and equally common phenotypical causality (what I call AMHypo).

Specifically, AMHypo develops secondarily to the growing volumetric influence of the small anterior tongue. A diminished tongue volume as it volumetrically expands has a negative impact on fully stimulating the volumetric "growth" of the surrounding anterior mandible. This has a causal negative effect on normal permanent tooth budding, on the normalized development of dental arch form, on an ideal occlusal relationship (most obviously the Class II malocclusion), and upon the development of dental crowding and dental impaction and isolated oligodontia. The smaller codevelopment of the anterior tongue and anterior mandible also displaces the posterior tongue, to produce the clinical effect of glossoptosis (see chapter 8).

In my view, AMHypo is really not about having a small jaw at all—it's about having a small anterior tongue—and it is very much about all the secondary anatomical problems that an embryologically small anterior tongue also brings.

There is likely a natural genetic incidence for the small anterior tongue and small anterior jaw present throughout human history, which through relatively recent selective female husbandry (< 8,000 years) is likely promoted by its Western cultural neotenic effect. (*Neoteny* is a deliberate breeding effect leading to an adult face appearing juvenile or childlike.) As with the cliff-edge model to explain increased survival for the human traits of narrow pelvis and large heads through the modern surgical obstetric intervention of Caesarian section,[3] so too is the advent of orthodontics, dental extractions, and modern medical management for the effects of glossoptosis also likely increasing broad community incidence for the small anterior mandible, as with the co-effect of predominantly Class II malocclusion.

CAUSAL PROPOSITION FOR AMHYPO

While there is speculation as to why AMHypo develops and true epidemiologic prevalence remains investigable, the predominant feature of a diminutive lower face is likely neotenic,[4] exemplifying esthetic sexual dimorphic distinctiveness[5] and satisfying Western-Grecian-Latin cultural and later European Renaissance artistic ideals of female beauty.[6] This would indicate that AMHypo is a product of culture and selective sexual breeding[7] and a feature of selection post–sexual maturation[8] rather than an attribute resulting from any phylogenetic or classical Darwinian evolutionary natural selection model.[1,2,9–11]

The notion of discoverability of regional breeding traits (as opposed to survival traits) arising in recent European populations has paleoanthropologic and credible scientific precedence. Recent discoveries in ancient population genomics indicate that modern European features of lactose tolerance, increased height (particularly in northern Europeans), and pale skin complexion are only relatively recent racial traits that have been very strongly favored by breeding selection over the past 20,000 years. While selection for the ability to digest milk sugars (*LCT* gene) in a developing agrarian culture was likely partially survival based, and pale skin (*SLC24A5* and *SLLC45A2* genes) may have allowed adaptation to lower UV levels at higher latitudes to stimulate dermal vitamin D synthesis, the appearance of blonde hair and blue eye color (defined by *HERC2/OCA2* gene) seems more certain as a trait cued by purposeful trait selection rather than by survival. DNA studies now confirm that blonde hair and blue eye color only emerged about 6,000 to 8,000 years ago in Europe, likely from a single common ancestor, and that the European

This would indicate that AMHypo is a product of culture and selective sexual breeding rather than an attribute resulting from any phylogenetic or Darwinian evolutionary natural selection.

trait of pale skin is of a similar age, implying a regional cultural foundation.[12,13]

When discussing the ontogenetic causation of AMHypo, it is clear that the condition becomes increasingly expressed only as dentate mandibular growth continues. Anterior tongue volume and anterior mandible codevelopment begins (embryologically) apparently normally. Despite this author's assertion that a diminutive jawline is due to a Western cultural appeal to femininity, the trait expression appears to occur with equal frequency in both

In essence, modern humans have created our own scourge: the small jaw.

males and females. It does not occur in all children of all families, though it appears to have strong familial Mendelian inheritance patterns. It appears to be very common in adult and adolescent Western populations, and though its primary Western epidemiology is unknown, it is likely not limited only to a discussion of Class II malocclusion incidence.

The prospective affected gene may be a regulatory or primary genetic one, affecting expression of the primary gene or gene set defining anterior tongue muscle volume and the embryologic conversion of the first gill arch. The likely affected muscles are the collective of mylohyoid, geniohyoid, and anterior belly of digastric, whereby anterior-hyoid-body to retrognathion/menton length is affected, and that of the genioglossus, which forms most of the dome and width and volume of the anterior tongue. The inheritance is likely autosomal and possibly recessive. Selection for the trait was probably sexual-cultural (neotenic) rather than survival based. In essence, modern humans have created our own scourge: the small jaw.

THE ORIGINAL HUMAN WOLF

There is a widely spread socioanthropologic proposition, and likely a misrepresentation, that it is the modern diet that has led to the small mandible, through reduced masticatory muscular use. This proposition imputes an epigenetic cause, whereby the environment over the individual's lifetime, or even in the mother's lifetime (through effects upon the ovum), may have diminished masticatory muscle size. In part, this idea builds upon an original idea by Begg[1] based on observation of Australian Aborigines, who maintained a larger jaw size than the European settlers in Australia. This idea was later promulgated by Corruccini by his observations of indigenous people of Chandigarh in India,[9] further built upon by subsequent socioanthropologic investigators such as Ungar,[10] and even given attention by the orthodontic great William Proffitt.[11]

Original evolutionary studies by Charles Darwin classically described differences in beak sizes in Galapagos finches. While diet was considered the influence that accounted for the differences he observed, his explanations involved timelines encompassing hundreds of thousands of generations and millions of years of evolution and supported the idea that genetic mutation was a rare event that gave either advantage or disadvantage to survival and was an ultimate driver to speciation. In the evolution toward the human jaw, it is known that a simple mutation of two letters in the myocin gene in part has led to smaller masticating muscles in humans compared with chimpanzees or gorillas,[14] which again involved similar timelines of evolutionary speciation postulated by Darwin. The argument of modern socioanthropologists represented by Begg, Corruccini, and Ungar that modern diet somehow leads to an unknown epigenetic change and epigenetic memory for a smaller jaw size, and only through a few or several generations, and which is based upon modernism, or an escape from ruralism, or cultural primitivism, seems incongruent to a more scientific and directly genetic rationalism of Darwinian evolution.

Nonetheless, these ideas persist in modern dentistry and orthodontics, to the point where the majority of clinicians espouse the notion that third molars have been made evolutionarily redundant for modern human function and in a timeline involving only tens of hundreds of years. In my mind there is no such thing as an evolutionary redundancy of human teeth or human tonsils. To say this is to misunderstand the Darwinian concept of evolution. Humans are naturally evolved to have a full complement of 32 adult teeth, and we should expect to carry them for our adult lifetime, in a Class I occlusion and free of crowding or impactions

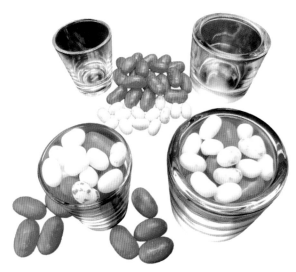

FIG 5-1 I use this jelly bean analogy to discuss tooth volume and necessity with adolescent patients and their parents. The jelly bean analogy has 20 large red jelly beans (representing unseen posterior teeth necessary for chewing) and 12 smaller white jelly beans (representing the anterior teeth that esthetically most parents want to keep). Given a choice between collecting 24 jelly beans (in a smaller shot glass) or 32 jelly beans (in a larger shot glass), a child will always select the larger option. Intermolar mandibular distraction osteogenesis (IMDO) surgery (to create the large shot glass whereby we keep all 32 teeth) is less invasive than having four premolars and four third molars removed (represented by removing 8 large red jelly beans and using the small shot glass). A smaller jaw also means having additional surgery for tonsil or adenoid removal (due to problems associated with glossoptosis and a reduced airway). The IMDO philosophy argues that crowded teeth, tonsils, or adenoids are not naturally redundant but are a consequence of abnormally and "neotenically" small jaws.

> Humans are naturally evolved to have a full complement of 32 adult teeth, and we should expect to carry them for our adult lifetime, in a Class I occlusion and free of crowding or impactions or airway collapse.

or airway collapse (Fig 5-1). Just like an East African human from 200,000 years ago—the face of the original human wolf.

Instead of our third molars or tonsils or adenoids being redundant because they "don't fit" in the jaws we have, it is our small jaws that are through inadvertent breeding (via cultural selection) inadequate. And this cultural ideal of neoteny combined with modern medical advancements that compensate for the underlying anatomical problem have led to the commonality of small jaws and the modern epidemics of snoring, obstructive sleep apnea, and dental crowding with malocclusion.

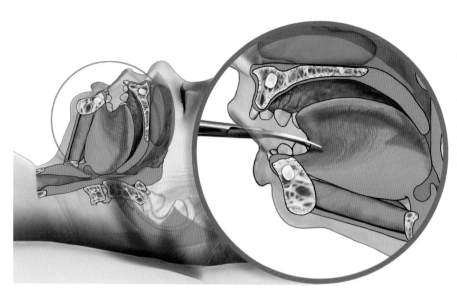

FIG 5-2 Snipping the tongue frenum has absolutely no therapeutic value in correcting for the sleeping child's tongue position. If anything, cutting it removes a key ligature holding the whole tongue forward. Glossoptosis and retroglossal airway obstruction is entirely linked to the phenomenon of the small mandible. In the hands of the nonspecialist surgeon, frenectomy is also a procedure fraught with complications.

Tongue tie

Another misconception in modern dentistry based on flawed logic is that snipping a lingual frenum in babies and children will somehow help the restless sleeping child breathe better, when in fact it does the direct opposite.

Snipping the lingual frenum in neonates or children (or adults for that matter) has absolutely no therapeutic effect on how a tongue functions at night when asleep, or in preventing airway collapse behind the tongue, or in allowing the jaw to grow to its full potential. If anything, it actually aggravates the poor tongue position by removing a structural attachment that helps to hold it forward (Fig 5-2)—much like cutting one end of an already short hammock.

The act in children is barbaric, without any scientific rationalism, and defies a rational interpretation of how glossoptosis occurs and of the anatomy involved. At best, any claim to therapeutic benefit is based in psychologic suggestion or wholly to satisfy parental request. Worse still is that in untrained nonspecialist hands, this procedure is also dangerous because of its potential for uncontrolled bleeding or irreversible trauma to the adjacent salivary gland ducts. The only time a lingual frenum should be snipped is for purely medical reasons and agreed to by a specialist surgeon.

And like a turtle's shell, the ultimate size of the front of the mandible is driven by internal forces that cause it to expand to accommodate the growing mammal within.

HOW THE MANDIBLE GROWS

In order to better understand how the mandible develops and forms from its relationship to soft tissue, it is helpful to look at other examples in nature. A turtle shell is a convenient model for comparison (Fig 5-3). The shell is made up of a back, or *carapace*, and an underside, or *plastron*. Its shape is made up of multiple plates, or *scutes*. The lines between these scutes enable the shell to expand. The animal and its shell start life together as a single interdependent unit. As the animal gets bigger, the individual scutes also expand, and the overall shell of the turtle seemingly grows.

Like a turtle's shell, mandibles start small too. And like a turtle's shell, the ultimate size of the front of the mandible is driven by internal forces that cause it to expand to accommodate the growing mammal within. In mammals, it is the tongue that grows (Fig 5-4). The front horseshoe of the mandible effectively acts like the turtle's carapace.

The front of the mandible, the anterior tongue, and the 16 teeth within the mandible are collectively one growth unit derived majoratively from the first gill arch. The jaw joints are a very small part of the overall jaw. Jaw joints have

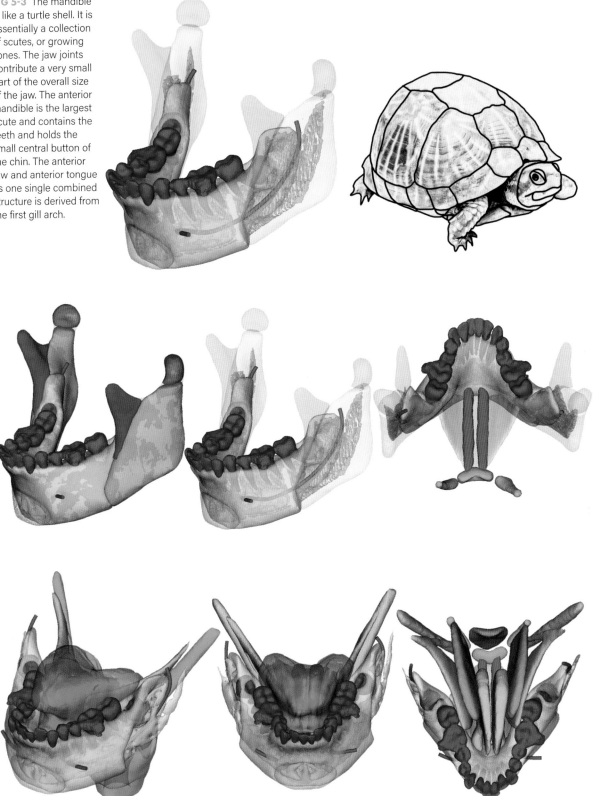

FIG 5-3 The mandible is like a turtle shell. It is essentially a collection of scutes, or growing zones. The jaw joints contribute a very small part of the overall size of the jaw. The anterior mandible is the largest scute and contains the teeth and holds the small central button of the chin. The anterior jaw and anterior tongue as one single combined structure is derived from the first gill arch.

FIG 5-4 The anterior mandible contains the attachments of the front of the tongue. As the volume of the tongue expands, it "grows" and expands the anterior mandible. A small anterior tongue produces AMHypo, which leads to dental crowding and impacted third molars. The small tongue indirectly causes almost the entirety of all forms of malocclusion and dental crowding patterns and random agenesis of single permanent teeth.

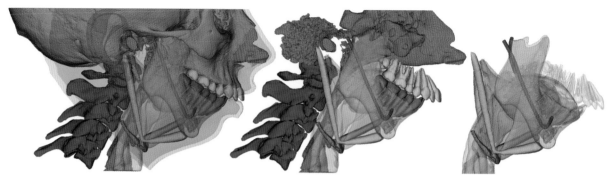

FIG 5-5 Destruction of jaw joints (in this case by juvenile rheumatoid arthritis [JRA]), leads to PMHypo, or a "vertical" form of Class II malocclusion. JRA is surprisingly frequent across all human races. It probably has an incidence approaching 1% of all populations and leads to massive facial disfigurement, significant dental crowding, and most importantly, severe airway compromise. Residual jaw joints are often abnormally forward. If a majority of all people with malocclusion have AMHypo, then a majority of all people with JRA will have AMHypo also.

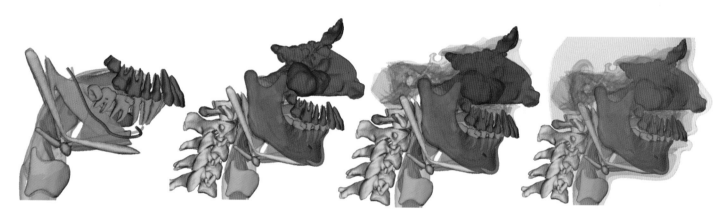

FIG 5-6 A reduced anterior tongue volume, which is a trait of white people, leads to reduced size of the anterior jaw. The associated "horizontal" form of Class II malocclusion (with increased forward prominence of the maxillary anterior teeth) is obviously seen as the adult dentition and malocclusion form. AMHypo leads to impacted third molars, mandibular dental crowding, and a reduced posterior airway space (behind the tongue). There may be a naturally forward-leaning head posture and a sense of reduced chin prominence with lack of defined jawline. The jaw joints are normal and normally located.

some innate growth within them, but overall they make up a very small proportion of jaw volume and equally make a very small contribution to postembryologic jaw growth or size. When embryology or postnatal disease destroys the jaw joints, it produces a particular type of jaw deformity. The primary feature of jaw joint loss is a reduced posterior vertical height of the mandible. I call the multitude and expressed range of conditions that affect posterior mandibular development *posterior mandibular hypoplasia*, or PMHypo (Fig 5-5). The range of condylar conditions and the diseases that cause them are found across all races and societies, and by comparison to AMHypo, they are rare.

Within the front of the mandible lie all the muscles and all the forward attachments of the anterior two-thirds of the tongue. The bone of the anterior mandible also contains all of the mandibular teeth. The "growth" of this largest jaw "scute" underscores the reality of how small or big the front of the mandible will become in adulthood (Fig 5-6).

As the anterior tongue "grows," its surrounding bony "scute" also expands, enabling the developing teeth to naturally erupt and form a full occlusion (Fig 5-7). If the front of the mandible is too small, dental crowding and dental impactions will occur. The small anterior tongue causes AMHypo, which leads to all the common patterns of malocclusion described in chapter 1.

The final scute is the chin. It is also connected to specific tongue muscles, called the *anterior digastrics*. A small chin, diminutive jawline, crowded teeth, impacted third molars, and malocclusion (with normal jaw joints) are all common associations of AMHypo.

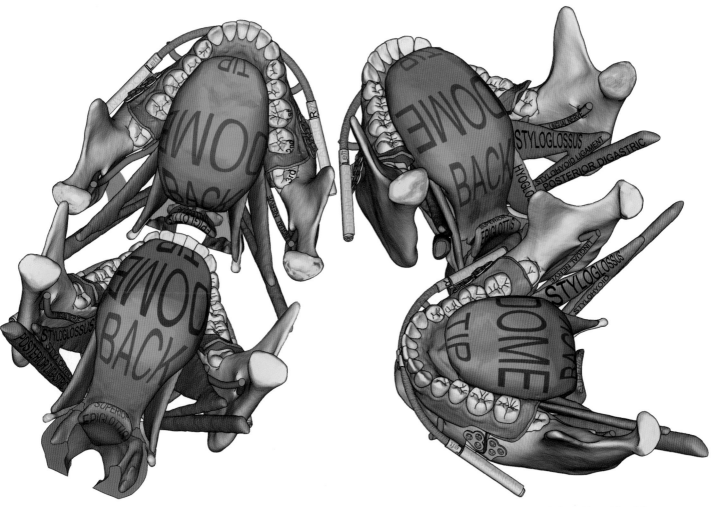

FIG 5-7 The anterior tongue and anterior mandible are one growth unit. IMDO uses tesseract distractors applied to either side of the mandible. By expanding and growing the mandible forward, it pulls the tongue with it, opening the airway behind the tongue. Creating new bone between the first and second molars allows for natural tooth eruption and maximal dental development.

CAN WE GROW THE MANDIBLE FURTHER?

The only true way to "grow" the mandible is to do so surgically. No orthodontic appliance will pull the mandible beyond its natural genetic potential. Many of the devices on the market instead restrict growth of the maxilla so that the jaws are proportionally small to eliminate the esthetic dental problem of significant overbite or malocclusion. But again, this is just a camouflage, and it only further limits the patient's function and overall tooth volume via premolar and later third molar extraction. The only way to truly extend the mandible to eliminate the same problem

> The only true way to "grow" the mandible is to do so surgically. No orthodontic appliance will pull the mandible beyond its natural genetic potential.

of significant overbite or malocclusion, not to mention poor esthetics, dewlap, and the more troubling consequence of AMHypo—glossoptosis—is through surgical intervention, most notably IMDO (see chapter 8). This is the only way to achieve a Class A orthognathic state (see chapter 1).

CONCLUSION

What likely began as an inadvertent cultural quest for female neoteny has transformed into a global dentofacial problem that many people are blind to because of its commonality and seeming normalcy, leading to ineffective therapies that further mask the underlying problem—AMHypo—and its inherent glossoptosis. As this book will continue to explain, jaw correction surgery is the only real solution.

REFERENCES

1. Begg PR. Stone age man's dentition: With reference to anatomically correct occlusion, the etiology of malocclusion, and a technique for its treatment. Am J Orthod 1954;40:462–475.
2. Mills JRE. Occlusion and malocclusion of the teeth of primates. In: Dental Anthropology: Volume V: Society for the Study of Human Biology. Oxford: Pergamon, 1963:29–52.
3. Mitteroecker P, Huttegger SM, Fischer B, Pavlicev M. Cliff-edge model of obstetric selection in humans. Proc Natl Acad Sci U S A 2016;113:14680-14685.
4. Zebrowitz LA. Stability of babyfacedness and attractiveness across the life span. J Personality Soc Psychol 1993:64:435–466.
5. Rhodes G. The evolutionary psychology of facial beauty. Ann Rev Psychol 2006;57:199–226.
6. Dillon S. The female portrait statue in the Greek world. Cambridge: Cambridge Press, 2010.
7. Berry B. The Power of Looks. Social Stratification of Physical Appearance. Farnham, UK: Ashgate, 2008.
8. Jones D, Brace CL, Jankowiak W, et al. Sexual selection, physical attractiveness, and facial neoteny: Cross-cultural evidence and implications (and comments and reply). Curr Anthropol 1995;36:723–748.
9. Corruccini RS. An epidemiologic transition in dental occlusion in world populations. Am J Orthod 1984;86:419–426.
10. Ungar PS. Evolution's Bite: A Story of Teeth, Diet and Human Origins. Princeton, New Jersey: Princeton University, 2017.
11. Proffitt WR. Contemporary Orthodontics. St Louis: Mosby, 1986:90.
12. Wilde S, Timpson A, Kirsanow K, et al. Direct evidence for positive selection of skin, hair and eye pigmentation in Europeans during the last 5,000y. PNAS 2014;111(13):4832–4837.
13. Matheison I, Lazaridis I, Rohland N, et al. Eight thousand years of natural selection in Europe. BioRxiv 2015. doi: 10.1101/016477.
14. Stedman HH, Kozyak BW, Nelson A, et al. Myosin gene mutation correlates with anatomical changes in the human lineage. Nature 2004;428(6981):415–418.

6

JAW CORRECTION PROCEDURES

Jaw surgery is as old as war. It is older than dentistry or even medicine. Anesthesia was invented for jaw surgery. Some of the greatest surgeons of history were jaw surgeons and dentists, including John Hunter, who helped found the oldest surgical club in the world (ie, the Royal College of Surgeons of England), and Hugo Obwegeser, the Swiss inventor of the bilateral sagittal split osteotomy (BSSO) operation in 1957. Modern stainless steel microplates and screws were invented for jaw surgery by Maxime Champy in Strasbourg, France, in the 1970s and championed by the instrument maker Karl Leibinger Surgical of Tüttlingen, Germany. The modern company of KLS Martin is now a leading manufacturer of titanium maxillofacial prostheses and also makes the intermolar mandibular distraction osteogenesis (IMDO) distractors illustrated in this book. The invention of jaw correction surgery and orthognathic surgery has as much to do with inspired surgeons as it has to do with creative and intuitive instrument engineers.

All maxillofacial surgeons begin their training in simple third molar surgery. After all, this is the fundamental foundation of all jaw surgery operations. Eventually, with good training, a maxillofacial surgeon will learn to master all the jaw surgery operations, which include IMDO, BSSO, LeFort advancement, LeFort-SARME (surgically assisted rapid maxillary expansion), genioplasty, GenioPaully, and the BIMAX. The operative location (Fig 6-1), the instruments we use, the staff that assist us, and the hospitals we operate within do not vary much between the various types of jaw surgery operations, nor does our experience with the patient. Figure 6-2 demonstrates a useful way of comparing patients' subjective experiences with each jaw surgery operation, from least invasive to most invasive.

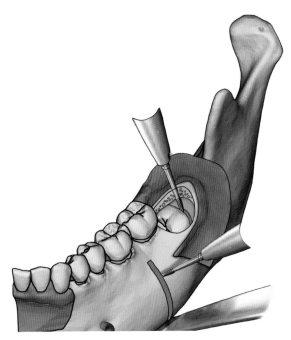

FIG 6-1 The BSSO and IMDO start off the same way, but the vertical superficial bone cut onto the outside of the mandible is the entire limit to the IMDO. By contrast, the BSSO has a significant surgical extension through the third molar, which requires its sacrifice. IMDO is less invasive than third molar surgery, removes virtually no bone, is easier to perform, and has less swelling and practically zero neural risk. IMDO also aims to prevent the third molars from impacting as well as gives an early cure to snoring and sleep apnea. To directly compare the IMDO and BSSO operation, refer to Fig 6-15.

Jaw surgery is as old as war. It is older than dentistry or even medicine.

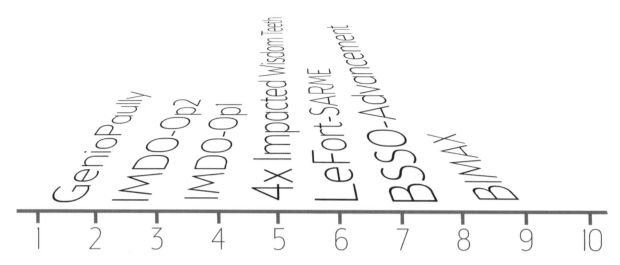

FIG 6-2 This simple line chart offers a useful way of comparing patients' subjective experience of each of the jaw operations (as long as they are performed by the same expert and in the same circumstances), on a scale of 1 to 10, with 5 being the experience of having four deeply impacted third molars removed under general anesthesia.

MAKING JAWS BIGGER

Bringing the mandible forward, with all of its teeth, such that the jaw joints remain perfectly neutrally positioned and healthy is actually very hard to do. Whatever you use to advance the front of the jaw has to permanently (and perfectly) overcome a force that wants to pull it backward to where it started.

Isaac Newton wrote his three laws of motion in 1687. His third law said that anything that tries to move in one direction is constantly resisted by an equal force that acts in exactly the opposite direction. In orthognathic surgery, we've renamed this third law the Law of Jaw Advancement. The problem with the Law of Jaw Advancement is that the further forward you advance the mandible, the logarithmically greater the force becomes that wants to pull it backward. That pull-back force comes from your skin and tongue, and it starts at a neutral zero. Eventually, you can only extend it so far, at which point the force is insurmountable. This point is called the maximal distensible limit.

All of us can find one form of our own maximal distensible limit quite easily. Just puff out your cheeks. Eventually there comes a limit that your cheeks cannot inflate any further. Thus your cheeks are acting like a leather purse. It distends, but it doesn't elastically stretch. There are only so

Bringing the mandible forward, with all of its teeth, such that the jaw joints remain perfectly neutrally positioned and healthy is actually very hard to do.

many things that you can stuff into it. There is a physical limit to the distention of natural skin.

Growing a mandible to tighten facial skin has cosmetic advantages. It really helps to define jawlines, and throughout this book, you can see examples of just how that happens. The biggest force resistance to moving the front of the mandible forward doesn't just come from the overlying skin. That force resistance also comes from behind and within the jaw, and therapeutically it's the most important force to overcome. That pull-back force comes from the tongue itself. It is called *glossoptosis* (Fig 6-3), and unless we as surgeons can fully overcome it, we are never going to fundamentally prevent or cure a patient of snoring—or its most serious disease effect, obstructive sleep apnea (OSA).

The amount of force needed to overcome glossoptosis and cure someone of snoring or OSA is determined by the distance we need to pull the front of the mandible permanently forward. I call this distance to permanently

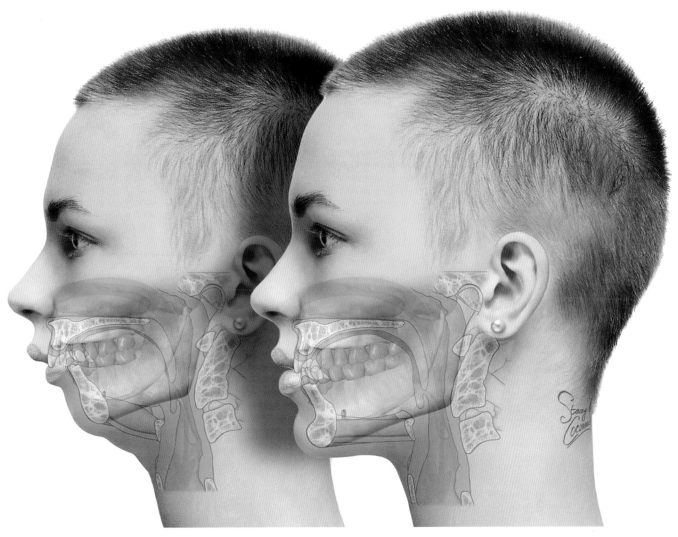

FIG 6-3 The most obvious sign of glossoptosis is a roll of fatty skin falling between the chin and neck. This fold is what orthognathic surgeons call a *dewlap*. The dewlap is actually your displaced tongue as it falls backward and downward under its own weight underneath and behind the small mandible. Seen from inside the face, this tongue displacement is called *glossoptosis*, and its collapse has its most important medical effect when you lie on your back and during sleep. Glossoptosis is the primary cause of snoring. Aggravated by weight gain, your dewlap may eventually lead to OSA. Because glossoptosis is related to the small mandible, it is also intrinsically linked to the presence (during adolescence) of adult dental crowding and bad bites. The normality of an open airway, facial profile proportionality, and a full 32-tooth dentition are all distorted in the "small jaw" condition.

overcome glossoptosis the *minimum distensible need*. Let me be clear that the minimum distensible need is imaginary. It's a guess. And what's worse, its length is going to be different for everyone (Fig 6-4). Nonetheless, the ideal jaw extension of the front of the jaw (with the jaw joints in a perfectly neutral position) lies somewhere between the *maximal distensible limit* and this *minimum distensible need*.

Of course, as well as curing a person of their glossoptosis, a surgeon must also gain a perfect bite relationship (with a maximum number of teeth) and an ideal facial proportionality. These three simultaneous things—bite, airway, and facial balance—are the three boxes that orthognathic surgeons and orthodontists, working together, must fundamentally tick.

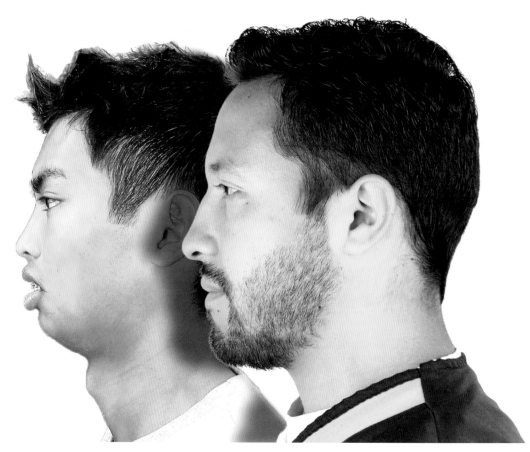

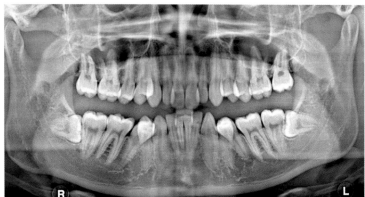

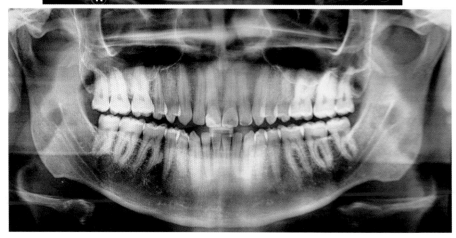

FIG 6-4 This figure shows two 25-year-old men of the same race. Both radiographs and facial profiles are in 1:1 proportion. The upper radiograph shows severe dental crowding of 30 teeth (the maxillary third molars were already removed). This patient has very small jaws, a small chin, a prominent dewlap, and severe snoring. The lower radiograph shows no dental crowding, a full complement of 32 teeth (which includes four third molars), naturally normal jaw sizes, and a perfect Class I bite. This patient has a normal profile, no dewlap, and no snoring, and he is a dentist by profession.

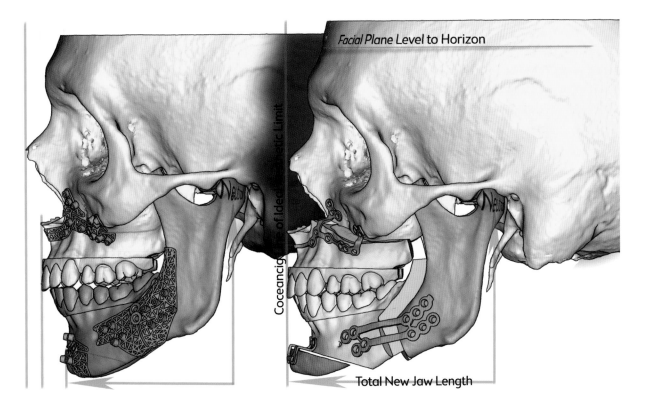

FIG 6-5A If I use a vertical line, drawn down from the tip of the nasal bone (which I call the Line of Ideal Aesthetic Limit), I find that I have a way of rationally combining an esthetic facial profile balance with an imaginary ideal length of the mandible necessary to overcome the underlying glossoptosis (through the associated pull of the tongue's geniohyoid muscle). This patient already had two maxillary premolars and four third molars removed as an adolescent. His school years were dominated by a "pull-back" style orthodontic treatment for prominent anterior teeth. At the time, little thought was given to the possibility that he may instead have a small mandible. He now snores intolerably as a 35-year-old adult and fundamentally wants a permanent cure, a better bite, and a better facial proportionality as well. To help, I used custom facial design technology and eventually bespoke titanium solutions combined with LeFort I, BSSO, and genioplasty advancements. This way I can also idealize the bite without relying upon classic orthodontics or intermaxillary fixation (IMF). While I cannot easily show the patient his tongue or how his facial look may change, making these hard tissue points meet this imaginary vertical line helps maximize smile and facial esthetics, while likely also passing the minimum distensible need of the tongue to overcome snoring. I have to pull the back of his tongue forward enough so that it doesn't collapse at night when he sleeps. Reaching a critical yet therapeutically unknown new jaw length is necessary to permanently overcome snoring and OSA. The jaw joints, meanwhile, need to remain perfectly neutral and balanced in their paired positions. The rigidity and precision of the custom titanium and predictability of the custom design process (mediated by the titanium cutting and drill guide jig shown at left), gives absolute predictability and long-term stability to the advancement distance achievable by this method. The achievable advancement distances are far further than I can predictably achieve through the use of traditional plate and screw systems. The argument of traditional genioplasty vs GenioPaully to overcome glossoptosis via the geniohyoid is discussed in chapter 7.

HOW TO ACCOMPLISH BITE, AIRWAY, AND FACIAL BALANCE

In my many years of surgical experience, aided by the fact that I 3D print the before and after facial skeletons of my patients, three simple trends of analysis have become apparent in all those cases that have successfully ticked all three boxes. First, it's become clear that we are capable of accommodating all 32 teeth. The adolescent combination of maxillary arch widening with an orthodontic HYRAX appliance and mandibular arch lengthening with IMDO (alongside a tooth-preserving style of orthodontics) is a very effective way of making both jaws just big enough to potentially accommodate all 32 adult teeth in perfect alignment.

Second, we can use a vertical profile line offset against the natural head horizon to determine the extent to which the mandible must be brought forward (Fig 6-5). The line is drawn against the tip of the nasal bone. Ideally the tip of the anterior nasal spine, the anterior surface of the maxillary central incisor, and pogonion all approximately sit on the same line, with the occlusion in an incisal Class

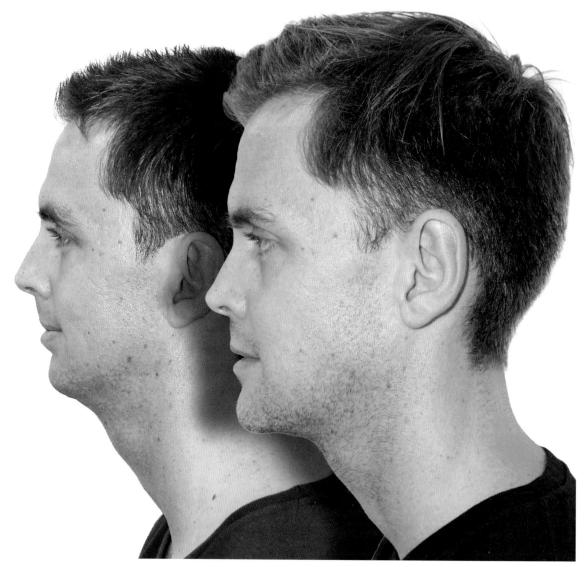

FIG 6-5B Clinical facial change to the patient's profile and the change to his dewlap as a result of surgical intervention by remedial BIMAX following adolescent extraction-based camouflage orthodontics.

I relationship. I use this line as a way of predicting how far I need to bring the front of the mandible forward. My goal is to find a balance between the practical extendable limit of each type of operation and the actual therapeutic and esthetic need of the patient. Falling short of the line potentially means that I have not reached the maximal therapeutic advantage that my operations could have reached in overcoming glossoptosis and snoring. If I do not reach the line, I risk not curing a person of their existing OSA or their future risk of developing it. Breaching the line means potentially compromising the personal esthetics or ideal facial proportions of the patient.

Third, we need to assess how well the airway is functioning. We all have three dynamic airway states. The first exists

while we're awake and erect but not exercising. People with a small mandible can develop a habit of holding their head forward to help them breathe in such a state. They normally do not know that their slouching habit is very much related to the smallness of their mandible and their underlying glossoptosis (Figs 6-6 and 6-7). If not addressed early, the slouching behavior can adversely affect how the cervical spine develops; it irreversibly entrenches the posture into adulthood (Fig 6-8). The classic methods of telling children to simply "sit up straight" or to "pull your shoulders back" or even using physiotherapy to help with back and shoulder muscular development do not really help very much.

The second dynamic airway type exists when we are running or doing some form of sustained aerobic exercise.

FIG 6-6 This patient has a small mandible and prominent anterior teeth. She also has severe glossoptosis. By subconsciously holding her head and neck forward, which also means that she has to round the shoulders forward (slouching), she is helping to open the airway behind her tongue. This neck posture, if not addressed early by fundamentally stretching her tongue forward by making her mandible longer, can become chronic and sustained. The abnormally small airway also compromises normal exercise development during adolescence. It is fundamentally difficult to run while slouching.

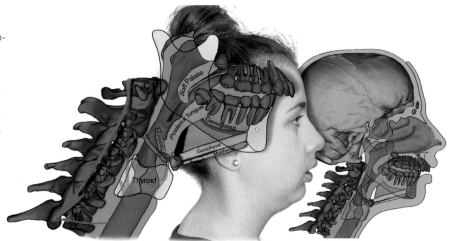

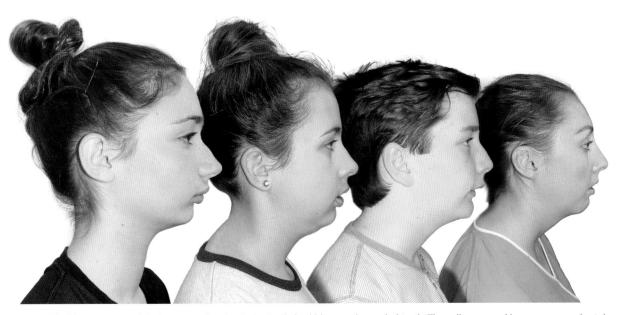

FIG 6-7 All of these young adults have prominent anterior teeth, bad bites, and crowded teeth. They all snore and have poor exercise tolerance. Each also has increasingly varying degrees of adverse adaptive neck posture to help overcome the breathing problems associated with their glossoptosis. These separate conditions are connected by the inherently small mandible and anterior mandibular hypoplasia (AMHypo) common to all of them.

FIG 6-8 This patient underwent camouflage orthodontics for her prominent anterior teeth as an adolescent. She also lost all four third molars. She cannot run and she cannot sleep on her back without completely closing off the airway behind her tongue. Her chronic forward head posture has also led to severe developmental problems in her cervical spine, which as an adult is now impossible to reverse. Using the Line of Ideal Aesthetic Limit, we know that to overcome snoring and her diagnosed OSA, her chin point and jaw length must forward advance by about 30 mm. Refer to Fig 13-7 to see this patient's profile after surgery.

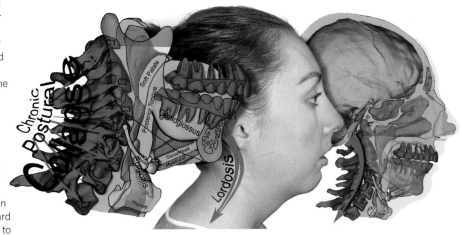

FIG 6-9 Following running, a child with a small jaw and who has inherent glossoptosis will adopt a common set of complaints and postures. First they will complain that they hate running moderate or long distances and thus they actively avoid it. Evidence for exercise avoidance can be seen by a sense of reduced muscular development of the thighs or calves. The second is that they will often complain of a "stitch" from running (which is a cramp in the overworked diaphragm muscle driving an increased rate and column of air through a reduced and high-resistance retroglossal airway). The third observation is for the effect of increased and abrasive and turbulent "dry" oral airflow through a restricted air column leading to a complaint of airway stricture behind the tongue or upper trachea, often relieved by combined prophylactic inhalation steroids with beta-adrenergic agonists like salbutamol. The fourth observation is the significant open mouth breathing, with the tongue and jaw held significantly forward and with hands on knees with head and neck hyperextended forward, all in an effort to maximally open the airway behind the occluding tongue to relieve the reduced-airway effects of heavy breathing. Adequately advancing the mandible and tongue during the active IMDO period can be measured against the subjective sensation of improved aerobic exercise tolerance and the elimination of airway complaints and of observed changes to adaptive postural effects.

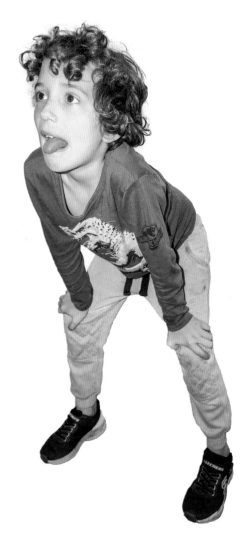

Exercising increases both the flow rate and volume of the air we breathe. Most people with small jaws and glossoptosis cannot open the mouth wide enough or take in air fast enough through their already reduced retroglossal airway to be able to easily sustain aerobic exercise (Fig 6-9).

The third dynamic airway state occurs when we are in deep sleep and lying on our back. During REM (dreaming) or slow-wave sleep, and when we are most relaxed, the muscles that are normally toned and contracted to hold our tongue forward during our waking state now become completely flaccid (Fig 6-10). For patients with a small jaw and glossoptosis, this relaxation of the tongue and the reduced patency of the airway lead to snoring. This is relieved by open mouth breathing or by lying on their side or belly during sleep, allowing gravity to help relieve the obstructed glottis. As they age and as neck fat closes the airway even further (the donut-hole effect), this initial primary snoring can progress to the deadly effects of OSA.

Entering light sleep can maintain general tone and help the tongue contract and prevent airway collapse.

The easiest way to maintain light sleep is through the brainstem's reticular activating system, which in turn is reflexively switched on by pontine clenching and tooth grinding neural cycles during sleep—a behavior classically associated with general restlessness, poor sleep quality, and daytime "stress."

While continuous positive airway pressure (CPAP) devices and mandibular advancement devices (MADs) relieve this nighttime collapse of the relaxed tongue into the supine airway, they do nothing to assist in the other two dynamic airway states and are not curative for OSA. For people trying to avoid surgery, CPAP is simply the last Band-Aid left in the drawer.

If jaw surgery is to be successful at lengthening a jaw and ridding someone of glossoptosis, it must improve neck posture, improve aerobic exercise tolerance, overcome snoring, and most importantly, eliminate OSA if it has already developed.

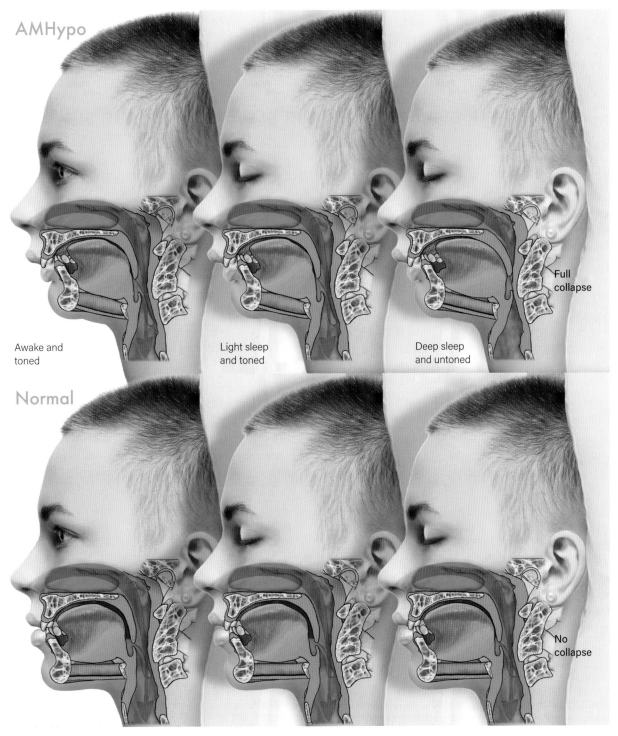

AMHypo

Awake and toned | Light sleep and toned | Deep sleep and untoned — Full collapse

Normal

No collapse

FIG 6-10 There are differences in the tone of the tongue that exist between our awake-and-toned versus our deep-sleep-untoned states (which occurs either during REM or dream sleep and with slow-wave stages of sleep). A small jaw is inevitably associated with both a fundamentally bad bite and glossoptosis. In order to comfortably breathe, the muscles underneath the tongue must contract forward, and with the lips naturally sealed, it enables unobstructed breathing through the nose. This forward contraction of the tongue muscles can only occur during awake-and-toned states. During REM or slow-wave sleep, the tone in the tongue is lost, and under the influence of gravity, the tongue will collapse backward onto the cervical spine, reducing or fully closing the airway. In the normal-sized jaw, a loss of tongue tone is not usually a problem, but in patients with small jaws and who have existing glossoptosis, this obstruction will at first lead to primary snoring. The sound of snoring is really the sound of turbulent air and of flaccid surrounding tissues that flutter around the stricture point. Primary snoring eventually transitions into frank airway obstruction, when it will lead to OSA. CPAP helps with this collapse and helps improve sleep quality, but it is not a cure by any means.

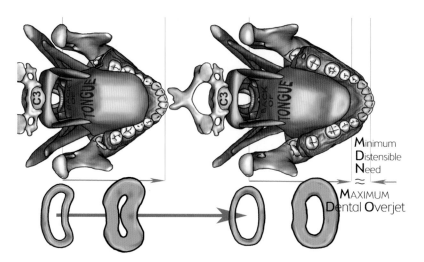

Minimum
Distensible
Need
≈
MAXIMUM
Dental Overjet

FIG 6-11 Extending a mandible forward stretches the muscles of the tongue and pulls the back of the tongue (and epiglottis) away from the cervical spine and from the back of the throat. Jaw extension literally tents and opens the airway, preventing inward collapse, much like pulling forward a thick rubber ring or torus. With age and as the neck gets thicker, the donut hole within also gets smaller. The combination of weight gain in older age and a preexisting glossoptosis is the fatal combination that eventually leads to OSA. Even if weight gain occurs, normalizing the jaw volume with IMDO or hyperextended BSSO using custom titanium should protect against the lifetime development of OSA arising from the combined effects of glossoptosis and neck obesity.

HOW FAR CAN WE EXTEND THE MANDIBLE?

As previously mentioned, most of the people I see for corrective jaw surgery are either *(1)* growing children/adolescents prior to any orthodontic treatment or *(2)* nongrowing adults who have already undergone camouflage or pull-back classical orthodontics. As they come with different body sizes, patients also come with a range of small-jaw sizes that fundamentally describe their baseline condition. My job is to plan an efficient strategy to minimize intervention but maximize benefit.

By coordinating the separate efforts of surgeon and orthodontist, we're trying to do several simultaneous things. First, we're trying to fit in all the teeth, or at least as many as

we can. Second, we're trying to stretch the tongue (and the airway behind it) far enough forward so that breathing is naturally comfortable—24 hours a day—with a normal head posture through the extremes of exercise and sleep (Fig 6-11). Third, we are trying to achieve a maximally normal bite that is matched to a maximally beautiful facial esthetic, alongside the elimination of any dewlap. Of course, a perfect smile and a perfect face are fundamentally subjective things. In the end, like any functional object, the face simply looks better, or more beautiful, if it functions best. And it functions best when it fits in all of the anatomy—all of the teeth, a normal bite, balanced jaw joints, an open airway, normal-sized jaws, lips that naturally meet, and a full profile with no dewlap (Fig 6-12).

FIG 6-12 *(a)* There are fundamentally two ways to look at big front teeth. Either you see them as due to a small mandible or you see them as purely a dental problem requiring only orthodontics. The airway is even easier to ignore, let alone the tongue and muscles that control that airway. Whatever treatment selected for a 14-year-old child, whether it involves camouflage orthodontics or fundamental jaw surgery, will affect that airway. But just remember that ONLY corrective jaw surgery can do anything to fundamentally and permanently correct glossoptosis. *(b)* Treatment by camouflage orthodontics and without extractions brings the anterior teeth backward and downward, giving a gummy smile, while training the mandible to come forward to get the teeth to meet. The primary problem with this medically speaking is that the moment the patient falls asleep, all tone is lost and the jaw naturally settles into its normal jaw joint position, recreating the glossoptosis night after night. *(c)* Bringing the anterior maxillary teeth back a little with orthodontics and then advancing the mandible through a classic BSSO procedure using normal plates and screws (where the stable limit of the forward slide is about 6 mm), together with a sliding genioplasty, improves the airway, but it is unlikely that the minimum distensible distance necessary to prevent snoring or cure long-term OSA is reached, and a partial dewlap inevitably remains. Some orthodontists prefer this method, as it maintains a "soft French look" to the female lower profile. This surgery can only be performed after the third molars are removed and usually after 18 years of age. *(d)* Formal reversal of the effects of camouflage orthodontics seen in *b* requires BIMAX using LeFort advancement and BSSO. Using custom titanium, greater and more predictable advancement distances are possible (up to 11 mm in the maxilla and mandible) without the need for IMF and splints as is used with the off-the-shelf BSSO plating system seen in *c*. The BSSO requires presurgical removal of the third molars, as does camouflage orthodontics, as the jaws are simply too small to allow their normal development. *(e)* IMDO does not require orthodontics in the traditional sense and is sparing of third molars. As with *d*, IMDO is combined with the GenioPaully in order to gain further pull on the tongue and maximize dewlap elimination (up to 10 mm). The combination spares the patient from prolonged orthodontics or dental extractions, and the aim is to gain a full 32-tooth dentition if surgery is conducted between ages 12 and 15 years old. IMDO can extend a maximum of 16.5 mm. *(f)* For adults where extreme advancement distances are required in order to breach the minimum distensible distance to overcome established OSA, previous IMDO (in *e*) can be magnified by custom titanium BIMAX in order to maximally distend the airway. The author's record when combining custom titanium BIMAX with previous IMDO and GenioPaully is a total forward pogonion movement of about 32 mm, at which distance the overlying skin is very tight. This hyperextension of the jaws, where stability and design are only possible with custom titanium, is what I call the SuperBIMAX.

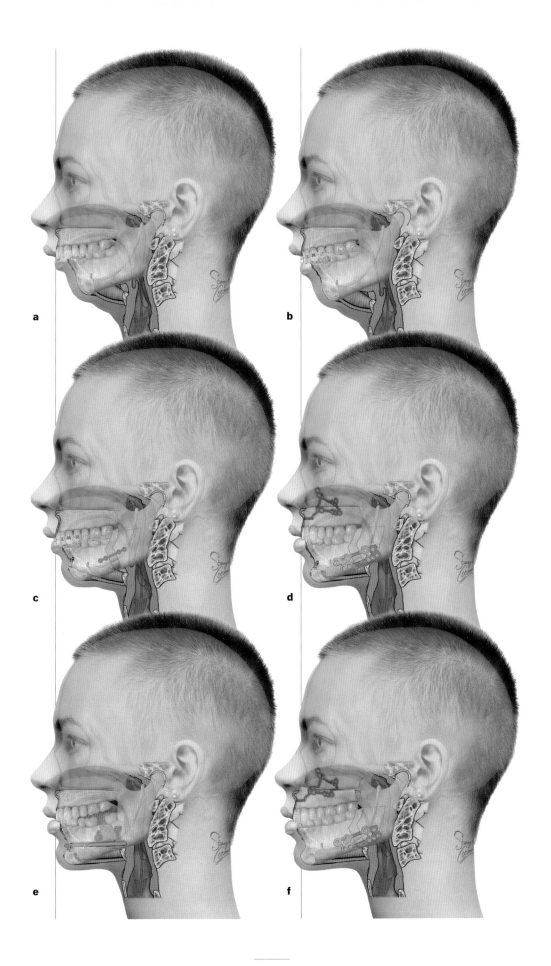

A good rule of thumb for determining how big a jaw needs to become is to think in terms of trying to fit in all 32 teeth. Ranking the size of patients' jaws is like giving them a par score on the golf course. Most of the 12- to 15-year-old children I treat are par 2 or 3. Some are 4. Almost all the adults I treat are par 5 and 6. Some are even an 8. The par represents the number of surgical operations or orthodontic steps that need to be coordinated. How I arrive at the par score I assign is sort of complicated; let me explain.

Most kids I see have already had pre-IMDO orthodontics, where they have achieved what I call a Class II, division 1 (orthognathic Class B) occlusion. The orthodontist, anticipating IMDO, has already expanded the maxilla and proclined the anterior teeth using fairly simple orthodontics in order to maximize the dental overjet. In two or three operations, I place distractors, then remove distractors, and I may also perform a GenioPaully. In the third operation, I remove the chin plate and recontour the chin button perfectly. IMDO is the simplest operation I have. It avoids third molar surgery, tonsillectomy, and adenoid removal. It makes orthodontics much easier. And by curing glossoptosis, it avoids a lifetime of other ill effects related to the development of OSA.

I call these kids a par 2, 3, or 4, meaning I take two or three surgical shots with orthodontics thrown in. I can use up to 16.5 mm of an IMDO distractor to advance the front of the mandible about 11 mm forward, which is titrated against their size and appearance and the relief from snoring. (Sometimes I ask that they run around the block each night during the distraction period and see if breathing becomes easier.) I then digitally design a piece of custom titanium for the forward chin button projection, which can extend the tongue another 6 mm. The final operation is a small bone graft to craft the chin button after I've removed the chin plate. Class I orthodontic mechanics can then be conducted several months later after the occlusion has naturally settled into a full Class I relationship. Finding the perfect balance between the maximal distensible limit and the minimum distensible need is normally easy and quick for these patients. And we tick all three boxes (bite, airway, facial balance) efficiently and predictably. Par 4 at the most.

Most adults I see have already had dental extractions and a period of camouflage orthodontics during their teens. They now snore, have already lost their tonsils and adenoids and up to eight teeth (from 32), and are desperate

It's far easier and simpler to treat kids before all the camouflage orthodontics happened in the first place.

for what is essentially life-saving treatment to cure them of OSA (Fig 6-13). They are obviously much bigger in overall size than the par 3 or 4 kids who are simply presenting for IMDO treatment. But these adults have exactly the same fundamental condition that the par 3/4 kids had. They all still have a relatively small mandible, and all of them still have primary glossoptosis. They obviously don't have dental crowding anymore, because the crowded and impacted teeth have already been long removed and their remaining teeth were long since "straightened" during their high school years. Their small jaw did not just lead to adolescent dental crowding. Their underlying glossoptosis has now transformed from simple snoring into full-blown OSA, whose secondary effects like hypertension, obesity, and diabetes make surgical treatment sometimes medically difficult. Their treatment is now super complicated. Now I need one operation to surgically widen the maxilla, one to extend both the jaws through custom titanium, and another finally to remove the plates that I used and recontour everything to take away any lumps or bumps. What was originally a par 3 or 4 is now a far more difficult course.

Because most adults are quite a lot bigger than 12-year-old children, the distances to "get to the line" are also proportionally bigger too. Instead of a 13-year-old needing a 13-mm IMDO to get 10 mm of pogonion advancement, these adults may now need 20 mm instead. To cure these people and to drag the whole weight of their tongue far enough forward (in order to get past their minimal distensible need), I need to plan a series of operations, each of which is increasingly approaching the maximal distensible limit of what is possible. Bigger people equal bigger pars. So what may have once required just an IMDO and maybe a GenioPaully now requires a posterior SARME, a huge forward advancement of the maxilla (up to 11 mm) with a custom titanium plate, IMDO to "grow" the mandible, a BSSO to gain further distance, and a custom GenioPaully. This is the SuperBIMAX. Par 8's like this are hard. It's far easier and simpler to treat kids before all the camouflage orthodontics happened in the first place.

FIG 6-13 This patient had two maxillary premolars extracted as a 14-year-old, with pull-back orthodontics on her maxillary anterior teeth to reduce their esthetic prominence. Later, she had her impacted mandibular third molars removed. Always a snorer as a child, which led to early tonsil removal, she is now 30 years old and finds lying on her back to be impossible for both breathing and comfortably sleeping. She also chronically grinds and clenches her teeth and has early jaw arthritis from this. According to sleep studies, she has a formal diagnosis of OSA, from which her parents and several relatives all suffer. She has been offered CPAP but just doesn't want it. Instead, she is returning for adult orthodontics to simply push (or procline) her maxillary anterior teeth forward again and to partially reverse her adolescent camouflage-orthodontic experience. Custom facial design and bespoke titanium allows for predictable advancement distances of her jaws in order to both overcome her glossoptosis and achieve a normal bite and ideal facial esthetic proportions. These photos are taken 3 weeks apart, and she states she is completely cured of her snoring (as confirmed by a nighttime snoring-detection app on her phone) and has a normal night's sleep. For the first time in her life, she feels that she can breathe through her nose and with her lips naturally closed. Overcoming her minimum distensible need meant a maxillary LeFort advancement of 6 mm, during which I also widened the dental arch with a concurrent posterior LeFort-SARME of about 3 mm and a BSSO of 10 mm with a GenioPaully of 6 mm, all using custom titanium. While this patient's priority was to overcome her snoring and to gain a better night's sleep, it was also rewarding to gain facial balance and harmony by not breaching the natural female esthetic line (which means we designed pogonion to fall 3 to 5 mm short of the line of maximal esthetic limit).

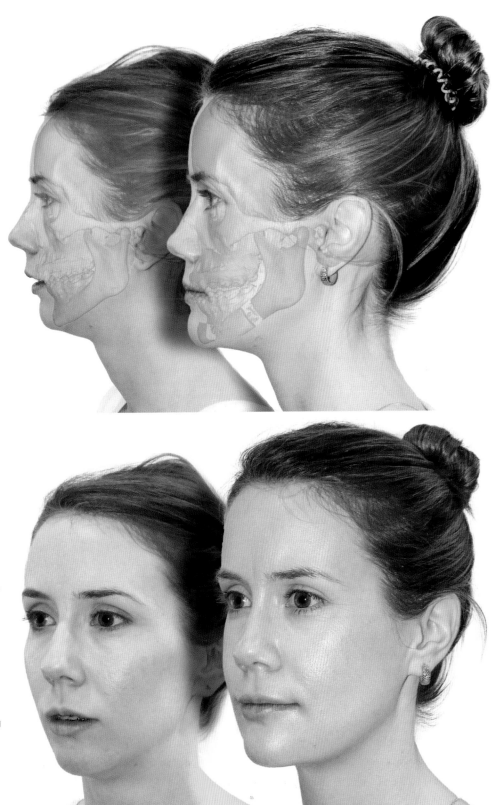

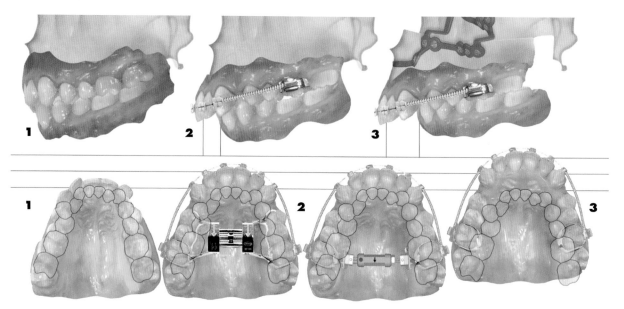

FIG 6-14 Maxillary expansion and proclination increases the circumference of the maxillary dental arch and maximizes the ability to contain all 16 maxillary teeth (including the third molars). Expansion can be performed in children and adolescents (up to 16 years in females and 17 years in males) using (2) a simple HYRAX appliance up to one-third of a millimeter per day (or 1/3 screw turn per day), conducted simultaneously with proclination orthodontics of the incisors using orthodontic springs. In adults, expansion is naturally difficult because the midline suture in the palate is fused and growth hormone secretion has ended. Using a Klapper-George Screw, modified by Mommaerts as a bone-borne device in an adolescent (2, shown in blue), prevents outward dental tipping (as it pushes directly onto bone and not teeth). It is also smaller and more tolerable than a HYRAX. As a medical prosthesis, the Klapper-George-Mommaerts is a device covered by medical insurance but only when inserted by a specialist surgeon. Use of a bone-borne expander also makes adjunctive orthodontics clinically easier, as it makes each modality of care independent of each other. For adults, maxillary arch expansion requires surgical re-creation of the palatal suture (also called a LeFort-SARME), and the proclination phase is neither fast nor nearly as clinically safe as for a growing adolescent. For adults, LeFort-SARME does not normally enable normal eruption of already impacted teeth. A formal LeFort advancement (3) can further increase the dental overjet (shown by the differences in the red lines), as well as open the airway behind the uvula and soft palate. The bigger the dental overjet, the greater the mandibular dental arch can be advanced. Maximizing the dental overjet gives opportunity to maximize the ability for IMDO or the BSSO to achieve the minimum distensible need to overcome glossoptosis and to eliminate snoring and OSA risk. See Fig 6-11 to help explain this relationship and Fig 6-12 to see how these lines relate to the Line of Ideal Aesthetic Limit.

THE DIRECT DIFFERENCE BETWEEN BSSO AND IMDO OSTEOTOMY

While it is possible to make the maxilla physically bigger by separating the midpalatal suture with a HYRAX device (Fig 6-14), there is no natural growth suture of the mandible. As explained in chapter 5, "growth" of the mandible occurs much the same way as a turtle shell grows. As the tongue and surrounding muscles get bigger, so does the mandible expand as a supporting strut. By the time the second molars have erupted, around the age of 12 or 13 years, the size of the mandible has already reached up to 95% of its eventual size potential.

Surgeons have two ways of making a small lower jaw "bigger." These two techniques are called the BSSO and IMDO. The BSSO is designed as a surgical "split and slide" of the vertical ramus of the mandible. The BSSO "telescopes" the tooth-bearing part of the mandible forward

in one advancement. It is a technically difficult operation; with traditional plate and screw systems, it cannot predictably advance the mandible very far, or in a perfectly stable way (Fig 6-15). The stable limit with off-the-shelf plates is probably only as long as a 6-mm slide.

The traditional BSSO is also very dependent upon extensive preceding orthodontics, and it usually relies upon having the third molars removed through a prior operation, as well as bite splints and jaw wiring. For many reasons and mainly due to orthodontic timing, the traditional BSSO is performed on adults 18 years and over and has a significant operative risk to the embedded nerve supplying the chin and lower lip.

IMDO describes a whole new method of treating small mandibles in adolescents. IMDO relies on surgically creating a "crack" or virtual growth suture that runs between the mandibular first and second molars (see Fig 6-15). This surgery is little different than the act of removing a

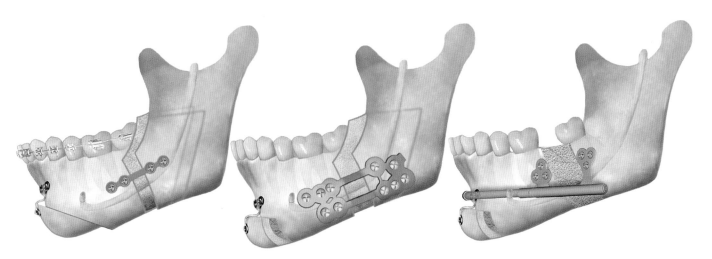

FIG 6-15 The BSSO uses plates and screws to telescope the mandible forward. We can use traditional off-the-shelf systems, which do not effectively advance the mandible very far or in a very stable way. The traditional BSSO is very dependent upon coincident orthodontics and the use of IMF and jaw splints. To improve the stability and extensibility of the BSSO, while avoiding IMF, we can use custom titanium to predictably advance the mandible body up to 11 mm. The IMDO procedure, on the other hand, can advance a total of 16.5 mm and can be used without braces and in adolescents (at which age the BSSO cannot be used). Unlike the BSSO, IMDO can prevent third molar impactions and allow for their preservation. GenioPaully is a means to further extend pogonion only and with it give enhanced stretch of the geniohyoid muscle as an indirect means of hyoid suspension and for prevention or cure of retroglossal airway collapse.

> IMDO is more conservative, cheaper, more sparing to teeth, easier to perform, produces less swelling, and carries far less surgical risk than either the BSSO or third molar removal surgery.

third molar. It produces relatively little swelling and, unlike the BSSO, has virtually no expressed risk of damage to major sensory nerves that run through the jawbone (eg, the inferior alveolar nerve).

Like putting a controlled crack in the glass of a window, the IMDO "suture line" produces no structural change to the mandible itself. The IMDO distractors displace the tooth-bearing part of the mandible forward—by up to 16.5 mm—in an extremely stable and predictable way. Because the extension advances only 1 mm a day, the amount that the tongue can be advanced is extremely controlled and can be titrated against eliminating snoring as well as in establishing a perfect bite relationship.

Unlike the BSSO, IMDO has no requirement for braces to be in place, and there is no requirement for elasticizing or wiring the jaws together after surgery. Surgery is also

cheaper, quicker, and leads to far less swelling. Kids go to school, and they can eat; talking and breathing actually improves as their jaws are grown. IMDO also creates room for crowded teeth to quickly unbuckle and unwind and aims to preserve all teeth, including third molars.

From an experienced surgeon's perspective, IMDO is more conservative, cheaper, more sparing to teeth, easier to perform, produces less swelling, and carries far less surgical risk than either the BSSO or third molar removal surgery.

But unless a surgeon performs IMDO and can directly compare it to the BSSO, they will never really know the truth of my assertions.

The following chapters describe the design and operations we can individually perform and blend in order to create an ideal face from an abnormal one. These six operations I call the 6Ways to Design a Face.

7

MANAGING THE CHIN AND JAWLINE
THE FIRST WAY

see sizable chin buttons in people with small jaws, and I see no chin buttons where jaw sizes are normal. I see chins that are excessively vertical, and I see chins that have no height at all. I see broad chins in girls who see them as unfeminine, and I see narrow chins in males who see them as unmasculine. I am told that chin clefts are inherited, but then chin clefts occur in individuals with no family history of the trait.

All in all, the chin is a confusing facial feature—to say the least.

FUNCTION OF THE CHIN

The chin is a natural esthetic point of focus, but few people give thought as to why they have one, or need one, or even how it relates to other parts, such as the upper neck or the lower lip (Fig 7-1). Most people will simply say "I don't have a chin" or "I have too much of a chin" or "I do not like my chin" or "Can you change my chin?" No matter the circumstances, this is a very fragile and personal conversation.

In my personal cosmetic opinion, chins have an esthetic centrality, giving balance to the sharpness of the nose and the angles of the jaws and cheek prominences, and an immediate relationship to the fullness (or not) of the lower lip. There is also an underlying relationship to the skin underneath the jaw and behind the chin (which I call the *dewlap*) as well as to the smoothness, symmetry, and slope or squareness of the jawline behind it. As such, it is my personal cosmetic view that chins should be centrally symmetric. They should lie neither too high nor too low, too far back nor too forward. A good chin is unnoticeable. A bad chin looks obviously odd.

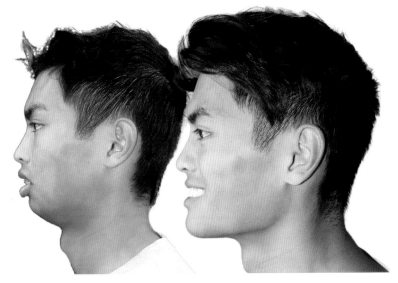

FIG 7-1 Managing the chin is about looking at the external (ie, the lower face, upper neck, and profile) as well as the internal (ie, the airway behind the tongue and the hard tissue foundations of the face). The functional combination of chin surgery with other fundamental jaw operations falls within the entire purview of the maxillofacial surgeon. The chin and jawline are inseparable. They are managed together. Refer to Fig 6-4 to see this patient's panoramic radiograph.

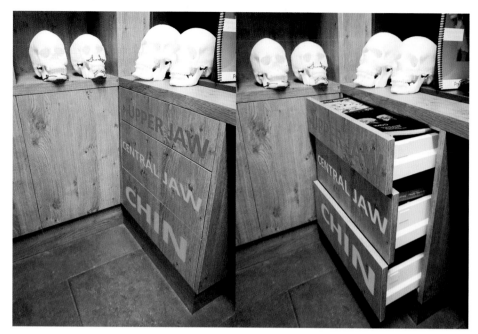

FIG 7-2 Moving jaws and the chin forward involves two surfaces. A front surface that alters the face, and a back surface that alters the airway. LeFort, intermolar mandibular distraction osteogenesis (IMDO), bilateral sagittal split osteotomy (BSSO), BIMAX, and GenioPaully are the procedures that simultaneously open airways and change facial profiles. Pushing a jaw or chin backward closes an airway. Here the drawers signify how both jaws and the chin must be advanced together to create a pleasing facial profile and improve the airway.

For me as a maxillofacial surgeon, a chin's purpose is to hold a tongue base forward, which holds an airway open.

But I am not a cosmetic surgeon. For me as a maxillofacial surgeon, a chin's purpose is to hold a tongue base forward, which holds an airway open. A chin button also holds up a lower lip, so that you can close the mouth, speak, and kiss. And yes, I agree that you can make a chin look really unexplainably nice. But I am purely a functional rationalist when it comes to chins, and everyone has their own ideal chin that doesn't belong on anyone else.

ANATOMY AND SURGICAL OPERATIONS OF THE CHIN

The chin has two surfaces, a front and back. The front surface gives outward lower facial soft tissue projection; the back surface pulls on the geniohyoid and anterior digastric muscles. The front supports and pushes the lower lip upward, both to maximize lip competency and give vertical facial balance; the back stretches the dewlap forward and stretches the diaphragm of skin and subdermal fat underneath the jaw. The front centralizes the natural center of the mandible and to the immediate sides symmetrifies the natural lines of the lateral jawlines (Fig 7-2).

It is rare to operate on the chin alone (Fig 7-3a). The cosmetic surgeon does this by adding a simple overlay silastic implant for the pure cosmetic objective of appeasing the client who requested it (Fig 7-3b). The esthetician does this with fillers and imagination. I occasionally will perform a custom-made onlay PEEK chin implant (Fig 7-3c). But even for me, the circumstances of doing this are very rare and completely without functional merit. Occasionally, a formal surgical advancement of the chin is performed alone, without the intermolar mandibular distraction osteogenesis (IMDO) or bilateral sagittal split osteotomy (BSSO) procedure. The esthetic circumstances that are satisfied by standalone genioplasty or Genio-Paully are extremely rare in my practice. But they can be performed alone to provide a defined therapeutic benefit to both lip competence and airway pull.

The chin wing, however, is designed to be performed alone (Fig 7-3d). And often. And often purely for cosmetic reasons. It became popular in Western Europe, where it was developed in Switzerland, because it overcomes the considerable cosmetic negative effects of camouflage orthodontics, namely poor lower facial profile. Thus, the adult European chin wing is the Band-Aid alternative to

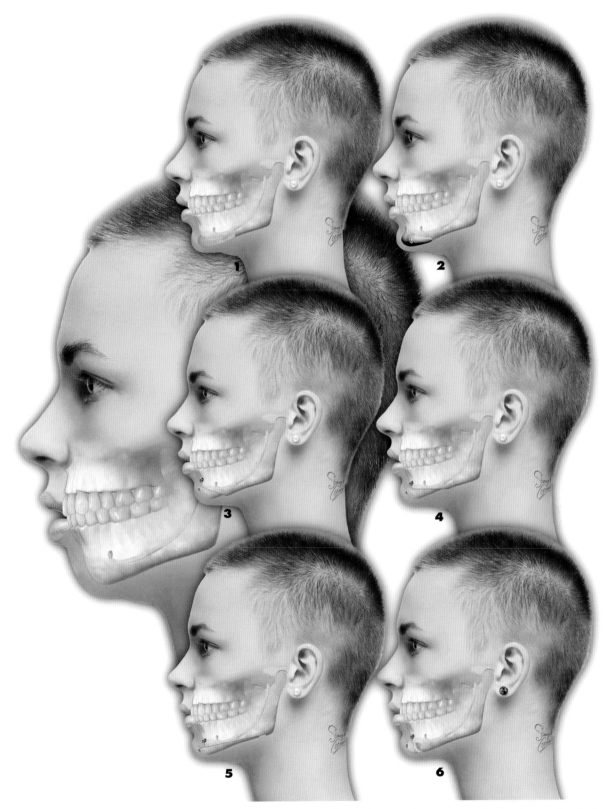

FIG 7-3A For people without a chin button (agenia), there are six general operation types that can correct for the shape and projection and position of a chin button. *(1)* The off-the-shelf silastic or expanded polymethyl methacrylate (PMMA) implant. *(2)* The custom-made polyetheretherketone (PEEK) implant. *(3)* The steep-sliding genioplasty. *(4)* The shallow-sliding genioplasty. *(5)* The chin wing. *(6)* The Genio-Paully. The following illustrations demonstrate these procedures on a model with a normal-sized mandible and a full complement of 32 teeth.

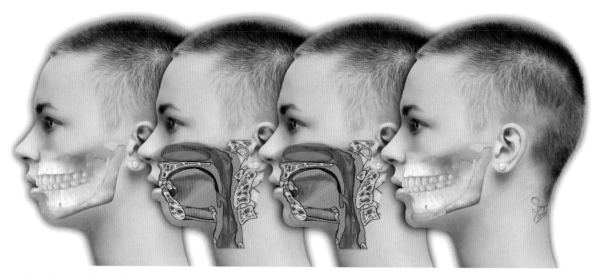

FIG 7-3B Silicone chin implants, as with expanded PMMA implants, come "off-the-shelf" and in a range of designs and sizes that are "eye-balled" to suit the cosmetic patient's self-described hopes and desires. They are notoriously hard to place, secure, fix, symmetrify, and facially balance. Along with migration, they also have high rates of infection, with inherent microporosity making any entrenched infection notoriously difficult to treat. They also do nothing to enhance airway pull and are very poor at providing lip competence. Chin implants are often co-performed with cosmetic nasal reduction surgery (rhinoplasty).

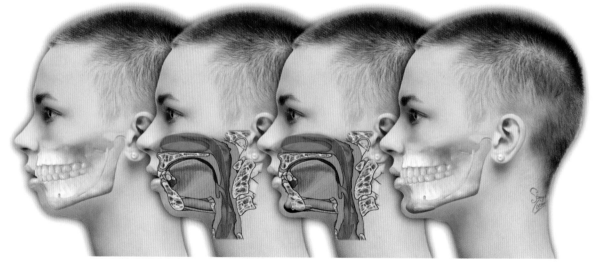

FIG 7-3C While completely tissue-inert and offering perfect tissue fitting and sculpting performance, the PEEK chin implant does absolutely nothing to correct geniohyoid pull or airway tenting. It has a marginal influence on eliminating dewlap but does provide improvement to lower lip competence. Unlike off-the-shelf prostheses, PEEK implants are designed and supplied with optimal bone-screw retention features in mind.

the adult remedial BIMAX. However, it does potentially give stretch to the geniohyoid if it is high enough, and in that it can be considered a therapeutic procedure. Nonetheless, in my opinion the chin wing is camouflage surgery for camouflage orthodontics. It serves as a cosmetic afterthought, and only as a surgical reaction to the negative facial profile effects of previous orthodontic treatment. It's

hard to validate it for the almost accidental therapeutic partial pull on the geniohyoid it may or may not give.

To discriminate a cosmetic chin operation from a functional chin operation is entirely based upon whether the primary drive is for esthetic (front surface) benefit or airway (back surface) benefit. The classic sliding advancement genioplasty popularized by Hugo Obwegeser is

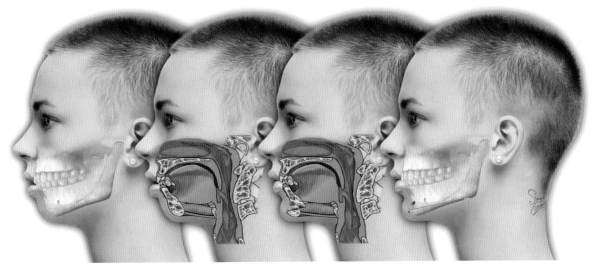

FIG 7-3D The chin wing captures the chin point and underside of the jawline below the major sensory nerve running through the mandible. It does capture the anterior belly of the digastrics to truly stretch the dewlap and may only partially provide some geniohyoid stretching effect. This series shows the effect of the chin wing with a full 32-tooth dentition, where the mandible size is normal but there is no true chin button.

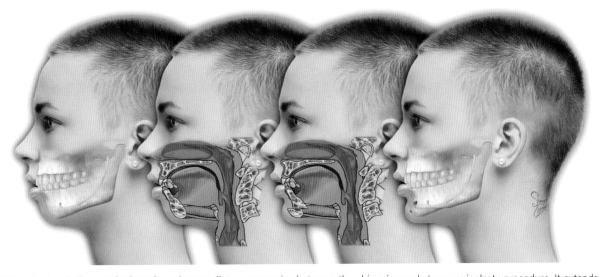

FIG 7-3E The shallow genioplasty is an intermediate compromise between the chin wing and steep genioplasty procedure. It extends backward a little to capture the underlying jawline, but considerable care must be exercised not to also nick or cut the pathway of the inferior alveolar nerve running toward its mental nerve exit and close to the cortex underside of the jaw itself. Being shallow, it captures more of the geniohyoid muscle but not completely.

designed to cosmetically improve the accompanying functional BSSO he developed, but only the shallow version captures the geniohyoid, and barely (Figs 7-3e and 7-3f). The chin wing, as previously mentioned, was designed to be entirely cosmetic. In a singular conversation of chins, particularly for cosmetic surgeons, the implication is that the chin is an entity alone to be corrected

alone. But for the maxillofacial surgeon, this is ideologically impossible.

By contrast to both the chin wing and advancement genioplasty, the GenioPaully is designed to deliberately capture the geniohyoid muscle (Fig 7-3g). The GenioPaully is purposefully designed to complement the IMDO and remedial BIMAX procedure utilizing custom titanium plates,

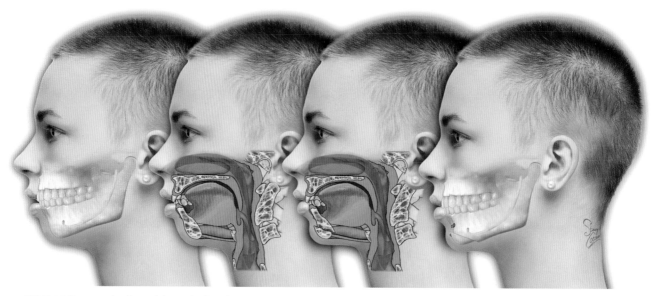

FIG 7-3F By capturing less of the underline of the jaw, the steep genioplasty is more sparing of risk to the inferior alveolar nerve and its mental nerve termination. It barely captures any of the geniohyoid muscle and has little effect on airway tenting. It does, however, partially relieve the dewlap. This can lead to a deep skin crease directly behind the chin, giving the appearance of a "witch's" chin defect.

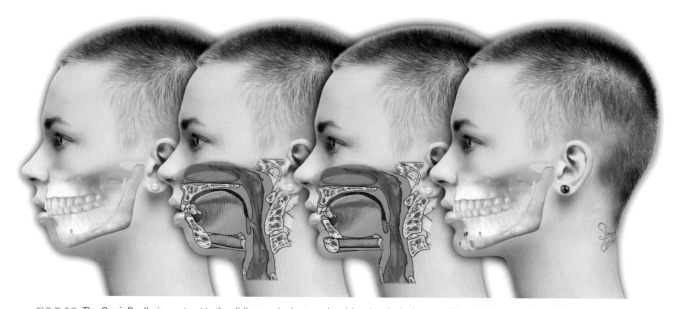

FIG 7-3G The GenioPaully, in contrast to the sliding genioplasty or the chin wing, is designed deliberately to complement the advancement BSSO and IMDO procedures, which both primarily contribute to mandible lengthening and tongue-pull effect. The aim of the GenioPaully is to deliberately and completely capture and stretch the geniohyoid and inferior digastric muscles, thus eliminating dewlap and maximally tenting the airway behind the epiglottis.

> Only the GenioPaully deliberately aims to pull the hyoid bone forward, and thus relieve glossoptosis, as well as correct lower lip incompetence.

in that it builds on the fundamental tongue-base advancement compounded by the design elements of both, and to complement the jawline esthetic. Even if the GenioPaully is performed alone, it is still considered a truly functional procedure for its effect on positive airway tenting behind the tongue (Fig 7-4). Only the GenioPaully deliberately aims to pull the hyoid bone forward, and thus relieve glossoptosis, as well as correct lower lip incompetence.

FIG 7-4A There are four pairs of broad muscle attachments on the inside of the anterior mandible: the mylohyoid, genioglossus, geniohyoid, and anterior digastric bellies. The osteotomy plane (brown) for the GenioPaully segment (light blue) attempts to capture the geniohyoid tubercles (also called the ante-pogonion or AntePo) and anterior digastric fossa and therefore the anterior geniohyoid and anterior digastric muscle attachments. Pulling on the forward-paired geniohyoid muscle attachments provides a direct forward pull of the hyoid bone behind it. The greater the anterior pull, the less contraction needed in the geniohyoid muscle to open the airway directly behind the tongue. The therapeutic effect of the GenioPaully is as a direct consequence of the forward movement of this pull and can be measured in midline CT radiology as a geniohyoid distance. A reasonable therapeutic clinical measurement is the difference of the anticipated geniohyoid distance (GH'-GH°), divided by the original geniohyoid distance ([[GH'-GH°] / GH° × 100), given as a percentage. The amount of geniohyoid pull has greater therapeutic effect upon opening airway than anything achieved through genioglossus forward carry obtained by either BSSO or IMDO. Any stretch on the anterior digastric muscle has the effect of stretching the dewlap or skin under the jawline. It is only with the GenioPaully that a controllable midline osteotomy can be made that evenly splits the BSSO mandible into two sides, without effect on the adjacent central incisor roots. Such midline osteotomization produces a five-piece mandible and is only perfectly controlled through the use of custom cutting and drill guides, precise screw lengths, and custom manufactured plates.

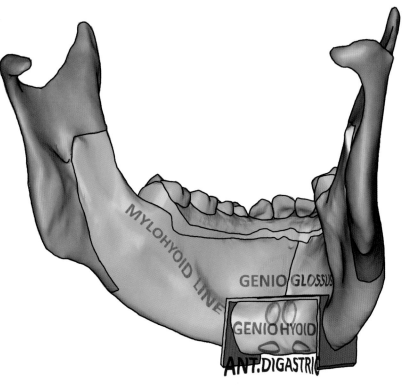

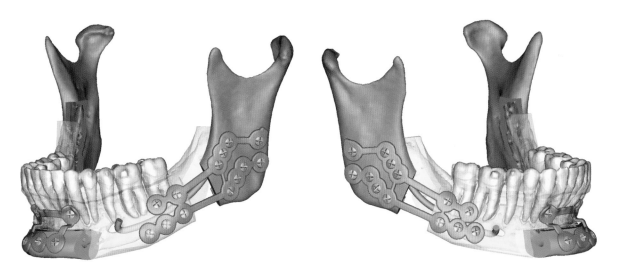

FIG 7-4B The GenioPaully is a highly modified box osteotomy of the central anterior mandible (green). The overall procedure is combined with shaving that occurs on both undersides of the anterior jawline of the tooth-bearing portion of the mandible (yellow). The precision of the cuts and the eventual placement of the central chin portion, its advancement, its rollout, the deliberate capture of the geniohyoid tubercles and the amount of hyoid stretch that occurs through the geniohyoid muscle, and the amount of vertical impaction to achieve lower lip elevation and roll are all highly designed. Outside of extreme surgical experience and exceptional talent, it is virtually impossible to perform the GenioPaully without the benefits of digital design and custom plate manufacture. The high horizontal and vertical parallelism of the lateral incisions must be accurately predicted in order to preserve the genu of the mental nerves and the root apices of the incisors and particularly the canines. Screw placement is also important in order to guarantee screw depth, orientation, and careful placement to avoid roots and nerves as well as to provide suitable torques and mechanical advantages that are designed to resist stretched skin and muscle. The GenioPaully also allows for the midline split of the central mandible, between the central incisors, which can enhance a combined BSSO procedure (blue ramus and yellow anterior mandible).

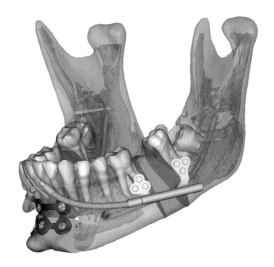
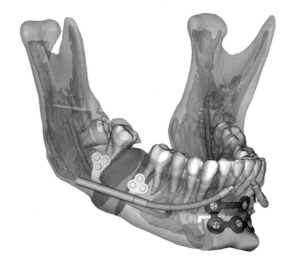

FIG 7-5 In comparing it to the combined GenioPaully-BSSO procedure, the GenioPaully-IMDO combination is used most effectively in an adolescent and prior to formal orthodontics. The red "osteoid" shows the amount of actual bone volume "grown" by IMDO and into which the second molar may migrate and more forward teeth may distalize and spontaneously decrowd. Forward migration of the second molar gives opportunity for the developing third molar to also naturally erupt and contribute to a full 32-tooth occlusion. The GenioPaully is designed after IMDO has been completed in order to maximize the esthetic, lip functional, and airway tenting effects that are possible through this procedure. The custom GenioPaully plate used with IMDO is a simple four- or five-hole trapezoid design.

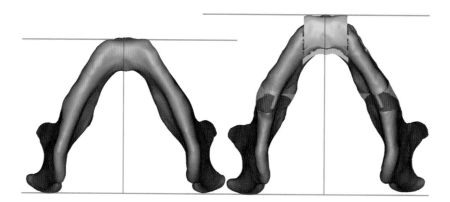

FIG 7-6 Digital comparison of the underside of the mandible before and after IMDO-GenioPaully in this nearly 15-year-old adolescent boy allows assessment of the influence of the GenioPaully-IMDO combination upon the volumetric jawline. While a bilateral 12-mm IMDO distraction was applied and the GenioPaully was advanced 5 mm, this gave an overall mandible length change of 10.8 mm based on an original horizontal mandible length of 81.8 mm—an overall increase of 13%. This increase in mandible length gave a therapeutic stretch of 9.4 mm of the original 29.9-mm geniohyoid muscle length, which was an overall gain of 31%. The adolescent was too young to subjectively complain of breathing difficulty during sleep prior to the procedure, hence the need for these linear assessments as objective measurements of change.

GENIOPAULLY

The chin is an extension of the jawline. It centrally merges the left and right halves of the jaw. You cannot manage a jawline without the chin, and you cannot manage a chin without considering the jawline. The jawline and chin must be managed together.

Making a jaw bigger by either IMDO or extension BSSO does not change or alter the shape or volume or projection or position of a chin. The GenioPaully is an add-on

The jawline and chin must be managed together.

procedure to craft the chin as both IMDO and BSSO have crafted the jawline (Fig 7-5). The GenioPaully gives additional proportionality. It works in combination with the IMDO or BSSO to enhance and balance and shape the lower face. The GenioPaully centralizes the chin point and twists and levels the underside of the anterior jawline (Fig

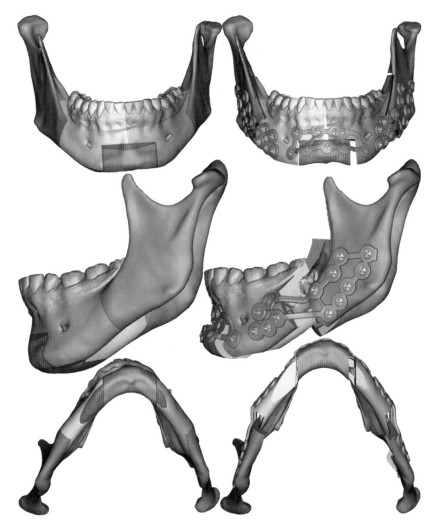

FIG 7-7 Combining the GenioPaully with BSSO under digital design conditions and specific customization of both cutting and plate guides allows the surgeon to maximize centrification and symmetrification of the jawline. The midline split of the mandible is only allowed for with the GenioPaully, which simultaneously also guides the degree of reduction to the underside of the anterior right and left halves of the central body mandible (shown in red). For many patients, there is one-sided developmental reduction in vertical ramus height that has contributed to the subsequent development of the asymmetric mandible. Whether it is by a childhood crush fracture of the condylar head or by embryologic diminishment of condyle and ramus size (such as Pruzansky Type 1 hemifacial microsomia, as in this case), the vertical height difference at the jaw angle and true posterior jawline symmetrification can only be remediated by an onlay custom PEEK implant following removal of BSSO titanium plates and osteotomy-site inlay graft, natural graft healing, and later repeat digital PEEK design and surgical insertion (see chapter 16). In assessing the mathematics of horizontal mandible length change for this 36-year-old woman (70.6 to 83.9 mm), there was a 19% increase, translating as a therapeutic geniohyoid length change increase of 16% (38.8 to 49.9 mm). Effectively, the overall therapy reversed her subjective complaint of snoring and nighttime breathing obstruction. It is difficult to provide mathematic standardization of the actual BSSO advancement distance, particularly in cases of asymmetry, in order to make meaningful interpatient comparisons. Whereas a unilateral BSSO advancement of 10 mm has a different effect between two different patients, a unilateral IMDO advancement of 10 mm is likely exactly the same as with any other person in a similar age group.

7-6). Because it is an inherently blind procedure involving many different structural elements, the predictable Genio-Paully can only be digitally designed; custom guides and plates are generated by that design and then transferred into the surgical space (Figs 7-7 and 7-8).

Obwegeser designed the genioplasty as a cosmetic procedure to complement the BSSO. It was always meant to be performed freehand and with off-the-shelf chin plates.

Figure 7-9 compares the realities of BSSO with sliding genioplasty (see Fig 7-9a), BIMAX surgery with GenioPaully (see Fig 7-9b), and IMDO with GenioPaully (see Fig 7-9c). IMDO with GenioPaully can be performed freehand or with custom titanium; either way it remains the most conservative, least costly, and quickest option to permanently, deliberately, and completely correct the adolescent small mandible and its accompanying glossoptosis.

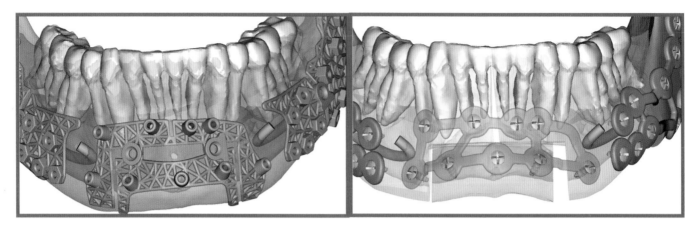

FIG 7-8 Performing a midline split between the mandibular central incisors can only be performed in combination with the BSSO and the GenioPaully procedure. The midline split allows the mandibular dental arch to be divided, thereby allowing for precise leveling and symmetrification of that arch as well as control of the outward roll, such that dental roots have symmetric angulation in this frontal view. The midline split is also not formally a cut channel, but more of a "window crack" (much like the IMDO osteotomy) that is three dimensionally controlled by the precise orientations, lengths, and torques of screws chosen to complement the custom titanium plate shown at right. In order to hold together what is essentially a five-piece mandible against the torsional, torque, and tension lines during the healing phase, nine screws are used, with three screws in each of the three central segments that comprise the midline division and GenioPaully. The plate itself has a large footprint in order to grip and control the bone surfaces. The osteotomy separations can be filled with bone graft alloplast such as particulate hydroxyapatite. The combined GenioPaully and midline osteotomy is a designed procedure with a designed plate and can only be precisely managed by the creation of a precision cutting and drill guide as shown at left.

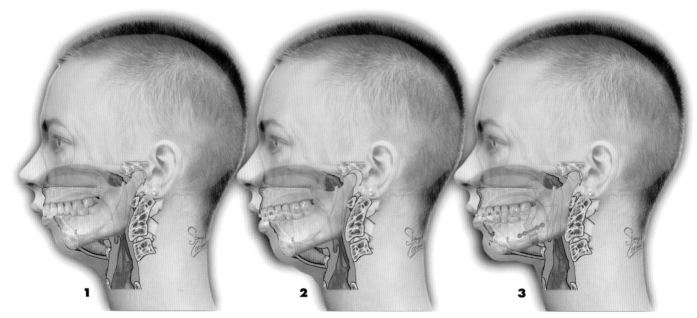

FIG 7-9A *(1)* Prominent anterior teeth are extremely common. *(2)* Unilateral orthodontic treatment is to pull back the maxillary anterior teeth and to train the mandible to be held forward. *(3)* The common remedial jaw surgical procedure to the resultant poor bite is the small BSSO and sliding genioplasty. This combination of therapy, from orthodontist to basic jaw surgery, includes third molar removal, takes many years, and does little to overcome the underlying glossoptosis associated with the small mandible.

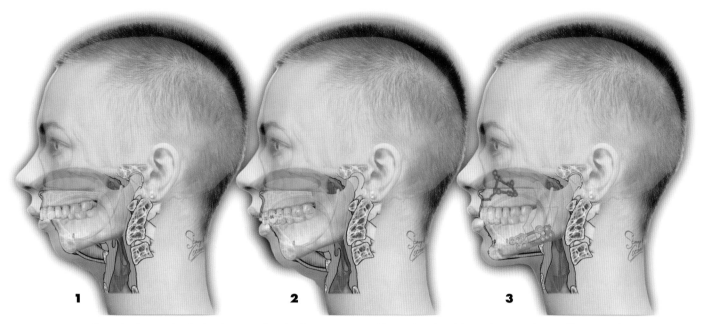

FIG 7-9B Where the degree of orthodontic camouflage has been extreme and is causing chronic jaw ache, excessive maxillary gumminess, and awkward smile dynamics, the counterclockwise rotation using custom titanium and double jaw surgery (BIMAX) with GenioPaully maximizes facial profile esthetics and overcomes the inherent glossoptosis of the original small mandible. However, this treatment takes several years and is extremely expensive. Third molar surgery is almost an inherent precursor to BIMAX surgery.

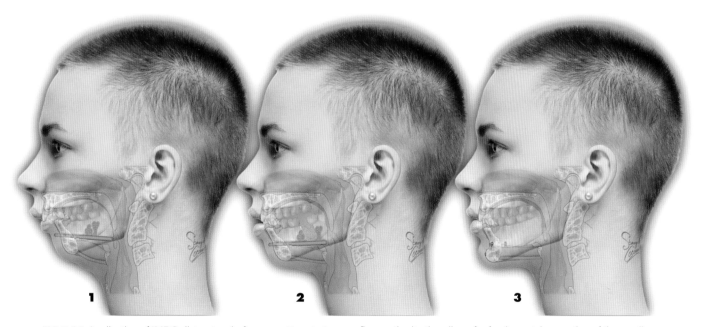

FIG 7-9C Application of IMDO distractors before any attempt at camouflage orthodontics allows for fundamental correction of the small mandible, which in combination with advancement GenioPaully maximally restores the normal size of the small mandible, preserves the full complement of 32 teeth in a natural Class I occlusion, and completely corrects for glossoptosis. This form of treatment is measured in weeks rather than months or years and significantly reduces overall treatment costs in adolescents with prominent anterior teeth.

8
EXPLAINING THE IMDO PROTOCOL
THE SECOND WAY

There are many known, though extremely rare, causes of an abnormally sized mandible, including hemifacial microsomia, Treacher Collins syndrome, and Stickler syndrome. More common are some still-rare medical conditions that can adversely affect how a child's mandible would have normally grown. Juvenile rheumatoid arthritis (JRA) can cause disruptive or even destructive effects to growing temporomandibular joints (TMJs). Vitamin D deficiency (rickets) or malnutrition can also affect how the mandible and teeth grow (Fig 8-1). A fall on the chin as a child can also bruise the TMJ and lead to asymmetric and abnormal growth of the mandible. But these rare causes do not explain the very high frequency of small mandibles that we see in most modern societies.

PIERRE ROBIN SYNDROME

Pierre Robin was the first person to really look at the phenomenon of the most common form of the small mandible in 1923 (Fig 8-2). A French stomatologist, he eventually became famous for helping other dentists, nurses, doctors, and young mothers learn to identify the "very small" mandible when it first starts to have noticeable effects—in newborns.

Of course, all babies have small mandibles. But they don't have teeth or bad bites to help you identify a *severely* small mandible from a normally small one. There is no measurement or clinical definition that defines normal from abnormal. But correctly identifying the severely small

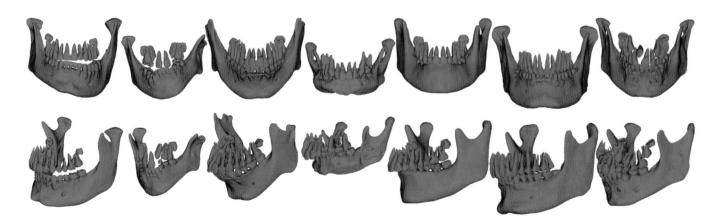

FIG 8-1 There are many forms of mandibular malformation, and the way jaws grow take on myriad patterns, including *(from left to right)* condylar hyperplasia, hemifacial microsomia, juvenile rheumatoid arthritis, Melnick-Needles syndrome, and anterior mandibular hypoplasia (AMHypo) Class B, C, and D.

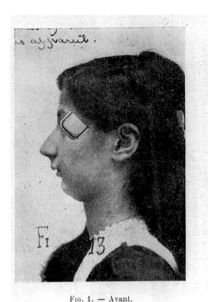
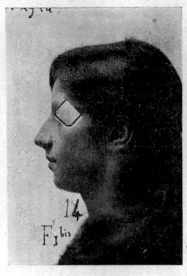

FIG. 1. — Avant.   FIG. 2. — Après.

FIG 8-2 Pierre Robin first described the small mandible in adults in 1923 and introduced the Monobloc snoring device that helped hold the small mandible forward.

mandible in newborns is very important. Early identification today helps to prevent cot death (or sudden infant death syndrome), as it did in the Paris of 1923. What Robin said was that "very small lower jaws lead to suffocation, especially when you lie the baby on its back." He even gave the phenomenon a new word: *glossoptosis*, or "tongue suffocation."

In Pierre Robin's time, all he could do was invent new feeding bottles and draw medical attention to the dangers of neonatal suffocation and feeding difficulties. Today, most modern major children's hospitals have neonatal surgical specialists who use distraction osteogenesis to help grow very small jaws (where it is clear the baby is suffocating) and thus help newborns with breathing and suckling (Fig 8-3). In Australia alone, about 15 children every year will have neonatal jaw distraction to help grow their severely small mandibles so that they can breathe and suckle normally. This means that for an Australian population of 22 million people, with an annual birth rate of 12.4 per 1,000 (or 275,000 babies a year), 1 in 20,000 babies will have the life-threatening form of Pierre Robin syndrome.

In Australian neonatal wards, however, doctors are only identifying and growing the *very* small jaws that are obviously leading to suffocation. There is no data on the true number of babies born with abnormally small jaws. We *do* know that the overwhelming majority of small jaws are just

> After all, a baby with a very small jaw looks just like any other baby.

not picked up by nurses or doctors at the time of birth. After all, a baby with a very small jaw looks just like any other baby. The only thing we know is that about 15 babies a year would otherwise suffocate because their small jaws are just so very very small. After they leave the hospital, babies will grow. Teeth will develop. And eventually the manifestations of the hidden small jaw will become obvious.

Today, most medical professionals would describe Pierre Robin syndrome as the small mandible found in neonates that leads to severe respiratory difficulty. But Pierre Robin syndrome is a disease found at all ages. In 1923, there was literally no way to help explain how adults snored or breathed or how they might even "obstruct" their airways. Less known was how small jaw size, a dental overbite, neck posture, a backward tongue position, or a compressed airway volume could be interrelated (see Fig 6-6). Nonetheless, Pierre Robin figured out these connections and even invented a jaw splint that helped hold the adult jaw forward (see Fig 8-2), which in turn opened the airway behind the "fallen" tongue. This "monobloc" is the basis for an entire industry devoted to antisnoring dental devices.

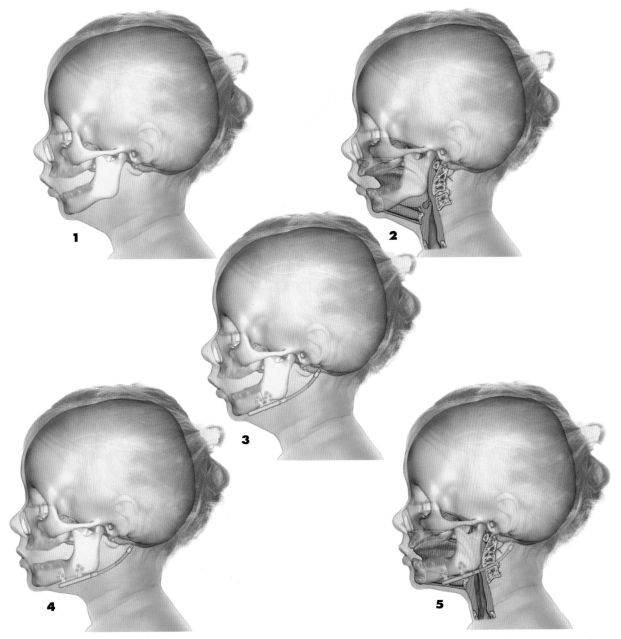

FIG 8-3 Distraction osteogenesis is an amazing fix for the life-threatening small mandible in neonates. Of course older children can also have small mandibles, as well as adults, but is it commonly recognized? The biggest problem with neonatal jaw distraction is the effect that surgery has on developing teeth and the future adult life. If at all possible, it is best to defer jaw distraction until age 12 years and to rely on methods Pierre Robin described to help with neonatal sleep posture and feeding.

Ultimately, what Pierre Robin discovered were these facts:

1. Small mandibles are very common (at least 40% prevalence by Robin's calculations).
2. Small mandibles are so common that no one sees them as abnormal.
3. The small mandibles leads to a bad bite, crowded and impacted teeth, and the esthetic sense of a lack of chin projection.
4. The combination of a poor airway volume and bad bite eventually lead to a distortion in facial proportion and cervical posture, which have systemic effects such as poor food intake, a lack of general physical health, and a general susceptibility to illness.

WHAT WE KNOW NOW

Medicine and dentistry have evolved greatly since Pierre Robin's day. Dental appliances, continuous positive airway pressure (CPAP) machines, and jaw osteodistraction surgery have evolved, not to mention the enormous advances in imaging technology. Quite frankly, it is amazing that this man and his insights existed in an age where today's technologies were so completely unimaginable.

What we know today is that the small mandible is indeed very common. Class II malocclusion, a major sign of the small mandible, is seen in roughly 25% of children. Dental crowding is seen in around 70% of children. Almost all adults over 40 years old have sleep-disordered breathing. And almost everyone has impacted third molars. All races of humans have people with small jaws, but the incidence is highest in those descended from white Europeans. At least 25% of white people have an obviously smaller mandible, and if you really look, the presence of small jaws is really much higher, and this prevalence is equal among males and females.

> What we know today is that the small mandible is indeed very common.

A small mandible is three dimensionally small. It isn't just short, but it is also narrow and relatively squat. Because of its smaller volume, it can contain fewer teeth. This means that many people with a small mandible have crowded teeth, impacted teeth (especially third molars), and worse, a bad bite, which dentists universally call a *malocclusion*. However, with modern medical imaging, we can now explain the link between the small mandible, bad neck posture, a receding profile, and of course the very real medical dangers associated with snoring and obstructive sleep apnea (OSA). There is a cure for what Pierre Robin described nearly a century ago, and it is called *intermolar mandibular distraction osteogenesis (IMDO)*.

THE IMDO PROCESS

The simple mantra of IMDO treatment is to **expand, distract, align.** IMDO treatment requires the close interaction and coordination of an orthodontic practitioner and an

> There is a cure for what Pierre Robin described nearly a century ago, and it is called intermolar mandibular distraction osteogenesis (IMDO).

oral and maxillofacial surgeon. Both need to be accredited in the IMDO process.

The pre-IMDO system typically begins with expansion of the maxilla. Expansion is done with a simple dental device—a HYRAX—placed by the orthodontic practitioner (Fig 8-4). Maxillary expansion opens the nasal airway and expands the dental arch length (Fig 8-5a). Orthodontic brackets are then placed on the maxillary anterior teeth to develop the front of the maxilla, creating the optimal amount of space to grow the mandible forward.

Active IMDO then lengthens, widens, and advances the lower jaw over a period of 12 to 14 days. This is done at home by a child's parents, with review by an IMDO-accredited specialist surgeon (Figs 8-5b and 8-5c). With this part of treatment complete, the teeth are allowed to naturally migrate, erupt, and settle into a natural bite relation. This is called the post-IMDO phase (Fig 8-5d).

Later comprehensive orthodontic treatment is usually delayed until facial growth is nearly complete to prevent any hindrance to normal facial development. It is usually simple Class I mechanics that is needed.

IMDO vs conventional jaw surgery

IMDO starts 1 to 3 days after surgery and proceeds about 1 mm per day, ending when directed by the surgeon and orthodontist. Distraction occurs at home. Orthodontic brackets and wires are not required during this phase because there are no surgical splints or intermaxillary jaw fixation during this time, unlike conventional forms of jaw correction surgery. Distraction can extend as far as 16.5 mm depending on the IMDO device manufacturer.

The creation of an artificial suture between the first and second molars is part of the surgical "art" of the IMDO operation (Fig 8-6). Credentialed IMDO surgeons are trained in methods to reduce physical risk to the inferior alveolar nerve that runs across this site. The nerve itself will grow as IMDO advances, though transient lip and chin numbness can occur due to this passive "growing."

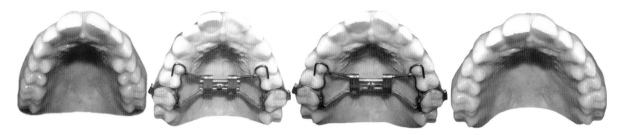

FIG 8-4 In the pre-IMDO phase, maxillary expansion occurs first using a normal orthodontic HYRAX appliance.

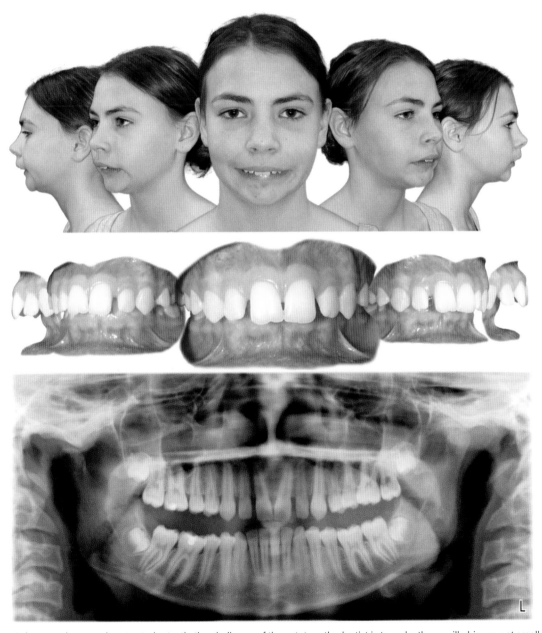

FIG 8-5A When treating prominent anterior teeth, the challenge of the astute orthodontist is to make the maxilla bigger, not smaller. Widening the maxilla enables maxillary teeth to disimpact and erupt normally, not to mention improve nasal airflow. The HYRAX is a common orthodontic appliance. Note the impacted third molars in this radiograph. There is a myth that third molars are vestigial and redundant in modern humans, but our aim as dentists should be to keep 32 teeth in full Class I occlusion. ⟶

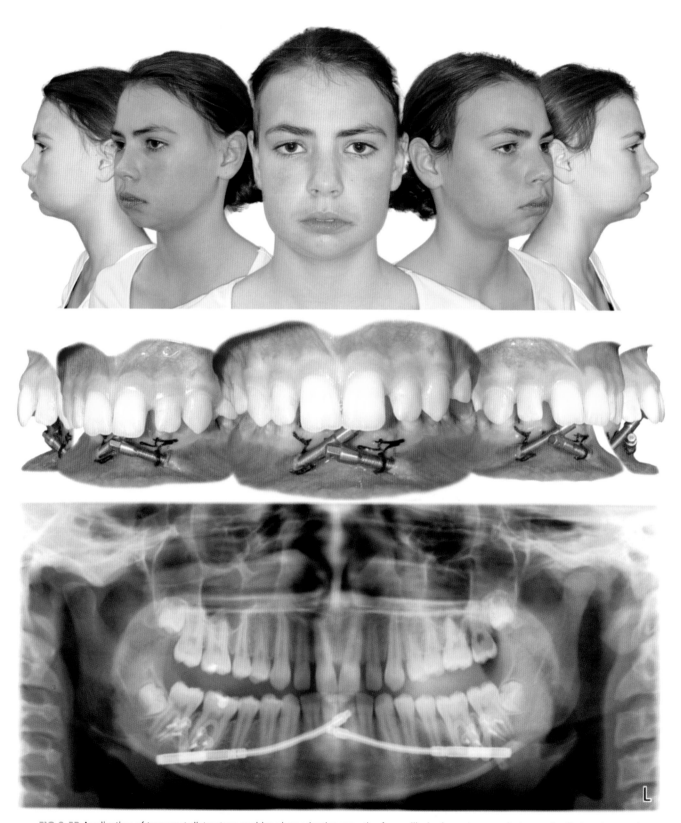

FIG 8-5B Application of tesseract distractors enables slow adaptive growth of mandibular bone to occur between the first and second molars and is performed by IMDO. Depending on the manufacturer of the IMDO distractor, advancement can be 14 or 16.5 mm.

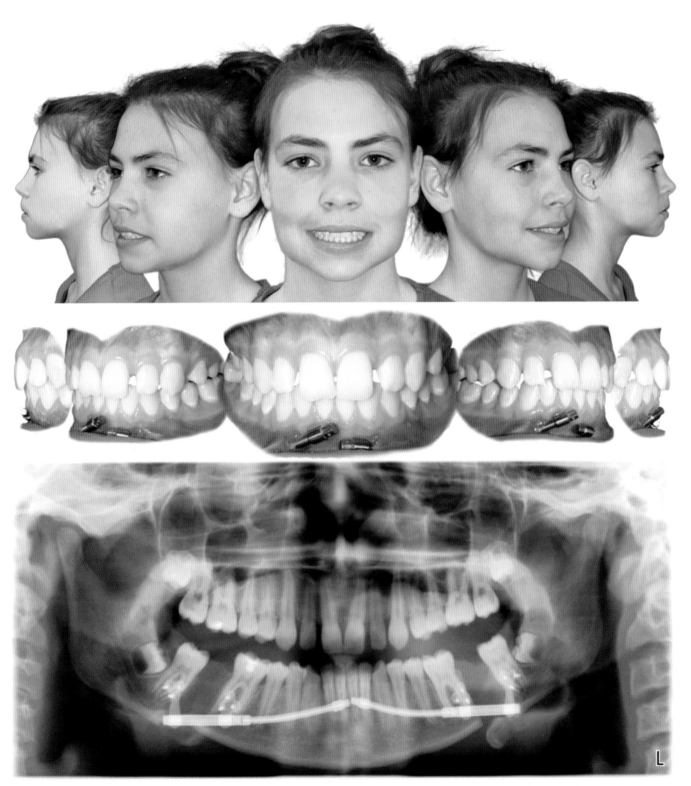

FIG 8-5C Home activation of IMDO (tesseract) distractors enables 3D volumetric change of the mandible and works much the same way as a maxillary HYRAX in expanding the maxilla. Orthodontics are not needed during this phase.

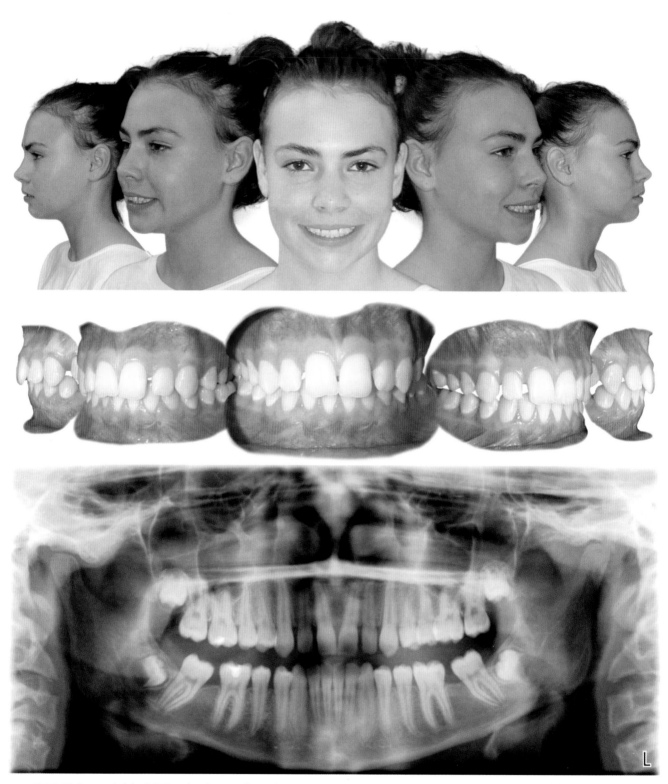

FIG 8-5D Removal of the IMDO and HYRAX appliances has enabled 3D growth of the maxilla and mandible using a combination of natural and surgically created growth sutures. The malocclusion is converted from orthodontic Class II, division 1 to Class I or from orthognathic Class B to Class A. Teeth are allowed to naturally erupt, develop, and disimpact. The ideal is a full complement of 32 teeth, a full Class I occlusion, and normalized facial profile with open nasal and retroglossal airways, without a future risk for snoring or obstructive sleep apnea (OSA) development.

FIG 8-6 There are two IMDO distractors that are attached to either side of the jaw in a specific direction. The directions are built into the design of the attachment devices. A small crack, which acts as an artificial "growth suture," is surgically created between the first and second molars. They are attached during a general anesthetic operation in a private hospital that is equipped to provide specialist orthognathic surgery. The amount of IMDO distance is a titrated measure given by the IMDO appliances.

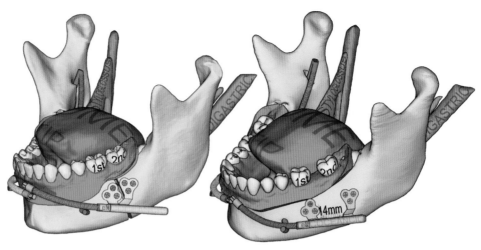

FIG 8-7 The IMDO distractors point slightly toward each other. Surgeons call this "vector collision," and it allows for simultaneous widening and lengthening of the mandible as part of the "tesseract changes" that must arise in normalizing the volume of the mandible. Access to turn the distractors are via distractor arms. These emerge from the gingiva and are hidden behind the lower lip. There is rapid migration of the first and second molars into the new bone formed within the distraction gap caused by IMDO.

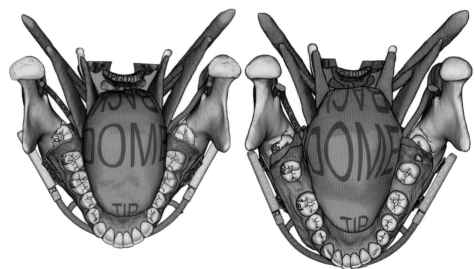

How does IMDO change the mandible?

As IMDO advances, the front of the mandible will not only lengthen but also widen across the midposterior width. In this way, the overall volume of the mandible will change (Figs 8-7 and 8-8), which will also affect the shape and position of the anterior tongue. As well as advancing the front of the mandible, IMDO creates dental space that the orthodontist can later use to help decrowd the mandibular teeth (Fig 8-9). Creating an increased dental arch helps prevent dental impactions, including those of developing third molars.

As IMDO advances, the front of the mandible will not only lengthen but also widen at the posterior.

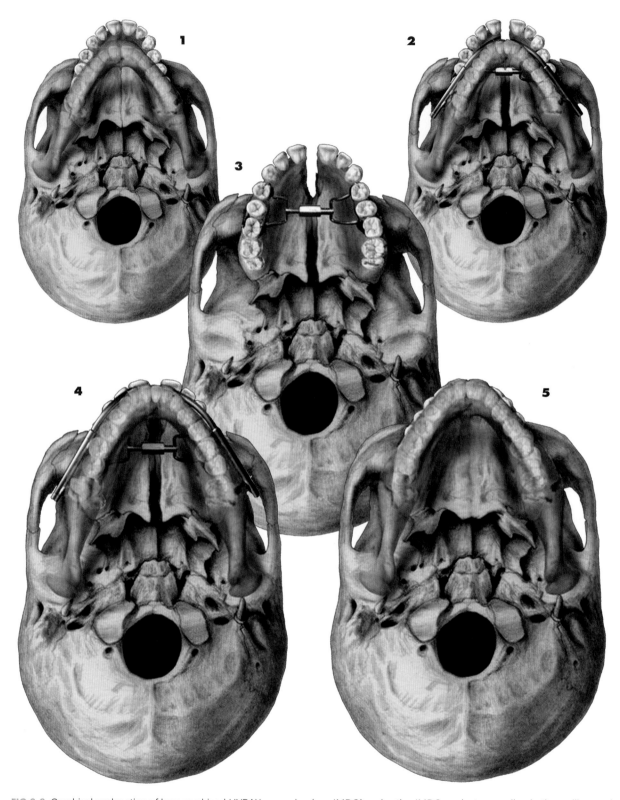

FIG 8-8 Graphical explanation of how combined HYRAX expansion (pre-IMDO) and active IMDO work at expanding both maxillary and mandibular jaw volumes. In the maxilla, the HYRAX takes advantage of natural midfacial sutures to help expand the middle face. Active IMDO uses surgically created sutures placed between the mandibular first and second molars to enable natural expansion of the lower face. This creates an overall pull-forward effect of the entire tongue and mandibular occlusion. All sutural separations, both natural and surgically created, are rapidly filled in with new bone, which in adolescents rapidly calcifies and becomes solid. (Credit is given to Andreas Reinhardt for assistance in drawing these figures.)

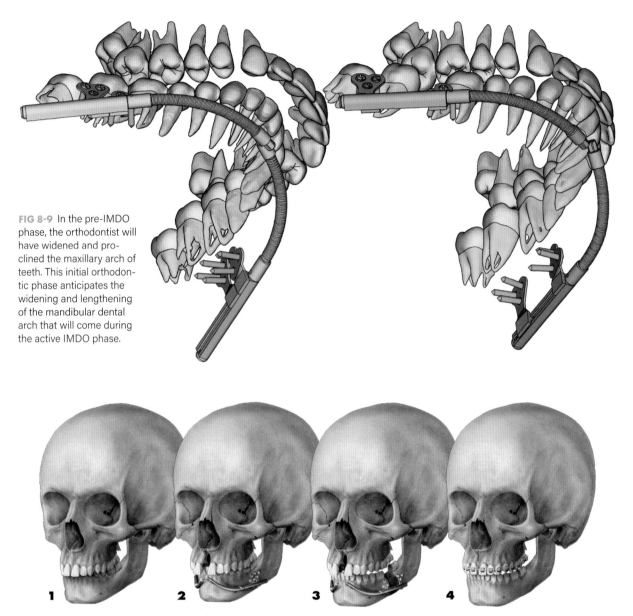

FIG 8-9 In the pre-IMDO phase, the orthodontist will have widened and proclined the maxillary arch of teeth. This initial orthodontic phase anticipates the widening and lengthening of the mandibular dental arch that will come during the active IMDO phase.

1   **2**   **3**   **4**

FIG 8-10 Maxillary expansion in the pre-IMDO phase expands the midfacial sutures and widens the nasal airway. Mandibular lengthening and widening by active IMDO corrects the AMHypo state and converts the occlusion from orthodontic Class II to Class I, enabling normal Class I orthodontics to proceed in the post-IMDO settling and orthodontic phase.

How will Class II occlusion change with IMDO?

In the post-IMDO phase, after the distractors are removed, teeth will naturally settle into a normal interarch relationship. This "settling period" is fastest during adolescence. Once dental settling is deemed complete, the orthodontist will then place fixed appliances to the teeth to further settle the dental arches into a fully interdigitating Class I occlusion (Fig 8-10).

How is dewlap eliminated by IMDO?

As the front of the mandible lengthens and the back of the mandible widens, the skin on the underside of the jaw also becomes tighter. This tightness increases as the IMDO distance increases. The greater the tightness, the greater the effect on dewlap elimination. By distracting regularly and in small increments, the associated increases in tension forces are gradually and gently overcome.

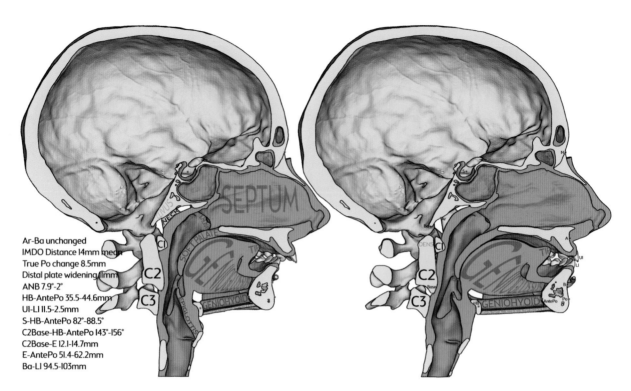

Ar-Ba unchanged
IMDO Distance 14mm mean
True Po change 8.5mm
Distal plate widening 11mm
ANB 7.9°-2°
HB-AntePo 35.5-44.6mm
UI-LI 11.5-2.5mm
S-HB-AntePo 82°-88.5°
C2Base-HB-AntePo 143°-156°
C2Base-E 12.1-14.7mm
E-AntePo 51.4-62.2mm
Ba-LI 94.5-103mm

FIG 8-11 It is difficult with plain radiology to precisely quantify the soft tissue changes that occur within and behind the mandible due to IMDO. The cephalometric values that you see in this diagram use new modalities, new points, and new measurements to amalgamate traditional and current forms of mathematic studies to objectively see the effects of IMDO.

How do cephalometric values change during active IMDO?

Lateral cephalometric values are of particularly great interest to IMDO orthodontists. Such measurements enable mathematic study of IMDO science. Cephalometry helps assess changes occurring in individuals and provides comparisons of the value of IMDO treatment compared to alternative-based splint therapies, more traditional forms of camouflage Class II orthodontics, or classical orthognathic-based surgical managements (such as the BSSO).

It is important to remember that IMDO involves complicated "tesseract geometry." A lateral cephalometric radiograph is two-dimensional. As a traditional form of assessment, lateral cephalometry gives only limited insight to the changing hypercube that occurs as IMDO advances.

Figure 8-11 gives some insight into what practical cephalometric values could be considered when mathematically analyzing IMDO.

What changes occur to the airway due to IMDO?

When a person is deeply asleep, it is presumed the tongue muscles relax, or lose their "awake tone." This potentiates the collapse of the airway behind the tongue, particularly when the individual lies on their back during sleep. It is difficult for doctors to make rational assessments of airway patency in awake persons. How small an airway becomes during sleep, behind a relaxed tongue and small mandible, is a very difficult medical assessment to make.

What we do know is that IMDO significantly and passively stretches the muscles of the tongue (Fig 8-12). This forward pull of the hyoid through tension of the inner chin muscles significantly prevents airway collapse during sleep. This process is called *airway tenting*. Probably the only way we can objectively measure this airway tenting effect is by using 3D radiology to assess changes in the digastric angle (see Fig 8-12a). An indirect (2D) way to assess airway tenting is by a lateral cephalometric measurement called the sella-hyoid-body-antepogonion angle, or S-HB-AntePo (see Fig 8-11).

Another more indirect measurement is change to the hyoid-antepogonion distance, as shown in Fig 9-7.

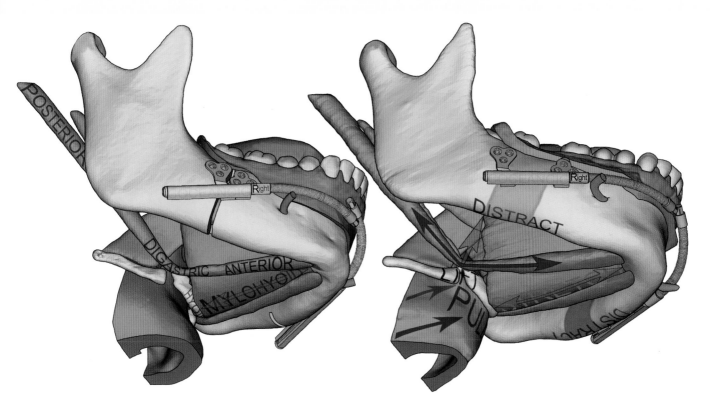

FIG 8-12A A small mandible is associated with a "fallen" hyoid bone. As distraction advances, the "digastric sling" or "digastric elbow" lifts the hyoid upward and forward, pulling the back of the tongue forward. The measurement of change in the "digastric angle" is probably the only accurate way to mathematically assess the effect of IMDO upon the airway structures behind the tongue, but it is almost impossible to practically measure in a routine way.

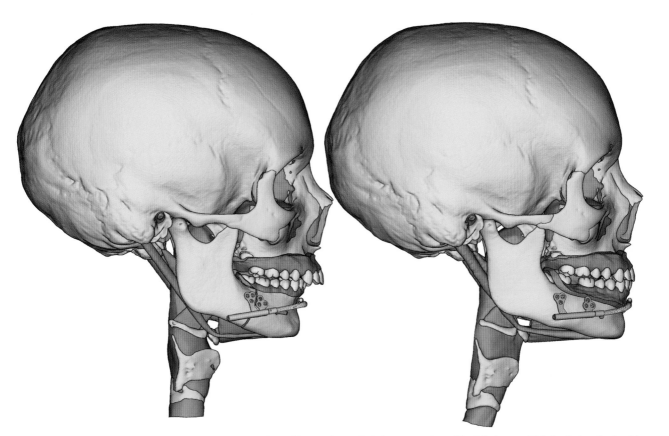

FIG 8-12B New 3D views enable the visualization of specific muscles and of airway structures. The full airway, which lies below the hyoid, acts as a weight that counterresists forward mandibular movement. Many muscles and tendons are involved that act much like mechanical slings and pulleys. Dental overjet, mandible size, tongue mechanics, and asleep-airway patency are all interlinked. ⟶

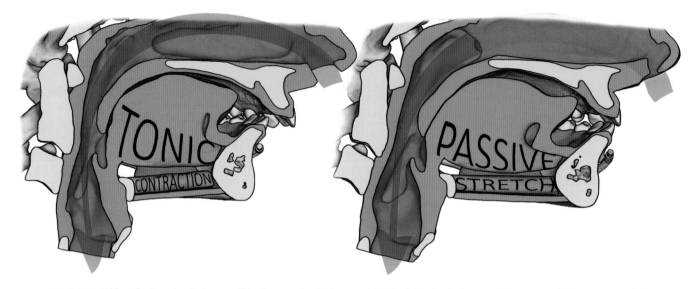

FIG 8-12C With a shortened anterior mandible, the muscles that connect the hyoid and anterior mandible must tonically contract to help pull the back of the tongue forward to maintain a patent airway. During sleep, these muscles relax and contribute to the effect of tongue collapse that contributes to sleep-disordered breathing. Lengthening the mandible through IMDO introduces a constant passive stretch to these tongue muscles. This in turn helps overcome hypotonic glottis collapse that occurs during deep sleep.

How does the profile change with IMDO?

The greater the dental overjet and matched maxillary arch widening that can be safely achieved by the orthodontist during the pre-IMDO phase, the greater the IMDO distance that can be safely attained to create a Class I occlusion during the active IMDO phase. The maximum IMDO distance that can be achieved is 16.5 mm (with some manufacturers and only 14 mm with others), which roughly translates to 10 to 12 mm of true mandibular incisor edge movement. In the case of the patient shown in Fig 8-13, who had a 14-mm bilateral IMDO, her mandibular incisal edge moved forward 9 mm, and her pogonion moved forward 8.5 mm. Her overall mandible widened 11 mm, measured across the posterior IMDO distractor plates (see Figs 8-14 to 8-19 for full treatment). Because the movements induced by the distractors occur in 4D space (a tesseract), traditional 2D trigonometry is not predictive of the linear measurements that occur within the 4D phase change.

The greater the dental overjet and matched maxillary arch widening that can be safely achieved by the orthodontist during the pre-IMDO phase, the greater the IMDO distance that can be safely attained to create a Class I occlusion during the active IMDO phase.

Esthetics and IMDO

It is not appropriate to validate IMDO surgery based solely on subjective esthetic or cosmetic facial changes. The social ramifications of the negative appearance of a small mandible, however, *are* a validated reason to consider corrective normalization of jaw size. Most dominantly, adolescents (and adults) have valid concerns that IMDO may abnormally affect their facial appearance through "overgrowing" or masculinizing the jaw line (especially young girls). Esthetic concerns should be raised with the treating surgeon, and while they should not be ignored, they must also be given reference to other wider medical and dental considerations too.

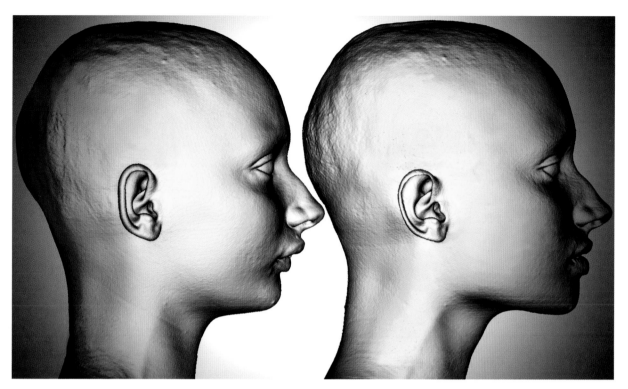

FIG 8-13A Profile changes (without distractors in place) approximately 3 months apart after 14-mm IMDO for correction of AMHypo and without chin surgery to convert orthognathic Class B to Class A. The fundamental facial soft tissue effects of IMDO are related to lower facial balance proportional to nasal tip projection, the creation of an esthetic jawline, the elimination of dewlap, and the creation of full passive lip balance. IMDO offers the ability to titrate mandibular growth to within masculine or feminine ideals.

FIG 8-13B Facial series demonstrating the facial profile before and after IMDO treatment.

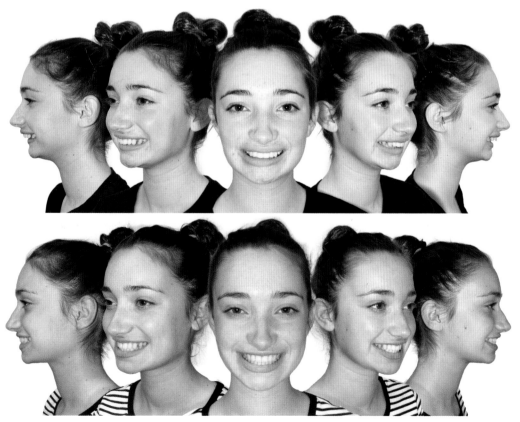

CASE 1

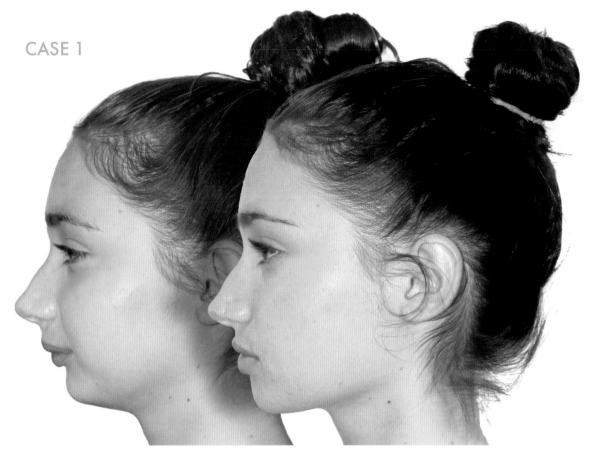

FIG 8-14 CASE 1. Adolescent patient before and after IMDO treatment for her AMHypo, shown at ages 14 years, 6 months and 16 years, 9 months. She had AMHypo and glossoptosis and was classified as orthognathic Class B. This section describes her treatment journey through pre-IMDO orthodontics and active IMDO phases of care and the complex anatomical changes that occurred along the way.

HOW IMDO TRANSFORMS AMHYPO IN THE ADOLESCENT

Case 1

This adolescent patient with AMHypo underwent IMDO treatment with preoperative and postoperative orthodontics (Fig 8-14). The pre-IMDO orthodontic process expanded her maxilla with a tooth-borne HYRAX expander (Fig 8-15). Maxillary expansion in the pre-IMDO phase reverses the compensatory narrow palate and widens the maxillary dental arch. Maxillary expansion is also orthodontically coordinated with incisor proclination to relieve dental crowding and better support the upper lip. By expanding the midfacial sutures, HYRAX expansion can visibly widen the intercheek bone distance while widening the nasal air passages and thereby making nasal breathing easier.

Because pre-IMDO orthodontics widen and lengthen the maxillary arch, this patient's existing prominent overjet

was increased further as a result (Fig 8-16). While this can appear to be the opposite of "normal" or expected orthodontic goals and processes, this creates the necessary room to then expand and lengthen the mandible in active IMDO.

IMDO permanently "grows" the front of the mandible into a stable forward position while retaining the normal TMJ position and function (Fig 8-17). It also creates a wider dental arch and mandible by creating new jawbone volume between the first and second molars. The effect also pulls the whole tongue permanently forward and resists collapse (and airway obstruction) during sleep (Fig 8-18).

Careful planning by the orthodontist in the pre-IMDO and post-IMDO orthodontic phases first prepares and then later consolidates orthodontic control of the occlusion into a full orthodontic Class I and orthognathic Class A state. This is all carefully coordinated before and after the active IMDO surgical process (Fig 8-19).

CASE 1

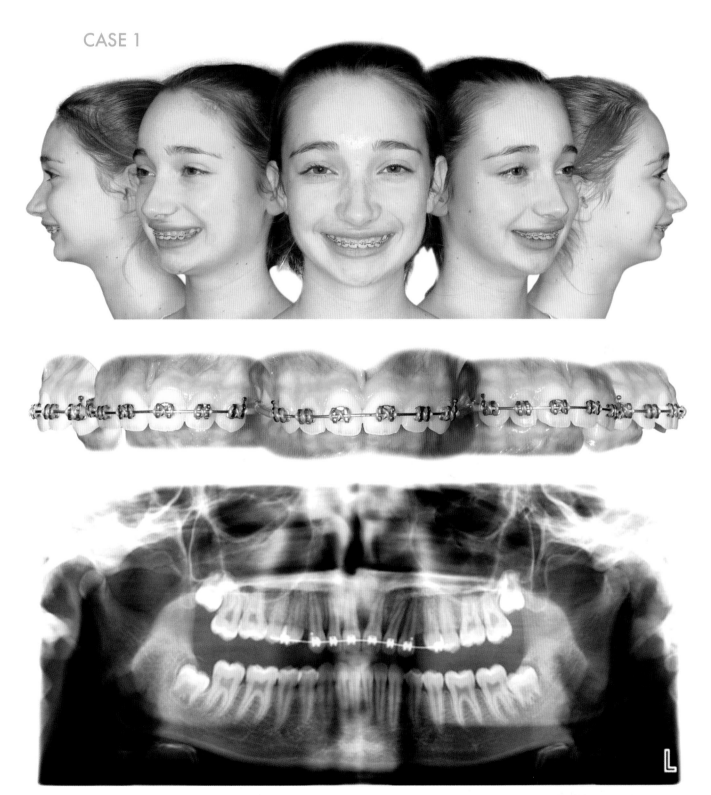

FIG 8-15 Patient at age 14 years, 6 months undergoing pre-IMDO orthodontics under specialist orthodontic care. It is important that any individual undergoing pre-IMDO mechanics is fully committed to undergoing the following active IMDO phase. The orthodontist should consider whether the parents have medical insurance before commencing pre-IMDO expansion orthodontics. Both the child and parents should first visit the IMDO surgeon to confirm a diagnosis of AMHypo.

CASE 1

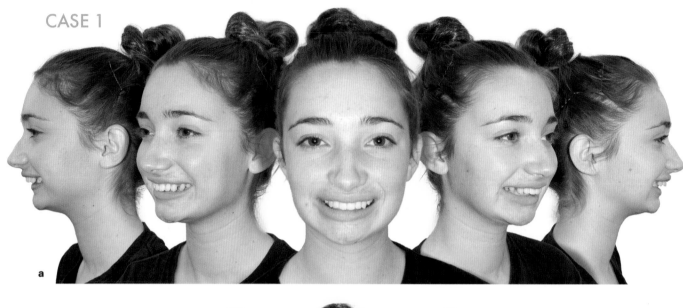

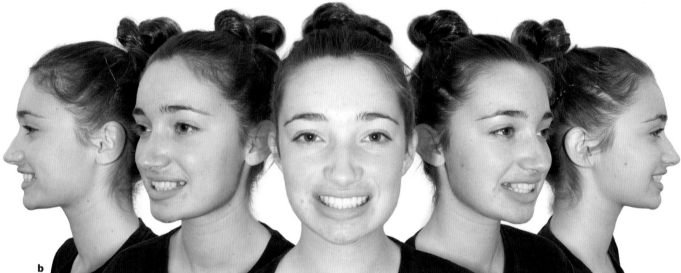

FIG 8-16 *(a)* Patient 12 months after removal of pre-IMDO orthodontics, shown at age 16 years, 4 months in a natural jaw position. She has learned to live with a full Class II, division 1 malocclusion, but eating, breathing, and sleeping are relatively difficult. *(b)* Patient artificially holding her jaw forward approximately 8 mm (taken the same day). This forward jaw position is often "trained" using dental or orthopedic jaw devices for its esthetic improvement, but it displaces the TMJs and can lead to temporal headaches and TMJ pain. This forward jaw position is also unsustainable during supine sleep, contributing to airway compromise. In Australia, this training of a child to hold their jaw forward and claiming the improved appearance as a result of the orthodontic therapy is given a name—the Sunday smile. Like wearing your best Sunday clothes, pushing the mandible forward also gives your best photographic appearance.

CASE 1

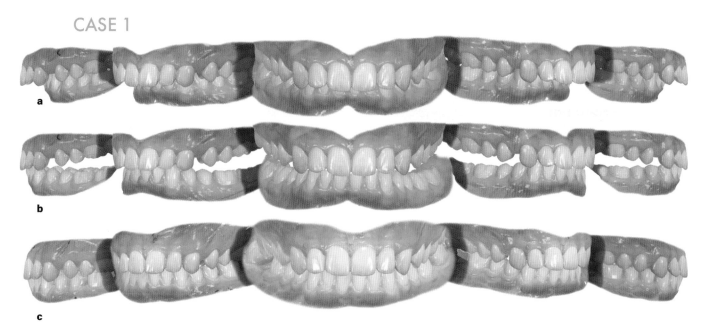

FIG 8-17 3D optical scans of the occlusion after pre-IMDO orthodontics with the TMJs in their normal (posterior) location *(a)*, after pre-IMDO orthodontics with full forward jaw posture (with the TMJs pathologically or unnaturally located) taken the same day *(b)*, and after IMDO treatment with the natural Class I bite achieved 3 months later with TMJs naturally (and posteriorly) located *(c)*. Note how IMDO allows the TMJs to stay in their normal position while advancing the front of the mandible into a stable forward position.

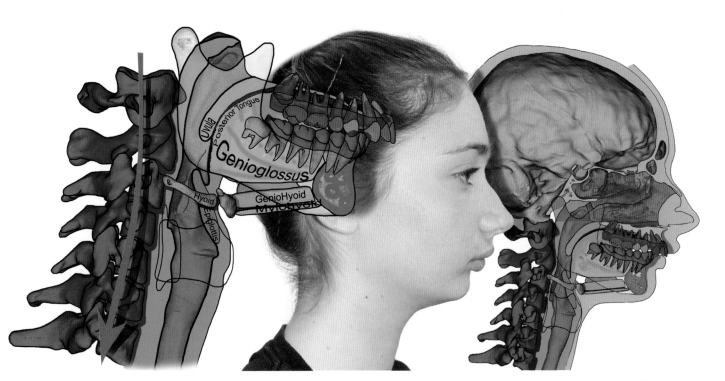

FIG 8-18 The relationship of cervical posture, airway, tongue tone, Class II malocclusion, and the small mandible. By bringing the mandible forward with IMDO, the tongue is also brought forward, preventing future collapse of the tongue into the airway and maintaining normal development and posture of the cervical vertebrae.

CASE 1

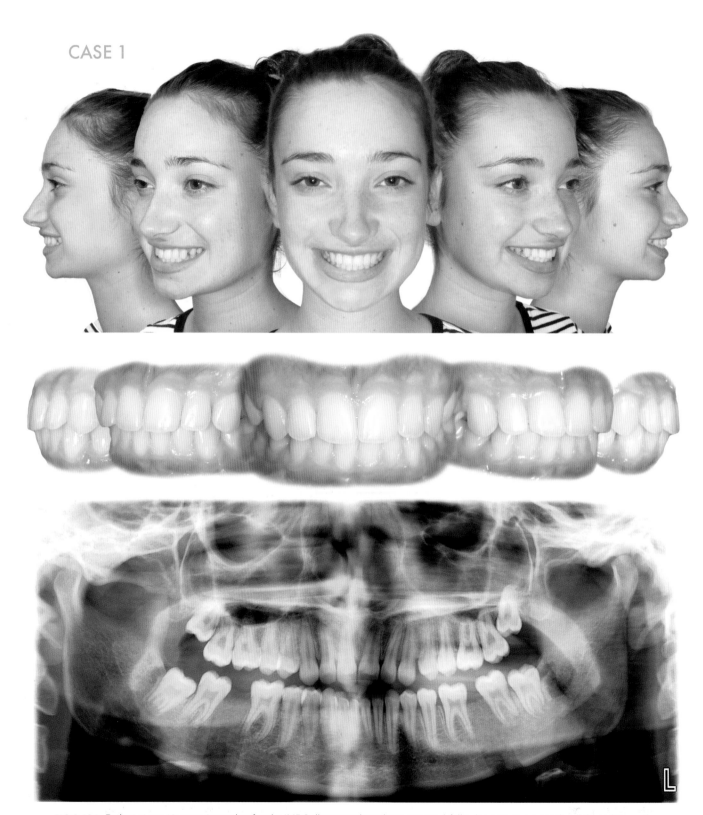

FIG 8-19A Patient at age 16 years, 9 months after the IMDO distractors have been removed, following a 14-mm extension (initiated 3 months previously). Following a period of natural dental settling, post-IMDO Class I orthodontics will be placed by her IMDO-accredited orthodontist. Dental spaces between the first and second molars rapidly close under natural eruptive forces but are best used in the post-IMDO phase to actively orthodontically decrowd and align the mandibular teeth. The new bone that has formed between the first and second molars will continue to consolidate, calcify, and mature over the next 3 to 6 months, before finally all evidence of active IMDO is lost. Eventually normal and simple Class I orthodontics will be used, and a full complement of 32 teeth in an orthodontic Class I or orthognathic Class A will be achieved, free of all risk of glossoptosis effects.

CASE 1

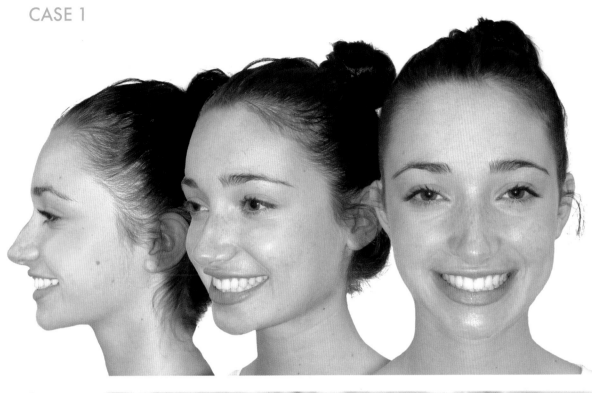

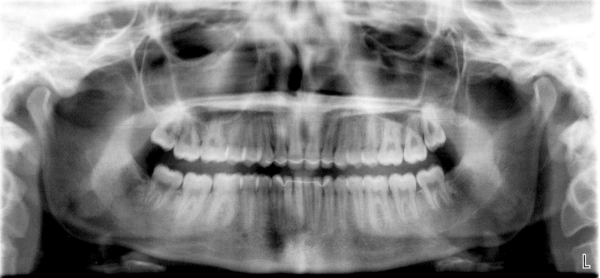

FIG 8-19B Final views and panoramic radiograph demonstrating 32 teeth after all orthodontic treatment was complete at age 19 years.

CASE 2

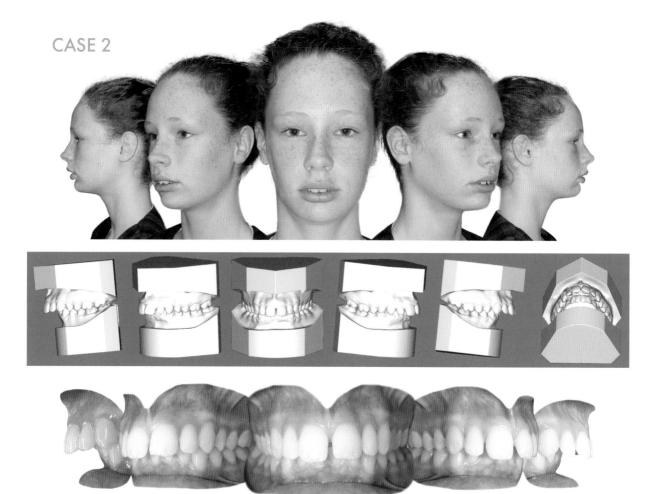

FIG 8-20 CASE 2. Orthodontic records of the patient at 12 years old. The casts and intraoral photographs show the Class II, division 1 occlusion, and the facial photographs highlight the small mandible. The panoramic radiograph revealed impacting third molars.

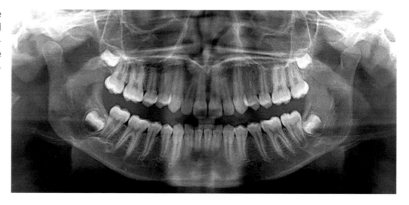

Case 2

This adolescent patient first presented to her orthodontist when she had just turned 11 years old for the orthodontic treatment of a classic dental overbite. Her complaint? She had big front teeth, and she didn't like them.

From a formal orthodontic analysis, she had an Angle Class II, division 1 malocclusion, with a narrow maxillary arch and retrusive mandibular position (Fig 8-20). But my orthodontist colleague Dr Peter Lewis recognized that the basic condition was her small mandible. To him, she had a horizontal growth pattern and still retained a high growth potential. From an IMDO perspective, she had classic AMHypo and was an orthognathic Class B. The patient complained of chronic jaw joint pain, tension headaches, and trouble running, all of which he felt could be resolved with IMDO treatment.

The first step in the pre-IMDO phase was of course to expand the maxillary arch (see Fig 8-4 for her HYRAX

CASE 2

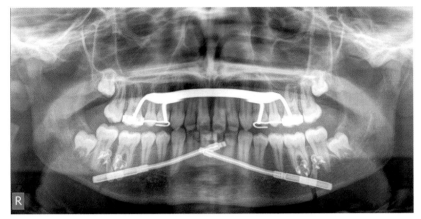

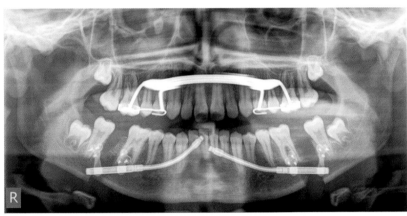

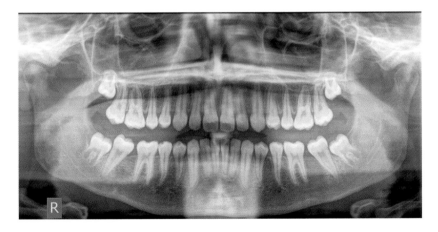

FIG 8-21 In the active IMDO phase, tesseract distractors were used to grow the mandible. Serial panoramic radiographs taken over 5 months (from age 13 years, 8 months to 14 years, 1 month) show the natural expansion of bone volume between the first and second molars. The third molars eventually developed and erupted normally. IMDO proceeds 1 mm a day; in this case, note that one side was advanced more than the other, for a total of 12 mm of IMDO advancement over 12.5 days.

expansion). This accomplished two goals: *(1)* It increased dental arch width, allowing for maximum opportunity to align the maxillary teeth and create a broader smile, and *(2)* it widened the upper airway, thereby widening the nostrils, improving nasal airflow, and broadening the midface esthetically. Tesseract distractors were then placed during surgery to initiate IMDO therapy (Fig 8-21). Once the IMDO distractors and orthodontic HYRAX were removed, the teeth were allowed to settle into a "natural" bite. This "hands-off" process usually takes 6 to 12 months and must occur before Class I orthodontic mechanics are applied for about a year (Fig 8-22). Figures 8-23 to 8-25 show the final results of treatment and the positive outcome achieved with the IMDO protocol.

CASE 2

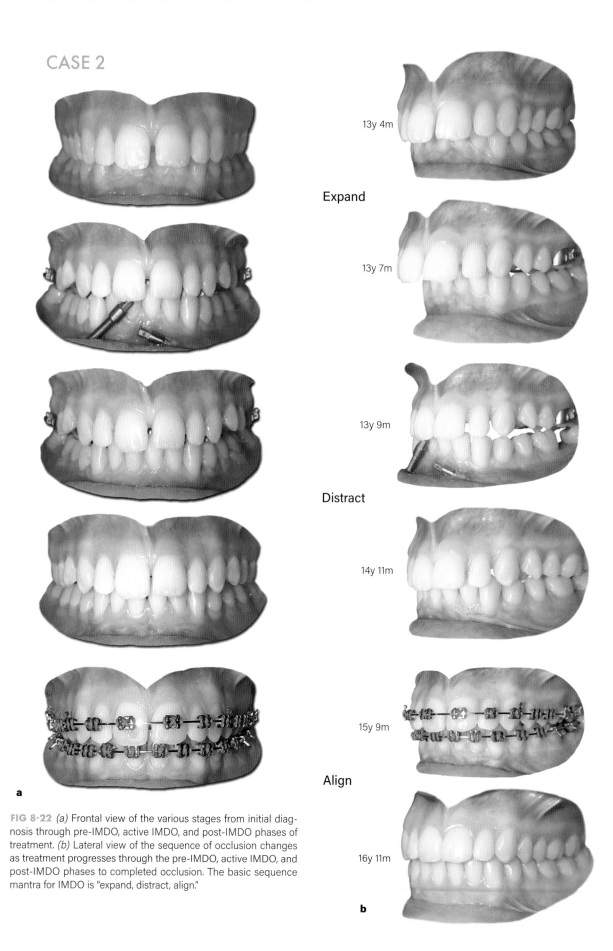

13y 4m

Expand

13y 7m

13y 9m

Distract

14y 11m

15y 9m

Align

16y 11m

FIG 8-22 *(a)* Frontal view of the various stages from initial diagnosis through pre-IMDO, active IMDO, and post-IMDO phases of treatment. *(b)* Lateral view of the sequence of occlusion changes as treatment progresses through the pre-IMDO, active IMDO, and post-IMDO phases to completed occlusion. The basic sequence mantra for IMDO is "expand, distract, align."

CASE 2

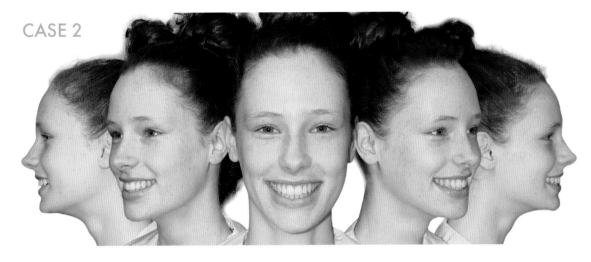

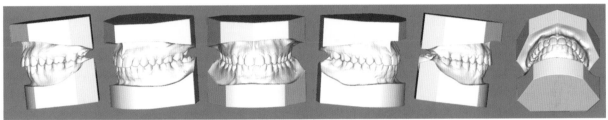

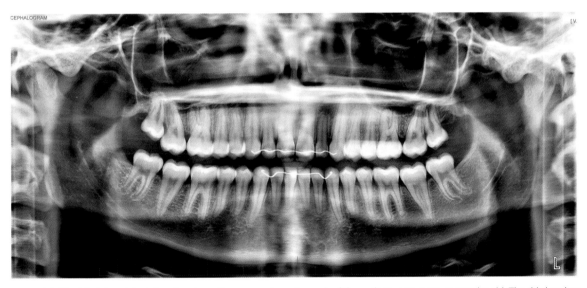

FIG 8-23 Final facial and dental cast series with panoramic radiograph of the patient at 16 years, 11 months old. The third molars have nearly completed their entry into a bilateral full Class I occlusion of 32 aligned teeth.

CASE 2

FIG 8-24 Of course we aren't treating to a photograph, a cast of teeth, or even a radiograph. Our patients have real lives and a real world that surrounds them. Beginning adult life with a full complement of teeth in a beautiful face with a beautiful smile and a full and open airway, free of the potential medical risks of having a small jaw, is a distinct advantage. That should be the ideal of orthodontic dentistry.

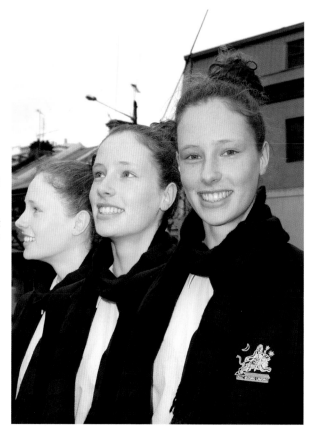

Before   After   Before

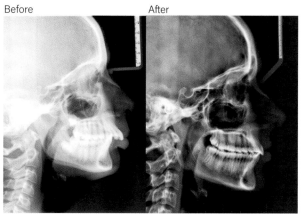
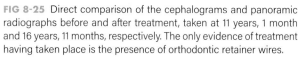
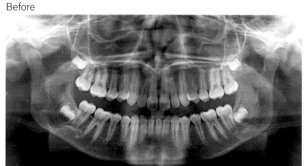

After

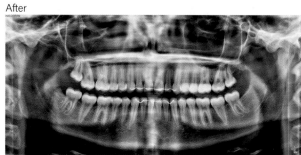

FIG 8-25 Direct comparison of the cephalograms and panoramic radiographs before and after treatment, taken at 11 years, 1 month and 16 years, 11 months, respectively. The only evidence of treatment having taken place is the presence of orthodontic retainer wires.

CASE 3

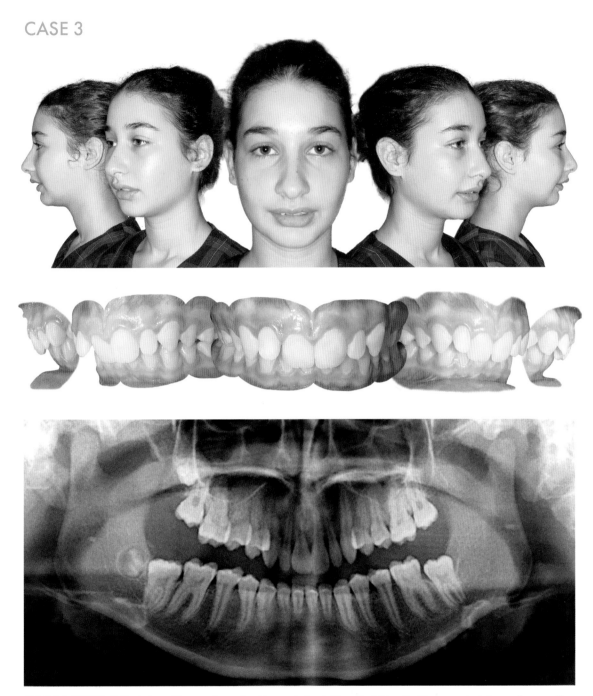

FIG 8-26 CASE 3. Patient at age 13 years, 9 months. Her occlusion is Class II, division 2 with severe dental crowding, maxillary incisor retroclination, and deep overbite. She also has AMHypo reflected in her reduced lower facial fullness. All of her second molars are partially impacted.

Case 3

For the collapsed anterior dental arch, the orthodontic aim is to maximally achieve the largest maxilla possible.

This adolescent patient presented with a Class II, division 2 malocclusion. But she also had AMHypo. Figures 8-26 to 8-32 document her journey with IMDO. She began treatment in an orthognathic Class C state.

> For the collapsed anterior dental arch, the orthodontic aim is to maximally achieve the largest maxilla possible.

CASE 3

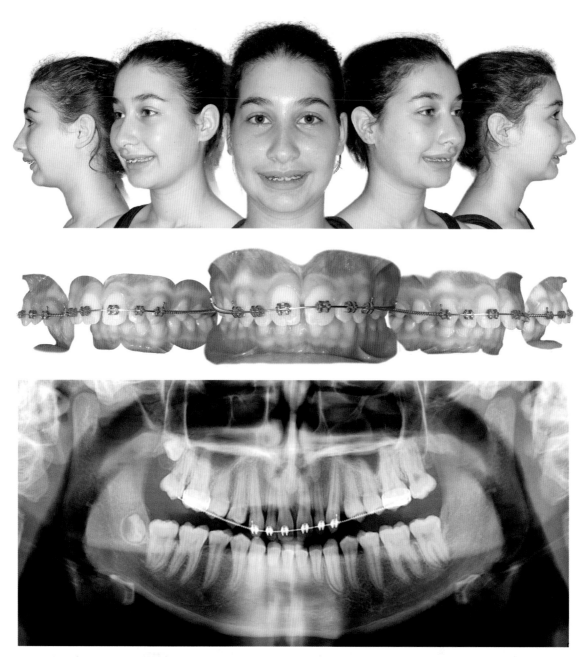

FIG 8-27 Patient at age 14 years, 7 months during the pre-IMDO orthodontic phase. During this phase, the maxillary arch is expanded, and the dental overjet is increased, providing greater support and fullness to the upper lip and improving the naso-labial balance. HYRAX dental arch expansion also widens the nasal base, improving nasal airflow. The orthodontic appliances should ideally be removed prior to the active IMDO phase.

CASE 3

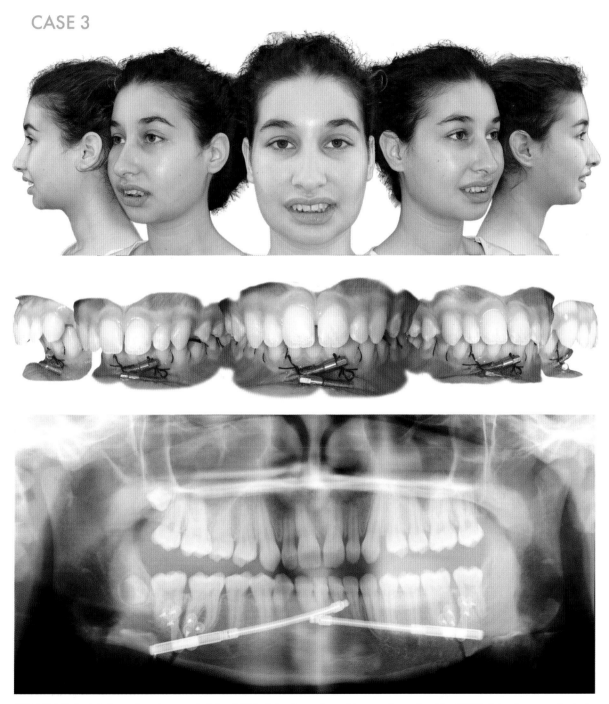

FIG 8-28 Patient 2 days after placement of the IMDO distractors, at age 14 years, 8 months. The IMDO distractors coordinate to produce a tesseract reformation of the mandible, which will help pull the posterior tongue forward. Swelling following this surgery is usually less than that observed following third molar removal, and the surgical procedure itself is less invasive. During active IMDO, lip sensation is normal, teeth are healthy, and the patient can attend school and undertake normal physical activities.

CASE 3

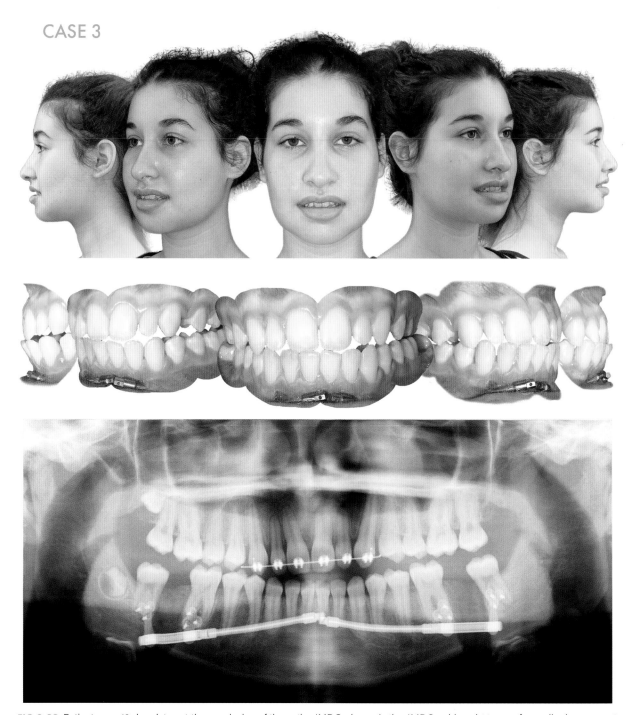

FIG 8-29 Patient seen 13 days later, at the conclusion of the active IMDO phase. Active IMDO achieved 14 mm of overall advancement, which has also widened the mandible significantly. The dentition has been brought into a Class III incisal relationship (where the mandibular teeth are now slightly beyond the maxillary anterior teeth). Distracting to this distance is determined by the surgeon and orthodontist and anticipates that the teeth will naturally settle into a normal Class I orthodontic relationship (the unnaturally proclined mandibular anterior teeth will naturally upright). While the distraction gap between the first and second molars looks dramatic on the panoramic radiograph, there is solid bone present and the distractors can be safely removed. This can be done under local anesthetic or in a hospital setting depending on local regulations.

CASE 3

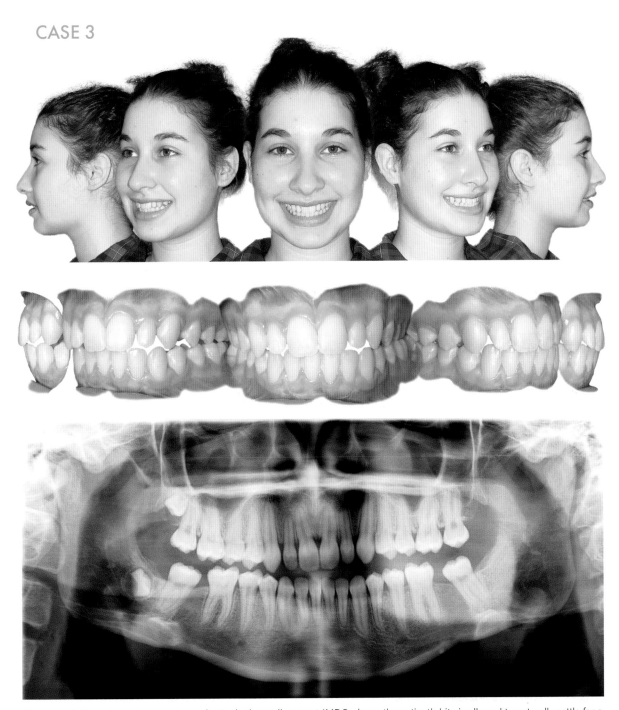

FIG 8-30 Patient at age 15 years, 2 months. In the immediate post-IMDO phase, the patient's bite is allowed to naturally settle for a period of approximately 6 months. During this time, she can eat and chew normally, which helps to settle the teeth into a natural bite. The mandibular second molars will naturally migrate into the new bone formed at the distraction sites. During this first 6 months, crowded teeth will move far more quickly and more gently under their own direction than can be achieved using active orthodontics. As anticipated, the mandibular anterior teeth have naturally uprighted and fallen behind the maxillary anterior teeth. Eventually, however, natural tooth movement reaches a physical limit. Class I orthodontics, either with Invisalign or classical brackets and wires, is always required to help with final movements. There is slight natural cant of the left maxillary dental arch upward, which can be improved orthodontically.

CASE 3

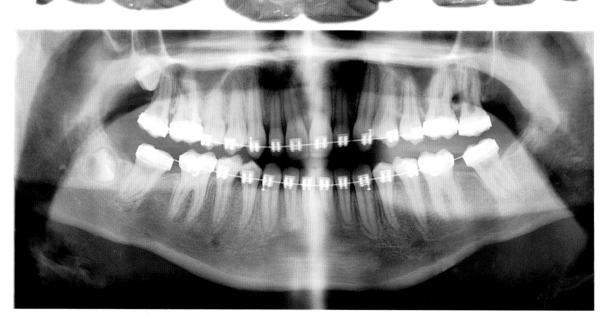

FIG 8-31 Patient at 15 years, 4 months. Active Class I orthodontics are applied to further settle the bite to produce an interdigitating occlusion. Orthodontic leveling is performed as well as final adjustments around the distraction gaps.

CASE 3

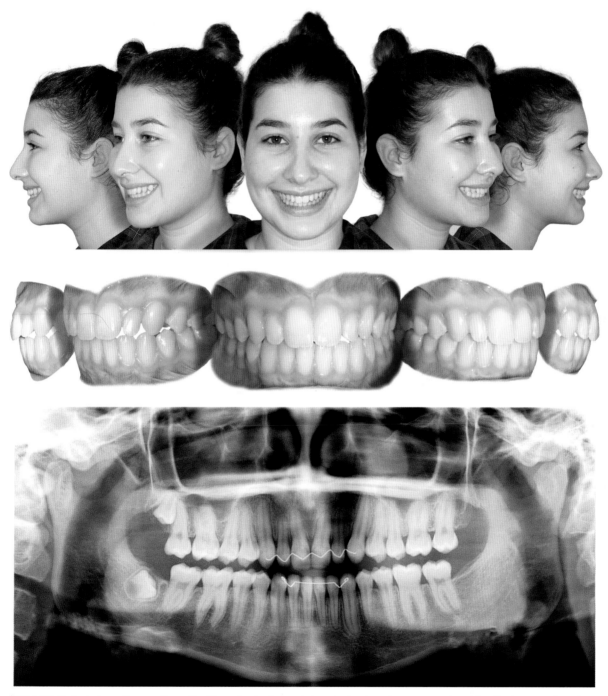

FIG 8-32 Patient at age 16 years, 11 months. The orthodontic brackets and wires have been removed, and fixed incisor retention wires have been in place instead for several months. There is normal bone development between the first and second molars, where active IMDO occurred just over 2 years previously. The third molars continue to develop and are on their way to normal eruption and function. The facial profile is normalized, and her airway is maximally patent, with no primary snoring or glossoptotic effects on aerobic breathing. The total treatment time from initiation of the pre-IMDO phase has been around 24 months, without dental extractions and with full facial and airway form achieved, reflected through a fundamental and demonstrable increase to the physical volume of the whole lower face.

9
DESIGNING FOR IMDO AND GENIOPAULLY

Designing for intermolar mandibular distraction osteogenesis (IMDO) and GenioPaully requires an understanding of intelligent 3D design, knowledge of sophisticated software, and application of the various STL programs and engineering processes within the custom titanium environment.

IMDO utilizes sophisticated tesseract distractors specifically designed for application to small jaws with anterior mandibular hypoplasia (AMHypo) and to the combined orthodontic and surgical protocols inherent to the IMDO system. An experienced bioengineer works with an IMDO-accredited surgeon to precisely locate IMDO distractors in a 3D state using segmented features of the teeth, gingiva, skull, and mandible and relative to achieving a patent airway and normalized profile.

IMDO SURGICAL INSTRUMENTATION

The following instruments and disposables are required (Fig 9-1):

- Smiths Osteotomy and Coceancig (inferior border) spreaders
- Epker slightly curved 4- or 6-mm osteotome with sharpening stone and surgical mallet
- Obwegeser channel, Kay-Austin, 5-cm Langenbeck cheek and adult Wieder tongue retractors, with medium-sized bite block
- No. 15 surgical blade and long surgical handle
- No. 9 Molt periosteal elevator
- 3-0 silk braided suture on tapered (trocar) 26-mm curved needle and fine 18-cm needle holder with fine 15-cm Adson's toothed tissue forceps

- Serrated 18-cm suture scissors with curved small mosquito forceps (to retrieve screws)
- Tapered fissure surgical bur drill 016HP (1.25 × 5 mm cut) used with surgical E-type handpiece Ø2.35mm
- No. 10 Frazier sucker with stylet & saline irrigation via blunt 18G needle (and 20-mL syringe)
- Four cartridges of 2.2-mL lidocaine with 1:80,000 adrenaline, 30G 25-mm sharp needle, and dental needle cartridge holder, and 4-mL 0.5% bupivicaine with 1:200,000 adrenaline delivered with 5-mL syringe with 30G 43-mm sharp needle
- Right and left IMDO tesseract distractors with hex driver for distractor arm activation in 14-mm (0.5-mm pitch) or 16.5-mm (0.4-mm pitch) lengths
- Ten 7-mm screws and two 5-mm screws Ø2.0 mm with screw driver handle and friction lock screw driver shank
- Short (7 mm) & long (transbuccal) drill bit
- Transbuccal trocar (rarely required)
- Two pairs of plate-bending forceps (rarely required)
- 4× (500-mm focal length) magnifying loupes

TESSERACT MANDIBULAR COMPONENTRY

The IMDO distractor has several titanium components (Fig 9-2):

- Hex activating end
- Spiral arm bendable distractor arm
- Distractor casing assembly (in 14-mm 0.5-mm pitch or 16.5-mm 0.4-mm pitch arrangements)
- Fixed short anterior plate and moveable long posterior plate, both with fixed offset (7.5 degrees)

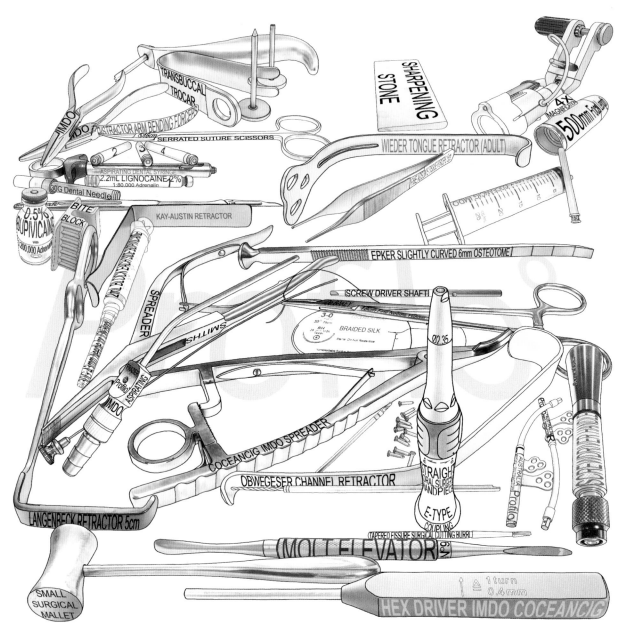

FIG 9-1 Surgical armamentarium for active IMDO procedure and insertion of tesseract distractors.

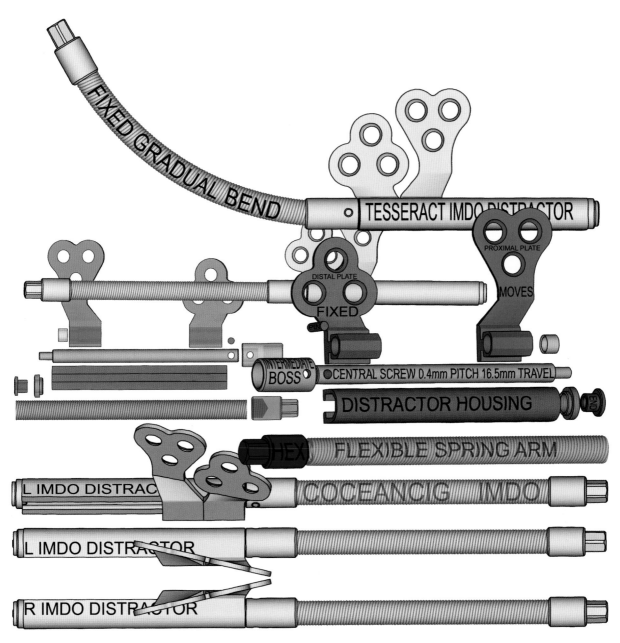

FIG 9-2 Tesseract distractor componentry and assembly. All is made from titanium medical-grade alloy. The distractor housing, containing the fixed forward (short) plate and movable distal (long) plate, are mirror pairs (right and left). The flexible distractor activating arm and internal screw thread are not mirrored, and both are designed to be turned with the right hand, using a hex screw driver, in a supination rotation. The plates are oriented to have a 60-degree angulation to the y-axis and 15-degree angulation to the z-axis of the linear distractor screw. The device is designed and manufactured such that both plates give permissive flexibility, with slight flap in the distal (moving) plate. The flexibility precludes any need for intraoperative adaptation by surgical plate bending. There is sufficient stiffness in the plates to resist mandibular forces in use while distraction is proceeding and during healing. The devices are designed for one-off clinical use, only in paired combination. The use of customized cutting drill guides is wholly provided upon prescription, design, and advice of the surgeon (see Fig 9-6). Depending on the manufacturer, effective distractor lengths are 14 mm (0.5-mm pitch) or 16.5 mm (0.4-mm pitch).

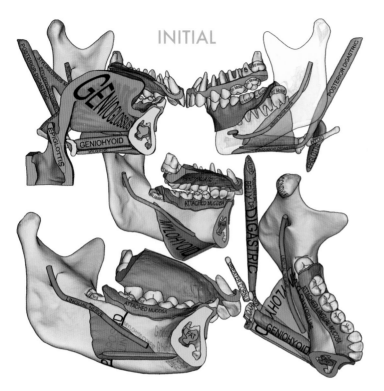

INITIAL

FIG 9-3A IMDO surgical protocol. The osteotomy line acts as a virtual "growth suture," which allows for stretching of the associated tongue muscles and volumetric extension of the horizontal mandible body by direct bone "growth."

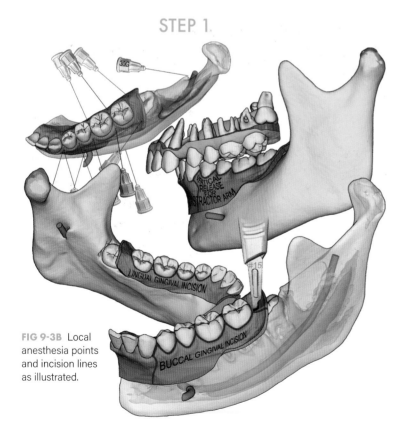

STEP 1

FIG 9-3B Local anesthesia points and incision lines as illustrated.

IMDO SURGICAL WORKFLOW

The operation is designed for full general anesthesia using nasal intubation and obstructive throat pack with ribbon gauze, full sterile draping, and with a single nurse assistant. Surgical loupes with central illumination (500-mm focal distance, 4× magnification) are essential for visualization. A surgical bite block is used with lingual retraction by a Wieder tongue retractor. The local anatomy of the osteotomy site assumes that the inferior alveolar nerve (IAN) travels within fat and loose tissue and that bony surgery is essentially cortical only. Irrigation is with 0.9% sterile normal saline. Blood loss overall is 40 to 100 mL for bilateral surgery. Total planned operating time is 40 to 60 minutes. For a right-handed surgeon, the left side is easiest to access (and vice versa).

The IMDO procedure aims to advance the anterior mandible forward and relative to the posterior mandibular rami. With distraction, the tongue is also advanced, pulling the whole tongue mass and hyoid-epiglottis complex forward and upward. Anterior tongue advancement is mediated by the bony attachments of the digastric, geniohyoid, and mylohyoid muscles (Fig 9-3a) and produces significant and logarithmically increasing retractive force as anterior mandibular advancement occurs. The lingual osteotomy line will directly cross only the mylohyoid attachment, midway along its lateral borders. The lingual nerve lies within the tongue mass, well medial of the osteotomy line. The bony operation is designed to proceed with or without custom titanium guides. What follows is a description *without* use of custom guides.

The surgical workflow is as follows:

1. Interpapillary (buccal and lingual) and subperiosteal insufflationary local anesthesia is given using 2.2% lidocaine and 1:80,000 adrenaline (total of 4.4 mL each side), followed by IAN and mental nerve blocks using 0.5% bupivicaine and 1:200,000 adrenaline (total 2.0 mL each side). Both use a 30G dental needle (Fig 9-3b). Buccal and lingual gingival incisions are made with a no. 15 scalpel blade. A 1.5-cm posterior mucosal relief incision is made along the external oblique ridge. A vertical 1.5-cm buccal anterior relief incision includes the canine to first premolar papillae, the base of which accommodates exit of the tesseract IMDO distractor arm for later activation.

2. The buccal and lingual periosteum is reflected with a sharp no. 9 Molt periosteal elevator (Fig 9-3c). Once the buccal periosteum is reflected, a periosteal releasing incision begins from the apical base of the anterior vertical incision, above and across the mental nerve exit and posteriorly and deeply toward the mandibular angle. This allows for safe reflection of the buccal flap for direct tangential view of the inferior mandibular border. The periosteal release limits significant stretch of the mental nerve at the mental foramen exit and increases the periosteal pocket volume available to accommodate the IMDO distractor at closing. The periosteal incision can lead to supraperiosteal spread of bruising and increased local facial swelling postsurgery.

3. A channel retractor is used to reflect the inferior border structures and to protect tissues from use of an oral surgical tapered fissure bur drill (under saline irrigation) to create a 1.75-mm wide cortical osteotomy cut, aiming toward the intermolar space. The cut is vertical, through the buccal cortex (Fig 9-3d). Inferiorly and below the IAN, the lower border of mandible is cut through to the lower lingual cortex. The cortex is roughly 3 to 4 mm thick. Do not use a bur to cut into intermolar crestal bone or through medullary bone or fat.

4. A slightly curved (or straight 4- or 6-mm) very sharp Epker osteotome is used to create a wedge indentation at the buccal superior border. Care is taken to avoid the adjacent periodontium of the first and second molars in the region of the interdental bone crest. The indentation is 2 to 3 mm deep (Fig 9-3e).

5. Preapplication of the closed distractor across the osteotomy is performed, parallel with the interplate line (Fig 9-3f). The activating arm sits above the root of the mental nerve, and distractor plates are affixed across the external oblique ridge, well below the crestal bone. Bending and adapting of plates is not required and extremely rare. Only the superior holes are screw retained (5 mm in anterior plate, 7 mm in posterior plate). The remaining holes are predrilled (anticipating screw flaring). The distractor and two screws are removed prior to progressing to the Smiths spreader.

6. With the distractor removed, a Smiths spreader is inserted into the buccal cut and used to initiate and complete crack propagation between the molars and tangentially across the mandible

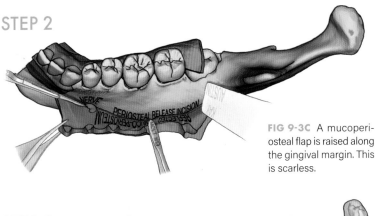

STEP 2

FIG 9-3C A mucoperiosteal flap is raised along the gingival margin. This is scarless.

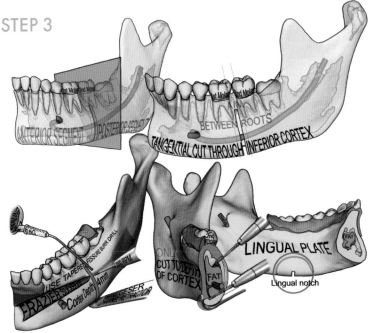

STEP 3

FIG 9-3D The crack line is between the first and second molars. The crack itself forms a growth plane, forming new bone as distraction advances in 0.5-mm or 0.4-mm increments twice daily.

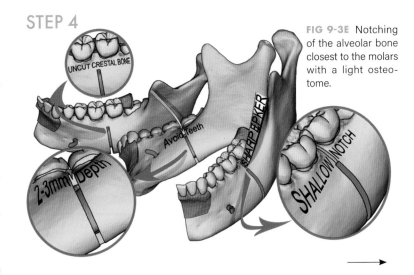

STEP 4

FIG 9-3E Notching of the alveolar bone closest to the molars with a light osteotome.

STEP 5

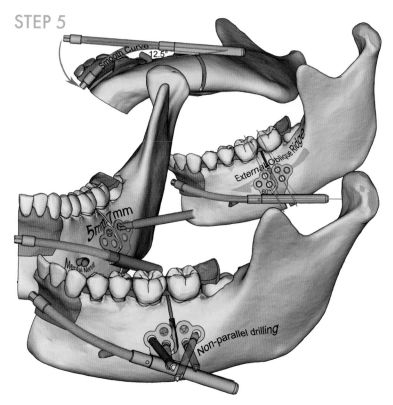

FIG 9-3F Once the outer osteotomy line is made, the distractors are aligned to it at the classic 30-degree angle. Specific custom guides can be prefabricated to provide further surgical orientation at this step.

STEP 6

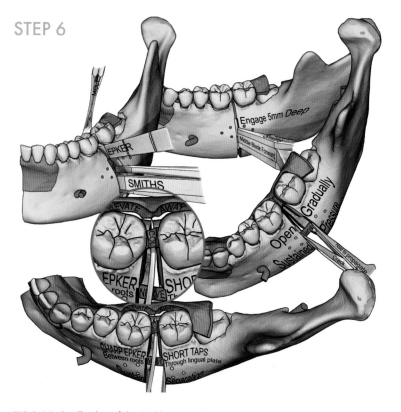

FIG 9-3G Application of the Smiths spreader allows for a controlled crack propagation to occur between the molars.

through cortical bone (Fig 9-3g). The osteotomy is complete when a discernable crack is heard and felt to occur through the lingual cortex. If the lingual cortical crack does not fully propagate, then a sharp thin Epker osteotome should be blindly introduced between the separated molar roots (this places the osteotome automatically above the IAN) and tapped through the upper lingual cortex. Taps are short and deliberate. The lingual gingiva should be elevated off the upper lingual cortex prior to this step in order to prevent inadvert cut-through by the osteotome. The lingual nerve is not anatomically at risk in this area. Widely opening the jaw with a bite block on the contralateral side also helps to propagate the lingual crack. Sustained, steady handgrip pressure (over a minute) on the Smiths spreader will achieve gradual crack propagation and eventual (usually sudden, accompanied with a "crack" sound) osteotomization. If too much pressure is needed for gradual separation to occur, the inferior border should be checked to reassess if the inferior lingual cortical bur cut has produced sufficient notch depth lingually. The IAN lies within fat and marrow and low-density cancellous bone and is very stretchable during this procedure. Proximal and distal segments should be vertically mobile and tested with finger pressure before proceeding to the Coceancig IMDO spreader instrument for inferior border stretching. The width of the buccal and inferior bone cuts is matched to the blade width of both the Smiths and Coceancig spreaders. Cortical bone separation occurs almost spontaneously in mature bone. In young teenagers, middle adolescence, or on repeat IMDO procedures (for extremely small mandibles), cortical bone can be frustratingly plastic. If lateral separation does not occur, wait 2 minutes, repeat the above steps, and aim to sustain a steady open pressure on the Smiths instrument. Do not progress to the inferior border (Coceancig) IMDO spreader until the Smiths separation is complete.

7. The Coceancig inferior border spreader is then used to further expand the inferior cortex and guarantee release of periosteum in the inferior lingual region (Fig 9-3h). This action enables even spreading of the osteotomy line during distraction and separates any remaining osseous and

periosteal tether point. Failure to use this instrument will result in anterior open bite and unpredictable mandible volume distortion as distraction advances.

8. The tesseract distractor is applied across the osteotomy using the predrilled screw holes (Fig 9-3i). Individual screws are lightly tightened in order to apply an equal tension of both plates across the mandible.

9. Prior to flap closure, the distractor is tested to assess for even opening of the intermolar distraction gap up to 5 mm (Fig 9-3j). Closure of the buccal and lingual flaps is made using interdental sutures (through dental papillae) with braided silk on a tapered (noncutting) 3-0 SH 26-mm curved needle. Use of such suture requires removal of suture material about 10 days postoperatively, which is preferred so as to reduce mucosal scarring and gingival infection and gingivitis risk. Flap design aims to minimize the amount of exposure of the distractor arm in the labial vestibule, maximizing comfort for the 45 days that the distractors are in situ while maintaining available exposure of the hex terminus for distractor activation.

COMBINING IMDO WITH GENIOPAULLY

The IMDO protocol involves three surgical procedures when combined with GenioPaully. In the first procedure, the tesseract IMDO distractors are precisely placed. These distractors are removed in the second procedure (about 42–70 days after insertion), and the chin button is advanced with a GenioPaully plate. In the third and final surgery, the custom GenioPaully plate is removed (about 3 months after surgery), and the local sites of the previous osteotomies are smoothed and contoured. These procedures result in full displacement of the tongue body forward as well as esthetic and functional balance for the patient profile (Fig 9-4).

Pre-IMDO orthodontics increases the esthetic balance, support, and projection of the upper lip (matched to the nose projection) and therapeutically widens and improves nasal airflow. Over just 14 days, active IMDO maximally reverses the patient's inherent glossoptosis and provides dental space to decrowd and naturally straighten the mandibular teeth, thereby

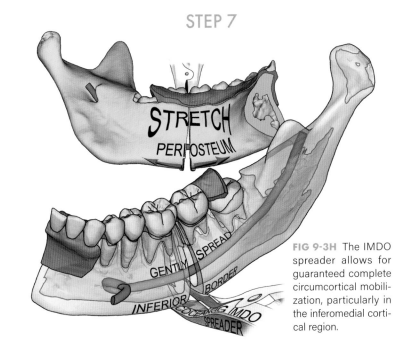

STEP 7

FIG 9-3H The IMDO spreader allows for guaranteed complete circumcortical mobilization, particularly in the inferomedial cortical region.

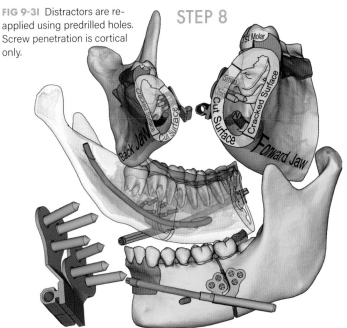

FIG 9-3I Distractors are reapplied using predrilled holes. Screw penetration is cortical only.

STEP 8

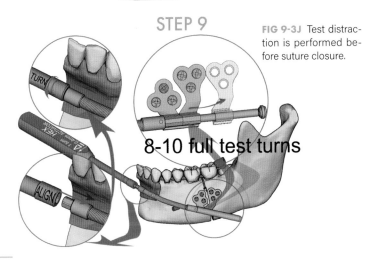

STEP 9

FIG 9-3J Test distraction is performed before suture closure.

8-10 full test turns

FIG 9-4 Before and after images of a patient treated with IMDO (see Fig 9-5) plus GenioPaully. Note the esthetic balance achieved. What you cannot see is the internal correction of her glossoptosis stemming from AMHypo, which can be inferred by the stretch of the underlying dewlap.

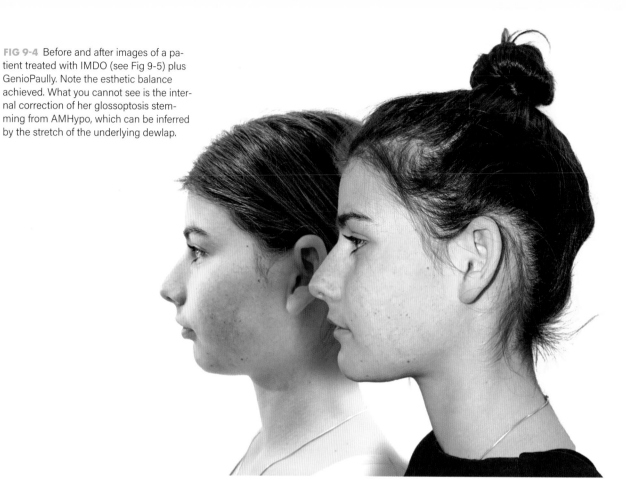

correcting the original malocclusion. The final Genio-Paully further refines the correction of the glossoptosis by completing the therapeutic stretch on the geniohyoid muscle, while also defining an esthetic chin button and providing functional support to the lower lip, thus eradicating the original lip incompetence and establishing nasal breathing and a permanently functional and therapeutically normal retroglossal airway.

SCANNING AND DESIGN OF HARDWARE

For complete design control, normal presurgical scanning and planning protocols for IMDO are established (Fig 9-5). Scanning enables the digital re-creation of the proposed distraction application and fabrication of custom titanium guides that settle the distractors into precise locations and orientations during the first procedure (Fig 9-6a).

> Manipulation of the chin button allows for precise control of lip competence and enhances tongue pull to completely reverse the original glossoptosis and tongue collapse inherent to the small jaw.

Once distraction is completed, scanning procedures are repeated, which allow for the creation of a formal chin button (Fig 9-6b). Manipulation of the chin button allows for precise control of lip competence and enhances tongue pull to completely reverse the original glossoptosis and tongue collapse inherent to the small jaw.

These design steps are not required where surgical experience with IMDO is already established or where surgical costs are intended to be minimized.

STEP 1

Following pre-IMDO
expansion and proclination

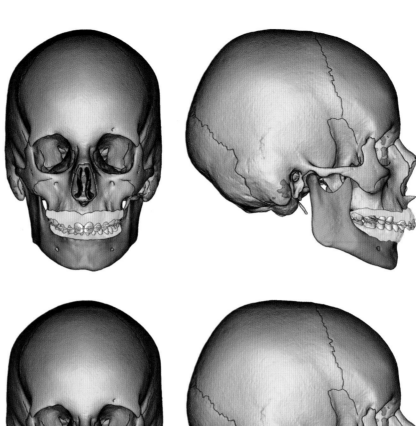

STEP 2

Custom guide production
for IMDO distractor location

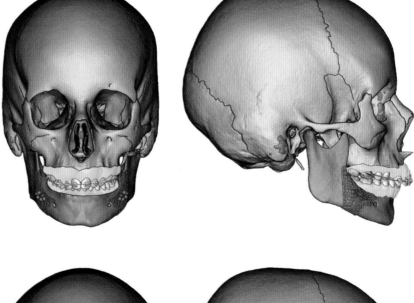

STEP 3

Operative placement
of IMDO distractors

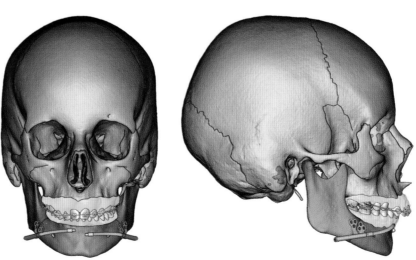

FIG 9-5 Overview of the combined IMDO/GenioPaully protocol, from pre-IMDO expansion to custom guide production, distraction, GenioPaully design and advancement, and final healing. →

STEP 4

IMDO distraction
up to 16.5 mm

STEP 5

Bone healing

Distractor removal
and GenioPaully are
conducted together at
around 42 to 70 days after
initial distractor insertion.

STEP 6

GenioPaully design

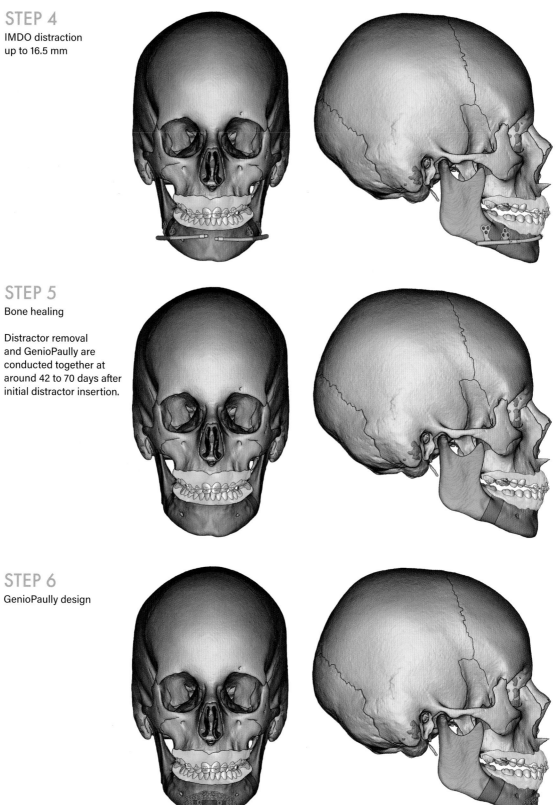

FIG 9-5 (CONT) Overview of the combined IMDO/GenioPaully protocol, from pre-IMDO expansion to custom guide production, distraction, GenioPaully design and advancement, and final healing.

STEP 7

Forward GenioPaully
advancement and undertrim of
anterior mandible

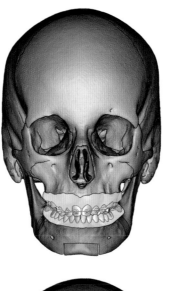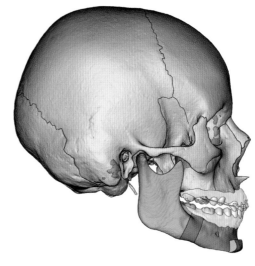

STEP 8

Custom GenioPaully plate
in place 3 months

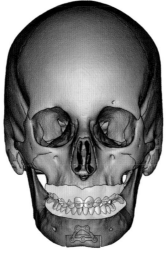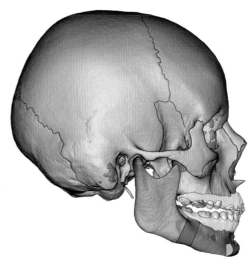

STEP 9

Final healed
extension of mandible

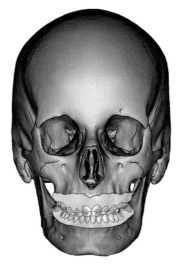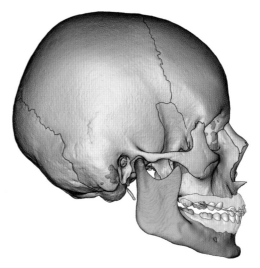

FIG 9-5 (CONT) Overview of the combined IMDO/GenioPaully protocol, from pre-IMDO expansion to custom guide production, distraction, GenioPaully design and advancement, and final healing.

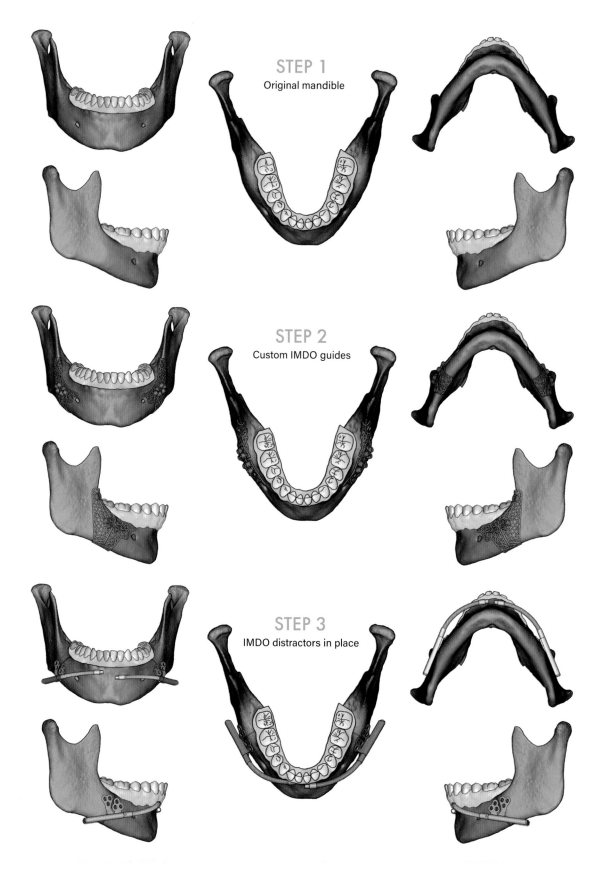

STEP 1
Original mandible

STEP 2
Custom IMDO guides

STEP 3
IMDO distractors in place

FIG 9-5 (CONT) Overview of the combined IMDO/GenioPaully protocol, from pre-IMDO expansion to custom guide production, distraction, GenioPaully design and advancement, and final healing.

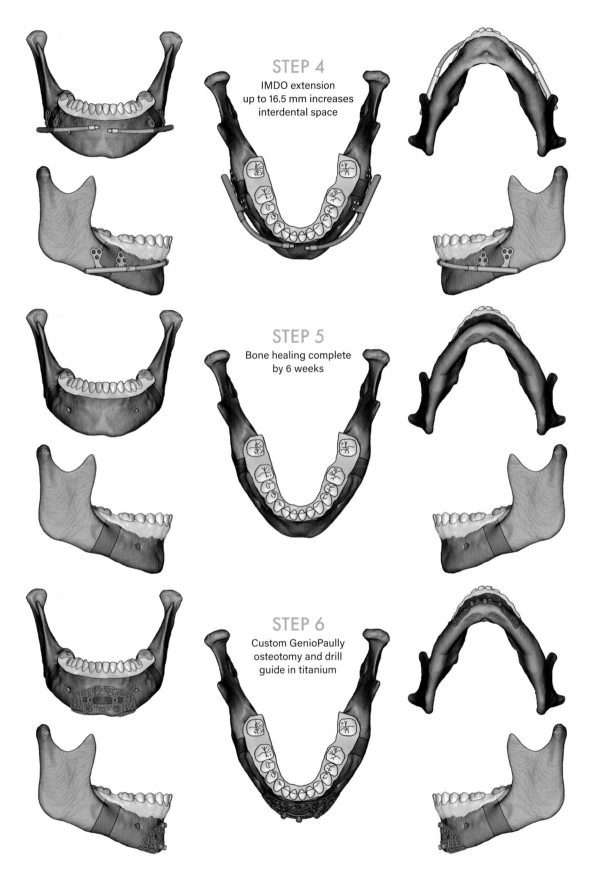

STEP 4
IMDO extension
up to 16.5 mm increases
interdental space

STEP 5
Bone healing complete
by 6 weeks

STEP 6
Custom GenioPaully
osteotomy and drill
guide in titanium

FIG 9-5 (CONT) Overview of the combined IMDO/GenioPaully protocol, from pre-IMDO expansion to custom guide production, distraction, GenioPaully design and advancement, and final healing. ⟶

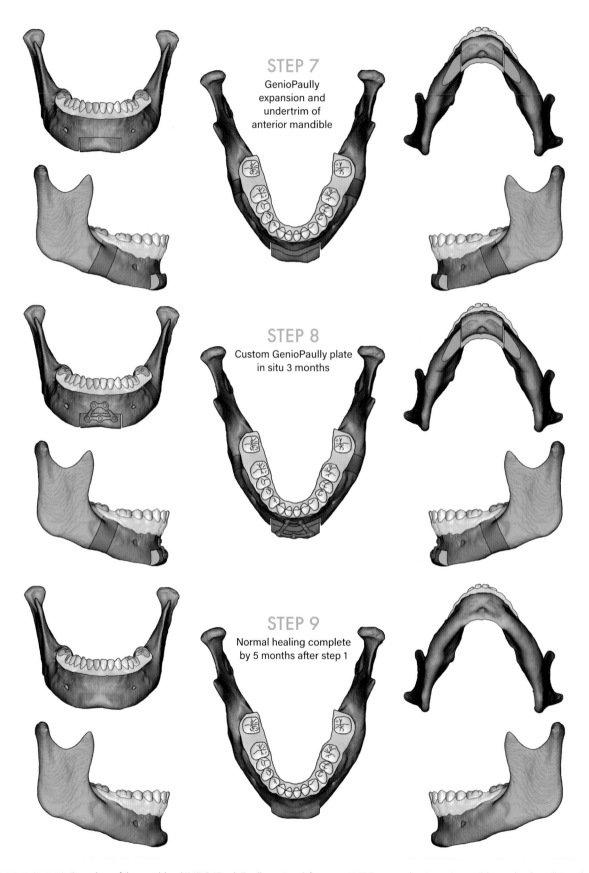

STEP 7
GenioPaully
expansion and
undertrim of
anterior mandible

STEP 8
Custom GenioPaully plate
in situ 3 months

STEP 9
Normal healing complete
by 5 months after step 1

FIG 9-5 (CONT) Overview of the combined IMDO/GenioPaully protocol, from pre-IMDO expansion to custom guide production, distraction, GenioPaully design and advancement, and final healing.

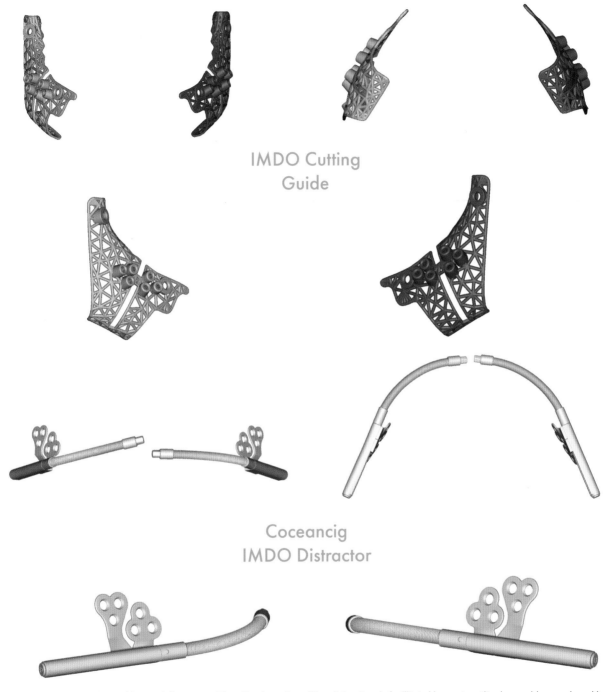

IMDO Cutting
Guide

Coceancig
IMDO Distractor

FIG 9-6A IMDO cutting guides and distractors. The 3D orientation of the distractors is facilitated by custom titanium guides produced by titanium 3D printing machines. The cutting guides facilitate creation and orientation of the intermolar osteotomy.

Custom titanium and GenioPaully

The GenioPaully procedure is a modified "box" genio-plasty that enables full cosmetic and functional control of the chin button, while also allowing for recontouring and reduction of the underside of the jawline. Used with custom design solutions (see Fig 9-6), the GenioPaully maximizes pull while elevating the lower lip to provide full lip competence.

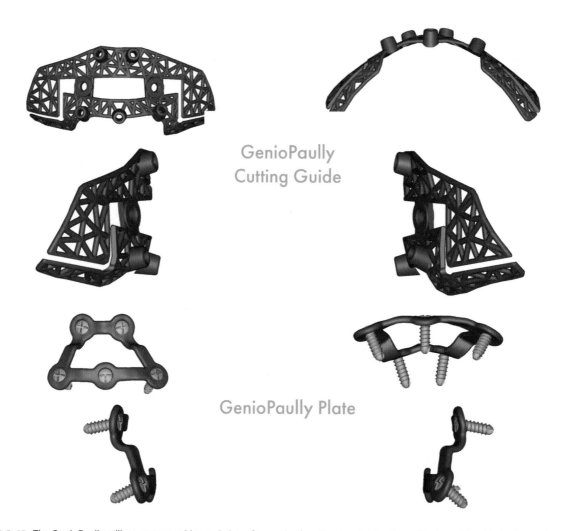

GenioPaully
Cutting Guide

GenioPaully Plate

FIG 9-6B The GenioPaully utilizes custom guides and plates for precise functional and esthetic positioning of the chin button and attached geniohyoid and anterior digastric muscles, maximizing tongue extension and improving lower lip competence as well as lower profile proportions. By contrast, the genioplasty has little or no effect on geniohyoid muscle pull.

UNDERSTANDING THE CEPHALOMETRIC CHANGE WITH IMDO AND GENIOPAULLY

A level and horizontal Frankfurt plane allows for a vertical drop line from the nasal tip and a means of establishing a vertical esthetic facial line. The ANS (anterior nasal spine) and anterior incisal face should aim to fall on this line if there is to be an esthetic balance of tooth projection matched to the upper lip and nose. If the maxilla is too short or the dental overjet is too small, a LeFort advancement can be combined at the same time as IMDO (see Figs 15-13 to 15-15).

Pogonion should also fall on this line in males or 5 mm short in females. Direct comparison should show the condylar poles in exactly the same position in their respective sockets, and thus a meaningful comparison and measurement of change in mandible length can be made (Fig 9-7).

Importance of the hyoid

The hyoid is an extremely variable bone and can easily move on swallowing, or breath holding, or with changes in neck position between scans. By using the original hyoid position, a meaningful measurement of geniohyoid stretch can be made between the original and postsurgical jaw sizes. The geniohyoid is the critical muscle that connects

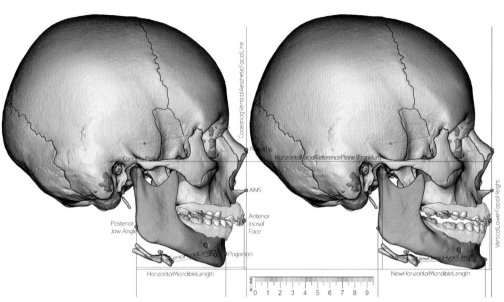

FIG 9-7 Lateral cephalometry for validation of the effects of active IMDO utilizes segmented 3D volumes derived from a combination of CT and intraoral optical scans. These "composite models" show the before and after changes resulting from the IMDO process. The hyoid bone remains artificially fixed in the original position for measurement and comparison purposes.

Before and after comparison of IMDO and GenioPaully

Sex = F Age = 13y 7m

	29.06.18	17.08.18
GenioHyoid Length	35.2mm	46.4mm
PoG - CVFRL	-46.8mm	-5.2mm
AIF - CVFRL	2.0mm	2.0mm
HML	73.6mm	88.9mm
VLFH (Nasal Tip)	93.6mm	94.8mm
SNB	79°	83°

Days in distractors	50 days
IMDO Net Distraction (R+L/2)	13mm
Net GenioPaully Advancement	4.4mm
Net Mandible Length Change	15.5mm
Net Facial Height Change	1.2mm
Net Pogonion AP Advancement	11.6mm
Net GenioHyoidMuscle Stretch	11.2mm

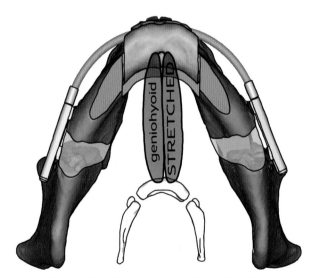

FIG 9-8 The double wishbone of the mandible and hyoid is connected by a single pair of muscles. Maximally and permanently stretching the geniohyoid muscle is the key to preventing airway collapse and curing OSA. Measuring the change in geniohyoid distance against a fixed hyoid before and after surgery gives a rational way of comparing different surgeries and their effects on airway patency.

the inside of the chin to the back of the tongue (Fig 9-8). Measuring the change in the geniohyoid distance (between antepogonion and original hyoid body) gives a meaningful understanding of how the combination of IMDO and GenioPaully therapeutically reverses the inherent glossoptosis associated with the small mandible.

The greater the change in the geniohyoid distance, the greater the chance of overcoming the "minimum therapeutic need" required for a patient to overcome snoring or risk of developing obstructive sleep apnea (OSA) due to glossoptosis. While orthodontists use the change in SNB angle to indicate how any interventional therapy may increase mandible length, the actual change in mandible length has better validity as an indirect means of assessing geniohyoid distance change. IMDO/GenioPaully increases jaw size in all three dimensions (Figs 9-9 and 9-10), rendering SNB assessment obsolete as a cephalometric measurement useful to understanding glossoptosis treatment.

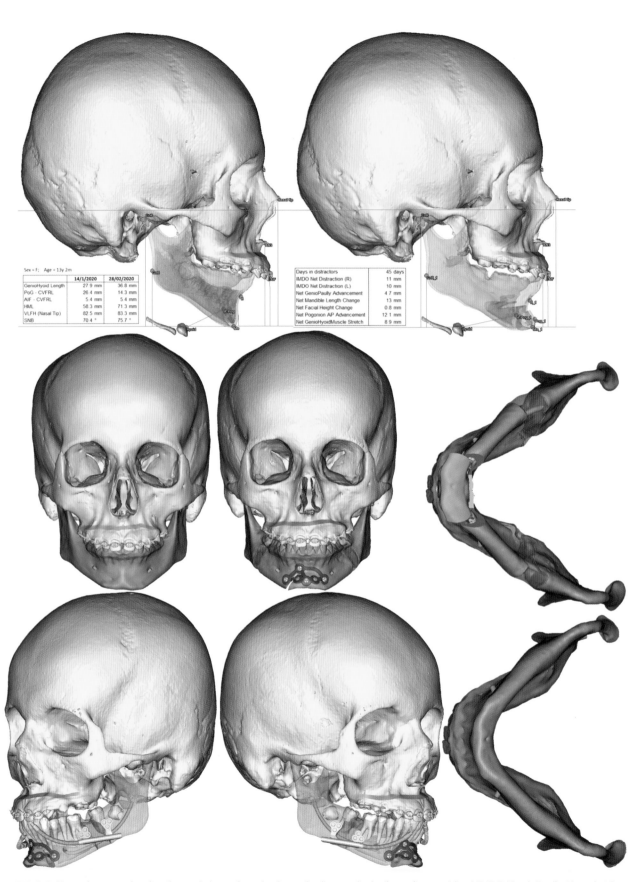

	14/1/2020	28/02/2020
GenioHyoid Length	27.9 mm	36.8 mm
PoG - CVFRL	26.4 mm	14.3 mm
AIF - CVFRL	5.4 mm	5.4 mm
HML	58.3 mm	71.3 mm
VLFH (Nasal Tip)	82.5 mm	83.3 mm
SNB	70.4 °	75.7 °

Sex = F; Age = 13y 2m

Days in distractors	45 days
IMDO Net Distraction (R)	11 mm
IMDO Net Distraction (L)	10 mm
Net GenioPaully Advancement	4.7 mm
Net Mandible Length Change	13 mm
Net Facial Height Change	0.8 mm
Net Pogonion AP Advancement	12.1 mm
Net GenioHyoidMuscle Stretch	8.9 mm

FIG 9-9 Example cases showing the cephalometric and volumetric changes in the face after combined IMDO/GenioPaully. Note that in every case, the mandible is increased in all three dimensions.

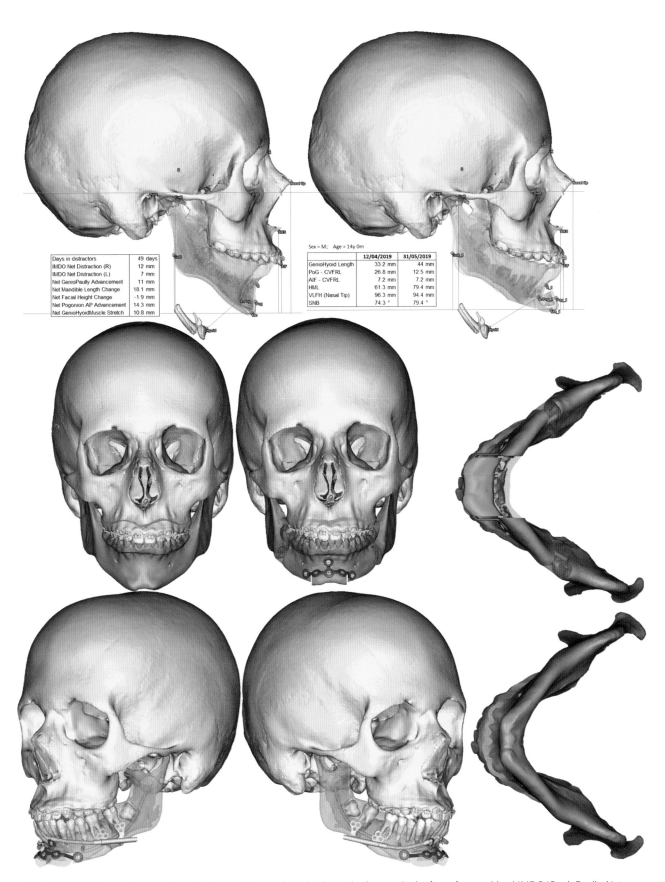

Days in distractors	49 days
IMDO Net Distraction (R)	12 mm
IMDO Net Distraction (L)	7 mm
Net GenioPaully Advancement	11 mm
Net Mandible Length Change	18.1 mm
Net Facial Height Change	-1.9 mm
Net Pogonion AP Advancement	14.3 mm
Net GenioHyoidMuscle Stretch	10.8 mm

Sex = M;   Age = 14y 0m

	12/04/2019	31/05/2019
GenioHyoid Length	33.2 mm	44 mm
PoG - CVFRL	26.8 mm	12.5 mm
AIF - CVFRL	7.2 mm	7.2 mm
HML	61.3 mm	79.4 mm
VLFH (Nasal Tip)	96.3 mm	94.4 mm
SNB	74.3 °	79.4 °

FIG 9-9 (CONT) Example cases showing the cephalometric and volumetric changes in the face after combined IMDO/GenioPaully. Note that in every case, the mandible is increased in all three dimensions.

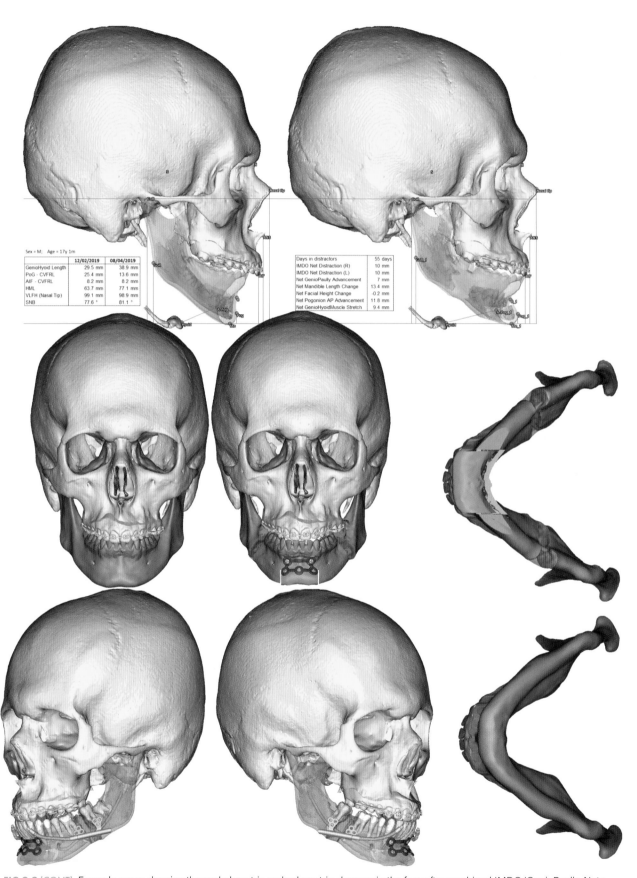

Sex = M; Age = 17y 1m

	12/02/2019	08/04/2019
GenioHyoid Length	29.5 mm	38.9 mm
PoG - CVFRL	25.4 mm	13.6 mm
AIF - CVFRL	8.2 mm	8.2 mm
HML	63.7 mm	77.1 mm
VLFH (Nasal Tip)	99.1 mm	98.9 mm
SNB	77.6 °	81.1 °

Days in distractors	55 days
IMDO Net Distraction (R)	10 mm
IMDO Net Distraction (L)	10 mm
Net GenioPaully Advancement	7 mm
Net Mandible Length Change	13.4 mm
Net Facial Height Change	-0.2 mm
Net Pogonion AP Advancement	11.8 mm
Net GenioHyoidMuscle Stretch	9.4 mm

FIG 9-9 (CONT) Example cases showing the cephalometric and volumetric changes in the face after combined IMDO/GenioPaully. Note that in every case, the mandible is increased in all three dimensions.

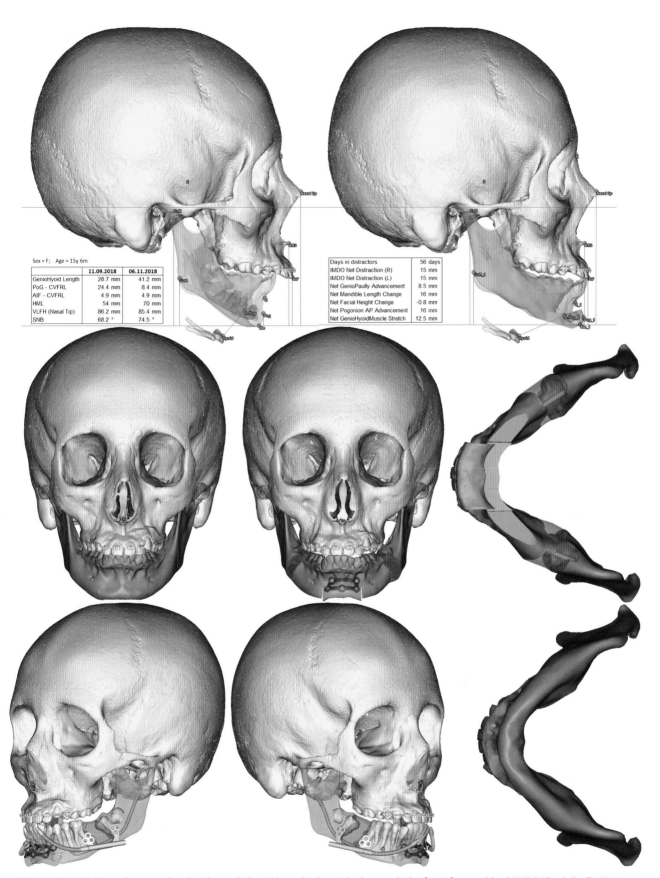

Sex = F; Age = 15y 6m	11.09.2018	06.11.2018
GenioHyoid Length	28.7 mm	41.2 mm
PoG - CVFRL	24.4 mm	8.4 mm
AIF - CVFRL	4.9 mm	4.9 mm
HML	54 mm	70 mm
VLFH (Nasal Tip)	86.2 mm	85.4 mm
SNB	68.2 °	74.5 °

Days in distractors	56 days
IMDO Net Distraction (R)	15 mm
IMDO Net Distraction (L)	15 mm
Net GenioPaully Advancement	8.5 mm
Net Mandible Length Change	16 mm
Net Facial Height Change	-0.8 mm
Net Pogonion AP Advancement	16 mm
Net GenioHyoidMuscle Stretch	12.5 mm

FIG 9-9 (CONT) Example cases showing the cephalometric and volumetric changes in the face after combined IMDO/GenioPaully. Note that in every case, the mandible is increased in all three dimensions.

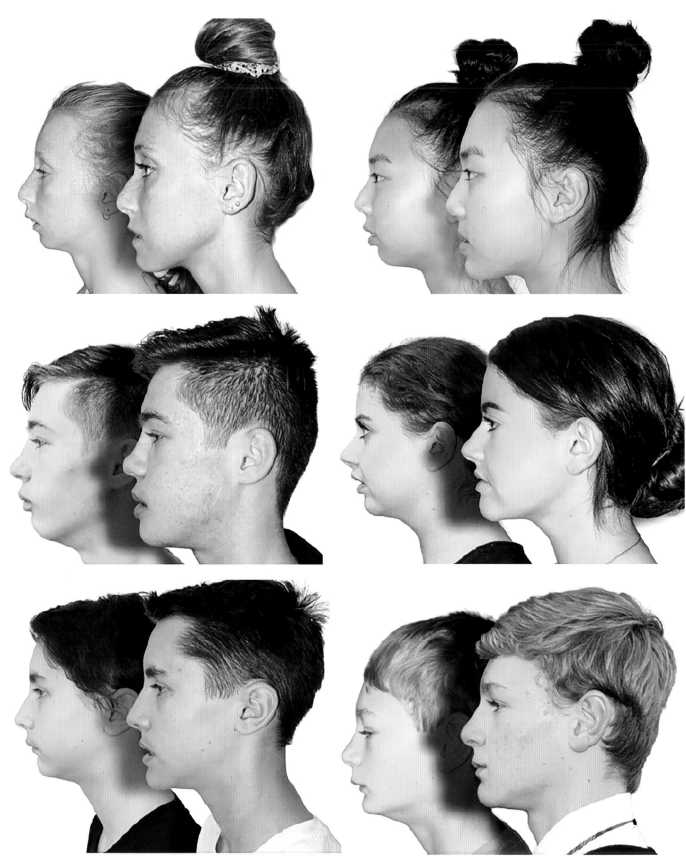

FIG 9-10 All of these patients were treated by a combination of IMDO and GenioPaully. Note the difference in jaw volume in each case as well as profile normalization. Follow-ups range from 2 to 10 years and demonstrate the long-term stability of this protocol into adulthood.

10
WHAT PATIENTS CAN EXPECT WITH IMDO THERAPY

This chapter provides specific information regarding what to expect both preoperatively as well as during the immediate postoperative period and active IMDO phase, including complications and medication use.

OVERVIEW OF IMDO SURGERY AND THERAPY

The intermolar mandibular distraction osteogensis (IMDO) surgical procedure creates an artificial growth suture that allows bone to grow across the distraction site. The artificial suture is created between the mandibular first and second molars. It exists like a crack in glass and extends through the outer shell of the jawbone. The inside marrow part of the jaw, which contains the main nerve, remains intact.

Until the distractors are opened, the "suture" remains closed and can very quickly heal. By turning the activating arms and gradually opening the distractors, the space within the crack is increased. New bone will deposit in this crack, and within a short time this new bone will harden and eventually calcify. Active IMDO works by continually opening the artificial suture to allow for more and more bone growth to advance the mandible (Fig 10-1). If left

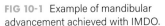

FIG 10-1 Example of mandibular advancement achieved with IMDO.

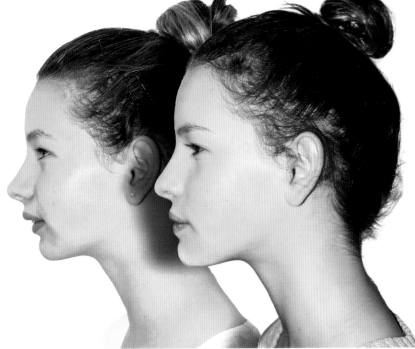

alone for only a few days, this artificial suture rapidly hardens, and ongoing distraction may not be possible. It is very important that full turns are continued two (0.5-mm pitch) or three times (0.4-mm pitch) daily in order to avoid premature fusion of the artificial suture.

> It is very important that full turns are continued twice or three times daily in order to avoid premature fusion of the artificial suture.

The turning may get more difficult as distraction continues, because the volume of new bone and level of forces pushing against the distractors are increasing. This may be uncomfortable or painful for the patient, but medications can be used to manage any discomfort (see section below). It is very important not to stop too early; it is always better to overturn than underturn. While distractors can be easily unwound if they go too far, it is much harder to open distractors against new bone that has already set.

Finally, the dramatic increase in jaw size during this active IMDO phase may be alarming to some patients or parents, but the actual underlying jaw shape will be very different once the distractors are removed and any swelling settles down.

LEADING UP TO SURGERY

What everyone should understand right from the beginning is that IMDO primarily applies universally to young adolescents. IMDO in adults is not as predictable in terms of bone maturation effects and is an agreed-only procedure with an experienced surgeon.

The requirement for preparatory orthodontics before IMDO can occur means that there must be a distinct understanding that IMDO will follow. Proclining the maxillary teeth and widening the maxilla is orthodontically irreversible and cannot be camouflaged if a parent or child elects not to proceed to surgery. Formal consent and agreement must be made between three parties—parent/child, orthodontist, and surgeon—before IMDO orthodontics can begin.

If the surgeon elects for custom IMDO guides, CT scanning should be performed only after the pre-IMDO orthodontics is completed. The pre-IMDO phase is usually very quick and progresses over 3 to 6 months only. A check with the patient's medical insurer should be made to adequately coordinate hospital timing and funding.

IMMEDIATE POSTOPERATIVE PERIOD

Mild to moderate lower facial and lip swelling may occur. This will gradually increase over the few days following surgery. Later, as swelling resolves, the jaw will also be growing, and the IMDO distractors will add to a sense of facial fullness. Swelling can be reduced with ice packs or wraps.

Mild to moderate face discomfort may also occur. This is made worse by mild throat discomfort, which makes swallowing difficult. Used with hot water, anesthetic mouth salts are very soothing for the inside of the mouth and can be used as a throat gargle.

It is important to keep the maxillary teeth clean with toothpaste and normal brushing. The mandibular teeth cannot be brushed because it will harm the surgical wounds and sutures. Chlorhexidine mouth soaks (using cotton balls) and hot saline mouth soaks can prevent plaque buildup and help soothe the gingiva. Avoiding sticky dairy foods also prevents plaque buildup and helps prevent later infection.

The lower lip will be numb for several days or even weeks. It may feel like pins and needles as recovery takes place. This is very normal. A small amount of saliva tinged with blood is also very normal but alarming to parents and child alike.

ACTIVE IMDO PHASE
First IMDO office visit

Distraction begins when the patient is ready to go home from the hospital, usually the working day following surgery. A visit to the surgeon will provide a baseline panoramic radiograph and everything needed for home activation of the distractors. A sterile screwdriver is provided to turn the screws, and this is easily cleaned with a soapy cloth or in the dishwasher.

Home turning

The distractors are turned twice or three times daily depending on the surgeon's direction. An IMDO distraction chart is given to the parents to document these turns so none are missed or forgotten (Fig 10-2). The child can perform the turns in a bathroom mirror, but strict adult supervision is required with the parent looking at the child, not in the mirror.

Profilo°
Surgical

IMDO™ DISTRACTION CHART

PLEASE BRING THIS CHART, THE SCREWDRIVER & A TOOTHBRUSH TO EVERY REVIEW APPOINTMENT

Patient Name:

Surgeon in Charge: PAUL COCEANCIG

Date of Surgery:

Start of Distraction:

Rotation/Activations per Day: LEFT | RIGHT

Type of Distractor: COCEANCIG IMDO™ PROFILO°

Distractor Location 1:

Distractor Location 2:

Next Check (Date)

Further Surgeon's Orders:

- Take ½ - 1 plain Panadol (Paracetamol) tablet, 30-60min before turning the IMDO™ distractor.
- Apply EMLA or numbing paste with cotton bud to gum around distractor arm behind lip 5min prior to turning distractor.
- 1x turn each side, morning, noon & night, in direction of arrow. Mark turns in boxes below. There are 3 full turns each day (1.2mm).

Date																								Total mm
Day	1			2			3			4			5			6			7			8		
Rotations	1	2	3	1	2	3	1	2	3	1	2	3	1	2	3	1	2	3	1	2	3	1	2	3
Left																								
Right																								
Notes																								

Date																								Total mm
Day	9			10			11			12			13			14			15			16		
Rotations	1	2	3	1	2	3	1	2	3	1	2	3	1	2	3	1	2	3	1	2	3	1	2	3
Left																								
Right																								
Notes																								

Please Note:

- Soak between lower molars and behind lip with cotton ball soaked in chlorhexidine (Savacol).
- Observe arrow direction when operating the distractor (you can get confused in a mirror).
- Be sure to follow a soft or purée diet during the entire distraction period. DO NOT CHEW.
- Careful oral hygiene is indicated during the entire treatment. DO NOT HAVE DAIRY PRODUCTS.
- Smoking/passive smoking can impair distraction results. Do not be near smokers.

Use photography to regularly update your surgeon via SMS.

FIG 10-2 IMDO distraction chart to be given to patients to record all turns of the distractors. Medication recommendations and further instructions are also provided for the patient.

Second IMDO office visit

The sutures used in the operation are usually silk, so they need to be removed after healing. Suture removal is usually timed for the approximate day that the surgeon determines that distraction will have nearly ended. Suture removal and distraction completion are usually predicted to occur between days 10 and 14. If the distraction required is great (12–15 mm), or if there is a great degree of asymmetry or dental crowding, then multiple visits to the surgeon and orthodontist during the distraction period may be required.

Note that it is easier and more predictable to overdistract and wind back than underdistract and readvance.

When distraction has ended, a date will be selected for the second operation to remove the distractors. If a GenioPaully is required, a new CT scan is arranged, and new engineering design is required. Generally distractors are removed between 42 and 70 days following the first operation.

Third IMDO office visit and second operation

The day or morning before the second operation, a post-distraction panoramic radiograph is taken to confirm the degree of bone healing and amount of physical move-ment of teeth that may have occurred. Unless there is a coincident procedure, such as genioplasty or insertion of orthodontic traction devices, the second operation to remove distractors is very quick and is a simple day-stay procedure. This second operation can be combined with a GenioPaully, which will necessitate a third operation to remove the GenioPaully plate.

Final and ongoing visits

Ongoing surgical monitoring of continual growth is encour-aged and not usually charged by the surgeon. If one child in the family is affected by AMHypo, it is likely that other children may also be affected by this inheritable condition. It is wise to maintain this relationship with the surgeon, as costs for treatment of additional children are generally reduced.

COMPLICATIONS

Some complications can occur following IMDO surgery or active IMDO therapy.

Numbness

An imagined complication is that the act of creating the artificial suture may cause damage to the inferior alveolar nerve (IAN), which passes through the jawbone across the surgical site. While this has never been known to occur, it is still considered a risk that the nerve may be severed by the operation itself. Nerve severance would lead to permanent numbness of the lower lip and chin on the side of the damaged nerve. If this occurs, it is irreversible and irreparable. It is important to stress that the operation is specifically designed to avoid this neurotmesis, but its theoretical chance is still an important focus for discussion.

> More commonly, it is possible to bruise or stretch the IAN during surgery or distraction therapy.

More commonly, it is possible to bruise or stretch the IAN during surgery or distraction therapy. This can produce transient numbness in the lower lip and chin, much like the pins and needles numbness that occurs when you hit the funny bone in your elbow. This numbness can take days or weeks to resolve; however, resolution is never noticed by the patient.

Loss of teeth

The most real common complication is the potential for the "crack" to affect the adjacent first or second molar, resulting in tooth loss. It is important to remember that the purpose of IMDO is to lengthen the tooth-bearing portion of the mandible, increasing the amount of room for already crowded teeth to erupt. Without such surgery, impacted teeth are almost always doomed to impaction and later surgical removal. Therefore, the small risk that crack propa-gation may lead to adjacent molar loss is matched against the inevitable risk that molar teeth are removed due to impactions or dental crowding. IMDO does not guarantee that all teeth will be kept or will develop normally, but it does dramatically increase the chance of keeping all the teeth.

Infection

Titanium is an inert biomaterial and is usually well tolerated by the body. However, the appliances themselves contain nooks and crannies where bacteria and food can hide and produce local swelling and potential infection. The chance of this complication is minimized with the daily use of chlorhexidine and hot saline mouth soaks and of course judicious cleaning of all teeth. Any infections that do occur, usually toward the end of the retention phase, do not cause any untoward or long-term issues and are easily resolved by either a short course of antibiotics or removal of the distractors 42 to 60 days after initial placement. If the patient suddenly develops swelling in the face unilaterally, the surgeon should be called.

Anterior open bite

IMDO works best in adolescent patients with a deep incisal overbite, long incisal overjet, and crossbite. IMDO corrects the incisal overjet very well but also acts to reduce incisal overbite. Anterior open bite can result if the patient already has a shallow overbite. However, this can usually be anticipated and managed appropriately either orthodontically (if minor) or surgically if necessary with LeFort-IMDO. In adults, IMDO is used to lengthen an extremely small jaw preparatory to SuperBIMAX therapy. IMDO in adults does not produce the same bite-correcting outcome as IMDO in early adolescence.

Failure of the distraction appliance

There are enormous pressures acting on the distractors, and these forces increase as distraction advances. It is therefore important to limit chewing and maintain a soft diet while the distractors are in place. The forces caused by chewing can cause physical attachments to pull away from bone or even break the metal of the appliances via metal fatigue. Furthermore, all contact sports should be avoided while the distractors are in place.

Developing third molars

Adolescent third molars will eventually develop and should be allowed to erupt. Rarely, these teeth may need to be removed, but such advice should be carefully considered with the IMDO surgeon.

Routine panoramic radiography monitoring

Panoramic radiography is the best way to monitor the distraction process and healing. It has extremely low radiation exposure.

MEDICATION USE

It is important to take all regular medications following IMDO surgery, and medications are recommended to manage pain and swelling during the active IMDO phase.

Antibiotic to prevent infection

Amoxicillin and clavulanate is the standard antibiotic provided to most patients after surgery. This antibiotic prevents postsurgical infection and can also be used to treat any infections during the active IMDO phase. For penicillin-allergic patients, clindamycin may be used instead.

NSAID to control swelling

A nonsteroidal anti-inflammatory (NSAID) such as piroxicam is provided after surgery to reduce swelling and pain in the 10 days following surgery. It is important to take the course for 10 days to control postoperative swelling.

Pain reliever

Acetaminophen is designed to prevent or ease pain during the active IMDO distraction phase. The first dose should be taken before the local anesthetic wears off, and dosing is every 6 hours for the first 24 hours. Regular acetaminophen use after this first 24 hours is not usually required. Active IMDO is not expected to be chronically painful, but general soreness may arise from local swelling and can be controlled with an NSAID. During the distraction phase, the patient should take one 500-mg tablet of acetaminophen 30 minutes before turning the distractors, depending on the child's weight.

Cream to prevent discomfort

EMLA cream (a eutectic mixture of lidocaine 2.5% and prilocaine 2.5%) is used in very small amounts around the distractor arms to prevent discomfort during the actual distractor turning process.

Extra pain management

Codeine is designed to provide extra pain relief for those who continue to experience discomfort during the active IMDO phase, despite regular use of piroxicam and/or acetaminophen. In those aged over 11 years, the safe dose is that given with cough mixture directions for breakthrough discomfort. Note that codeine commonly causes nausea and constipation with overuse.

Anesthetic throat lozenges or spray

Sore throat is a common postoperative side effect of IMDO surgery. Therefore, anesthetic lozenges including benzocaine (8.2 mg/lozenge) or lidocaine (10 mg/lozenge) may be used to control this unpleasant side effect. Benzydamine throat sprays can also be used to treat sore throat or any oral ulcers that may have developed as a result of surgery.

Mouth and wound care

Anesthetic mouth salts containing benzocaine (100 mg in 30 mg plain salt) can be used in a ratio of 1 teaspoon to half a glass of hot water to soak wounds. This is prescribed by a compounding pharmacy. It is safe to use this solution as regularly as the patient desires, but three times a day is the recommended protocol. This solution can be used starting 24 hours after surgery. This is to be used as a soak, not a rinse, and it should NOT be swallowed.

Oral surgery mouth soaks containing aqueous 0.2% solution of chlorhexidine in a 200-mL bottle are also used three times a day (morning, noon, and night) to clean the

Mouth soaks should NOT be rinsed, because they may open fresh wounds or cause bleeding.

wounds. This solution prevents bacterial colonization of the wounds. The anesthetic mouth salts should be used prior to this soak because chlorhexidine solution may contain a minimal alcohol content and may sting otherwise. Again, this should NOT be rinsed, as this may open up fresh wounds or cause bleeding, or swallowed.

The teeth are gently brushed with toothpaste after the sutures are removed. Chlorhexidine-soaked cotton balls are applied between the separated molar teeth and behind the lower lip three times daily until the distractors are removed.

Other

Anti-nausea medications and dietary supplements may also be prescribed by the treating surgeon during the postoperative period.

BONE HEALING IN THE DISTRACTION SITE

Using IMDO during growth and up to early adulthood predictably grows normal jawbone. However, as we age, bone marrow changes, and our bodies' ability to quickly heal means that adult IMDO requires much longer periods for bone healing to occur. Therefore, in adults, the surgeon may require use of bone grafting, local miniplate use, and prolonged periods of antibiotics to help maximize healing over longer periods of time.

11

INTRODUCING CUSTOM BIMAX
THE THIRD WAY

As orthodontics has developed, more people have come to appreciate the interrelationship between a perfectly functioning bite and facial harmony. Recent refinements lie in how we can very precisely create a full and esthetic smile matched with ideal facial balance and symmetry. People also appreciate the importance of eliminating nasal airway obstruction, snoring, and late-adult obstructive sleep apnea (OSA) risk. In the past, there was little practical attention given to absolutely normalizing the face and airway. Today we have access to modern medical computed tomography (CT), digital bite records, surgical planning software, full facial 3D scanning, and full airway analysis to help us determine the best treatment options to create both esthetic and functional long-term outcomes.

Designing the ideal face and ideal smile for a given patient combines the digital expertise of the orthodontist, surgeon, and bioengineer. Ideal form matches ideal function. We want our patients to have perfect symmetry, perfect balance, perfect chewing, and perfect breathing. Custom titanium offers all of these options. We have done away with inherently inaccurate plaster casts of teeth through the use of digital scanning solutions that are matched with full head CT imaging combining full virtual reconstruction of airway structures, soft tissues, teeth, and facial bones. Surgical engineers then use sophisticated planning algorithms to predict ideal facial proportionality and long-term stability, using 3D titanium printing technology to provide custom surgical guides and surgical plating solutions.

The result is a real paradigm shift in how orthognathic surgery can be performed. To a surgeon it means less surgery time, less swelling, faster recovery, fantastic surgical predictably, and greater stability, not to mention greater

> *We want our patients to have perfect symmetry, perfect balance, perfect chewing, and perfect breathing.*

accessibility and affordability for patients, as medical insurance often covers prosthetic and hospital costs. To the orthodontist it also means the elimination of heavy archwires, brackets, and bite splints and an easier working relationship with the surgeon. Custom titanium also means that surgery can be performed without braces at all, or in combination with simpler orthodontic solutions such as Invisalign, or as a "surgery-first" bite solution matched to prosthodontic and esthetic dentistry planning with the cosmetic dentist.

WHAT IS CUSTOM BIMAX?

BIMAX is a surgical procedure whereby both jaws are significantly advanced using custom-engineered titanium plates in conjunction with GenioPaully to augment the chin (Figs 11-1 to 11-5). By bringing both jaws forward with LeFort 1 and bilateral sagittal split osteotomies, the nasal tip is turned upward, the lips are better supported, the lower facial height is improved, and the jawline is defined. Most importantly, the tongue is pulled forward with the mandible, thereby eliminating any glossoptosis that could later develop or has already developed into OSA. BIMAX surgery is generally reserved for adult patients, most of whom have already unsuccessfully undergone camouflage orthodontics (see chapter 12).

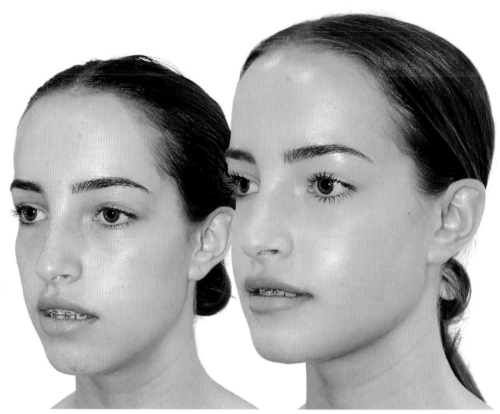

FIG 11-1 This 15-year-old patient has been in braces for 2 years to help correct her dental overbite. She has primary anterior mandibular hypoplasia (AMHypo). She has not had dental extractions, but her third molars are impacting. She has difficulties with natural nasal breathing. At the end of her sophomore year of high school, she has chosen treatment with bimaxillary orthognathic correction surgery (BIMAX) using custom titanium and custom facial design. Custom titanium offers the solution of combining bite correction with facial proportion optimization. Proper planning aims to maximize airway patency to normalize nasal breathing, eliminate snoring, and prevent late-adult OSA risk. Surgery includes LeFort 1, bilateral sagittal split osteotomy (BSSO), and GenioPaully, combined in an orthognathic process called *counterclockwise BIMAX*. These photographs were taken 6 weeks apart, before and after the BIMAX surgery.

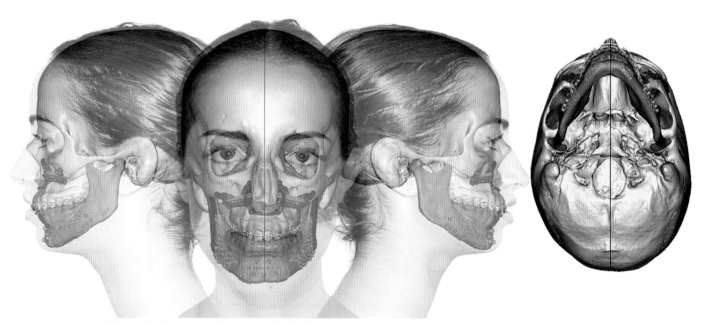

FIG 11-2 Red areas indicate areas of custom skeletal adjustment related to the surgical guide. An anterior nasal floor (piriform) reduction and rim of LeFort 1 relief allows for impaction of the maxillary arch of teeth, reducing the gummy smile and opening the anterior nasal area to provide nasal airway patency. Slight advancement of the maxilla rotates the nasal tip upward and broadens the nasal valves, simultaneously improving nasal esthetic balance while giving nasal airflow clearance and providing fuller upper lip projection. Esthetic control is given to eliminating the gummy smile, filling the buccal corridors on full smile, and creating passive incisor display that helps fill and support the upper lip. The underside of the chin is also trimmed as part of the GenioPaully procedure. The overall facial effect is to provide frontal symmetry and skeletal balance. By also providing a chin advancement, there is stretching of the skin underneath the chin, eliminating dewlap and feminizing the jawline. A passive lip competence is also obtained, facilitating natural mouth closure. The amount that the maxilla can be impacted without also constricting the nasal air passage is determined by segmenting the nasal mucosa (see Fig 4-20).

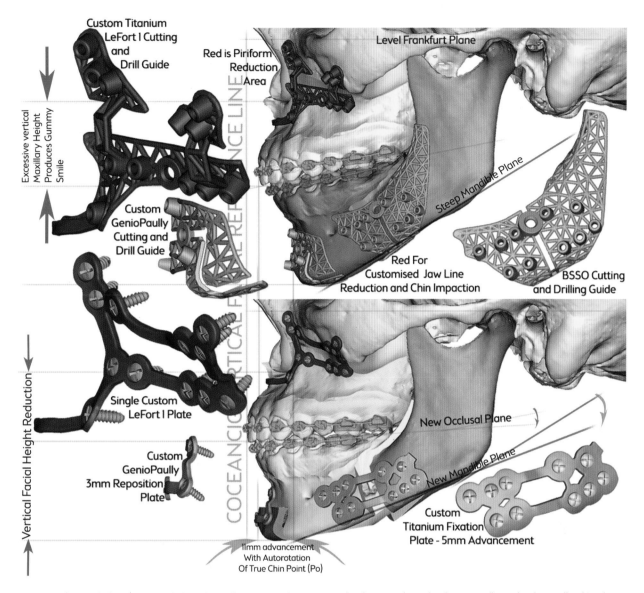

FIG 11-3 Before and after guides and plates in 1:1 direct proportion. Custom titanium uses inert titanium-vanadium-aluminum alloy (Grade V or XXIII titanium), sintered in a titanium laser-printing machine to produce complex 3D shapes. Custom guides (top left) guide specialized fine bone cutting tools in precise locations (red areas in top right), as well as locations for screws of specific depth, width, and direction, in order to avoid underlying teeth and neural structures. Because plates and screws only engage previously located screw holes and are precisely adapted to the surface topology of the bone shape, precise repositioning of dental arches and jaw joints is achieved, eliminating the need for bite splints, intermaxillary fixation, and further fixed orthodontics (though normal orthodontics are currently present in order to facilitate postsurgical orthodontic bite settling). In total, four cutting guides, four plates, and 48 screws are used (56 elements), all of which are eventually removed. There is an overall 18-mm maximum advancement of the chin point (pogonion, Po) that can be achieved using the BSSO (10–12 mm) and GenioPaully (6–10 mm). For very small jaws, where there is a requirement for further advancement of the chin point and tooth-carrying portion of the jaw beyond 18 mm (Po), the patient should consider combined utilization of IMDO. Combined custom titanium and IMDO can advance pogonion by up to 40 mm, well beyond the traditional limits of the BSSO procedure alone.

Dependence on precise data and segmentation protocol

For custom BIMAX to be effective, and for design to work, the collation and manipulation of accurate CT and dental data scans is extremely important. Once scans are obtained, no further orthodontic adjustments are allowed until surgery and healing are completed.

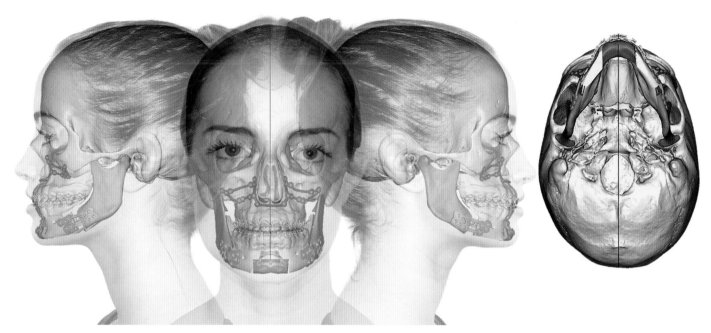

FIG 11-4 Before and after soft tissue overlay of advanced jaw segments, using custom surgical guides and shown with custom titanium plates in place. Surgery is performed entirely inside the mouth and has little difference to other jaw surgery procedures, such as removal of deeply impacted third molars. Once the chin point button is advanced maximally, it stretches the inner tongue musculature to pull the back of the tongue forward and relieve future risk of snoring or OSA development in late adulthood. The plates are removed 4 to 8 months after surgery to eliminate all evidence of surgery.

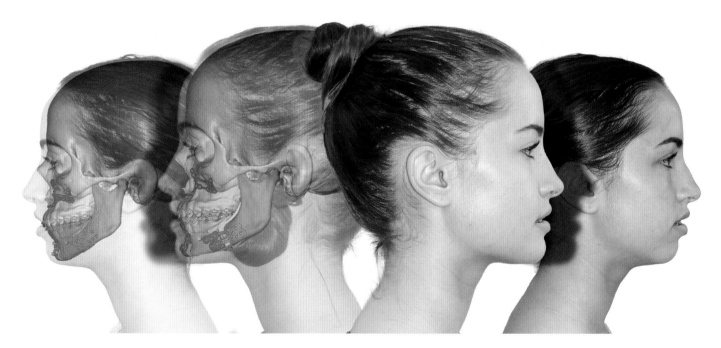

FIG 11-5 Custom titanium and bespoke facial design maximizes facial esthetics, bite balance, and airway patency. Jawlines can be maximally feminized or masculinized, but the aim is always to eliminate dewlap and restore lip balance and functional facial proportion—matched to a perfect smile. When BIMAX is used with forethought and interdisciplinary coordination, there is rarely a requirement for intermaxillary arch wiring or elastics, and orthodontic processes are maximally made efficient. Without planning and without coordination, however, BIMAX is a reactive event—and rarely proceeds happily.

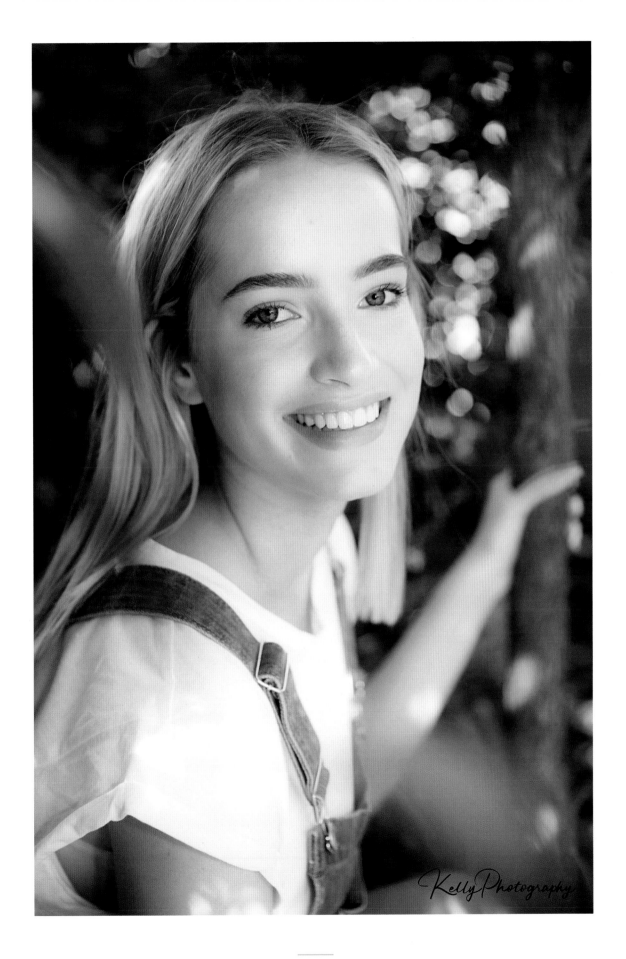

12
THE REMEDIAL BIMAX

When a person comes to me to have remedial BIMAX, they are scared. They are also usually angry. They are scared because I'm a surgeon, and they are angry because, up to this point, everyone has promised everything to avoid me. Jaw surgery is invasive. It has profound risks. It has a bad reputation. It isn't conservative. It involves breaking jaws. It's extremely expensive. It's very painful. It makes you uglier, at least for a while. And most importantly, it represents a failure of every previous promise made. Previous experts have offered better, more conservative, less invasive, more

What makes remedial BIMAX surgery particularly difficult on a psychologic level is that it involves a person's face—a person's outward identity.

benign, less risky, cheaper, more predictable, and more cosmetic alternative treatments that fundamentally didn't involve surgery.

And none of it worked.

FIG 12-1 This 27-year-old patient presented to my office complaining of lethargy and sleepiness that she associated with an emerging snoring pattern. Since adolescent orthodontics for a reverse underbite (orthodontic Class III malocclusion or orthognathic Class E) moved her mandibular teeth backward, there has been a sense of a retracted smile and thin lips, and clinically her profile form is what orthodontists call "concave." The etiology of Class III malocclusion and the small maxilla is almost always the result of anterior mandibular hypoplasia (AMHypo) and glossoptosis. Essentially, the small mandible leads to the small maxilla. Remedial BIMAX surgery is a simple, massive advancement of both jaws using custom-engineered titanium, with a slight GenioPaully reduction, in conjunction with Invisalign. Overall we upturn the nasal tip, filling out the lips and maintaining lower facial height, while defining a feminine jawline and simultaneously preserving a Class I occlusion. Most importantly, by making the mandible longer, we pull the tongue forward and eliminate snoring completely, eliminating the risk of developing obstructive sleep apnea (OSA) later in life.

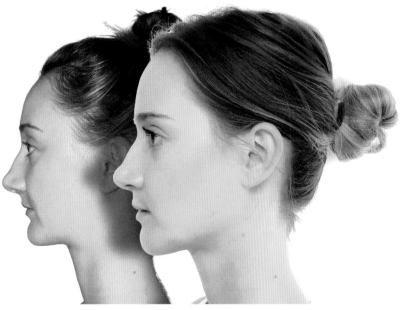

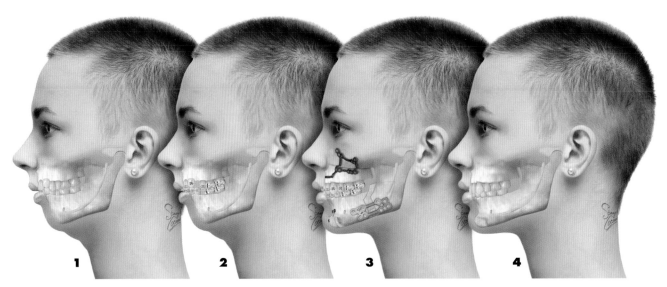

FIG 12-2 The classic camouflage orthodontics first and remedial BIMAX second sequence. *(1 and 2)* In this philosophy, impacted canines or severe orthodontic Class I dental crowding implies a condition that is entirely dental. Premolar extractions and eventual removal of the impacted third molars create room for the remaining teeth to decrowd and become dentally aligned using classical orthodontics, in a process called *camouflage orthodontics*. *(3 and 4)* The resultant orthodontic outcome of a "straight bite" with a greatly reduced dental mass is then advanced in a remedial BIMAX procedure using custom-engineered titanium plating systems to open the airway and restore the patient's profile. The final result provides a "normal" facial profile but at the expense of having undertaken some years of adolescent and then repeat adult orthodontics, the loss of about 30% of the normal dental mass, and at least four formal jaw surgery operations (including previous tooth extractions and separate third molar removal).

What makes remedial BIMAX surgery particularly difficult on a psychologic level is that it involves a person's face—a person's outward identity. Seeing me about a face is not like coming to me about your kidney or your lung or your throat or your toe. Our faces are not some abstract, unknown part of us. They are private and personal yet public and scrutinized by anyone we meet. So if I say I can fix it, it implies that it is already broken. And to have a broken face is usually internalized as having an ugly face.

There is an almost infinite complexity to the face. It changes every day, year to year, decade to decade. Our face holds an objective functionality and yet an indecipherable beauty. It expresses our emotions and inner thoughts. And when it is broken, or imperfect, or imbalanced, we can only stare at ourselves in the mirror and imagine the differences and myriad convoluted potential journeys to an indescribable personalized ideal.

But no one gets referred for remedial BIMAX surgery for esthetic reasons. Jaw correction surgeons are not cosmetic surgeons. We are fundamentally functional. Having said that, it is not ethical to offer remedial BIMAX surgery without also maximizing every opportunity that this surgery provides. After all, most patients seeking remedial BIMAX for orthodontics have already had braces, and sometimes they are in their second or third round. By the time a referral is made, it is usually by a general dentist who has listened to

the patient, and both are deeply frustrated with the years of failed orthodontic treatment. Any conversation about surgical bite correction with an adult who has been subjected to years of appliances and social embarrassment will therefore involve esthetic demands as well, because adult patients want a perfect smile. They don't want gumminess. They want a level and central and symmetrically wide smile, with white teeth that meet, function, and chew normally. They want full lips, a normal chin, and a balanced nose.

But they also want to breathe better, and remedial BIMAX surgery is an acknowledged and scientifically proven, curative therapy for OSA. So if I want to achieve levelness and yaw correction, maximize symmetry and smile esthetics, and open the airway, I need to see all parts of the face—not just teeth, occlusion, and facial bones but the airways and mucosa, muscles, and neck and facial tissues—frontally and upside down and inside out.

CAMOUFLAGE ORTHODONTICS

A child with dental crowding or a dental overbite will normally be taken by their parent to see a family dentist, who will usually refer that child to an orthodontist for correction. From the start, the idea of dental crowding or a dental overbite or a dental malocclusion defines the

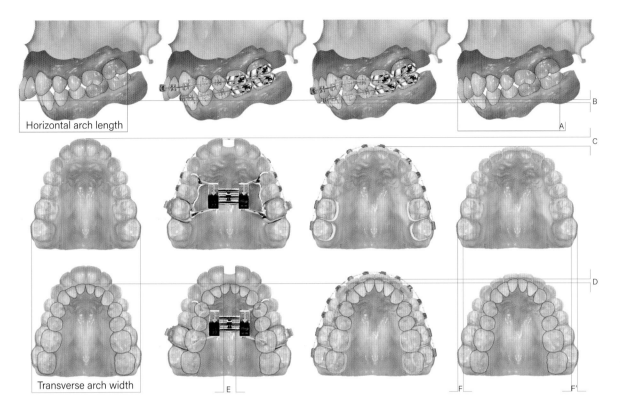

Horizontal arch length

Transverse arch width

A - Reduction in horizontal arch length
B - Increase in vertical incisal height
C - Retraction of maxillary incisal edge backward
D - Proclination of mandibular incisal edge forward
E - Expansion of midline suture
F + F' - Combined increase in transverse arch width. Should equal E.

FIG 12-3 Camouflage orthodontics: The nonextraction method of treating prominent anterior teeth. To avoid premolar extractions, the orthodontist relies on maxillary arch widening using either a removable splint (see Fig 12-4) or a fixed HYRAX orthodontic device. By also using a fixed orthodontic wire, expansion of the posterior dental arch enables the maxillary anterior teeth to be pulled backward and downward. The mandibular anterior teeth are also orthodontically proclined forward to reduce the dental overjet. The overall effect is to convert a Class II to a Class I occlusion, but at a significant negative effect to facial balance and lip competence.

child's dental condition as a dental problem of too many teeth. The logic says that it has an obvious dental origin and that ultimately everything from assessment to solution is to be provided by a dentist (or specialized dentist, the orthodontist). But the pure idea of describing malocclusion as a dental condition is only one end of a spectrum of philosophies. At the other end lies the medical concept of the primacy of small jaws and the phylogenetics of small tongues and small airways and small lower faces, all of which give rise to bad bites and crooked and impacted teeth.

If the "purely dental" child is seen to simply have prominent anterior teeth or crooked teeth or teeth that are too big, then the underlying small jaw is entirely ignored, and any subsequent orthodontics will only camouflage this underlying condition. In referring to this dental basis of assessment and care, corrective jaw surgeons use the term *camouflage orthodontics*. Camouflage orthodontics is very effective at making the upper jaw smaller to match it to the existing or anticipated size of the already small lower jaw (Figs 12-3 to 12-9).

Let me be clear that this book is not a critique of the classical dental methodology of orthodontics. I am the first to admit that orthodontists are very very good at straightening teeth. But when orthodontic treatment is used to camouflage an underlying and more fundamental anatomical

FIG 12-4 Full sequence showing how the gummy smile results from camouflage nonextraction orthodontic treatment of orthodontic Class II, division 1 malocclusion (orthognathic Class B) using a combination of jaw splints and subsequent fixed orthodontics. *(1)* Appearance of Class II, division 1 malocclusion featuring a long dental overjet and deep incisor overbite. *(2)* Splint therapy is engaged to both widen the maxilla and open the bite, reducing the dental overbite and training the child to hold the mandible forward ("posture training"), which reduces dental overjet. *(3–6)* Preferential splint height reduction allows the molars to overerupt, thus leveling the posterior bite and facilitating a transition to full fixed orthodontic appliances. *(7–9)* A combination of growth restriction on maxillary jaw development introduced by constant appliance wear, chronic forward jaw posture training, and use of Class II elastics eventually reduces the incisor overjet but at the expense of both retracting and pulling down the maxillary anterior teeth. The overall effect increases vertical maxillary height (the "gummy smile"), increases lower facial height, and produces extreme lip incompetence and chronic and abnormal forward jaw positioning.

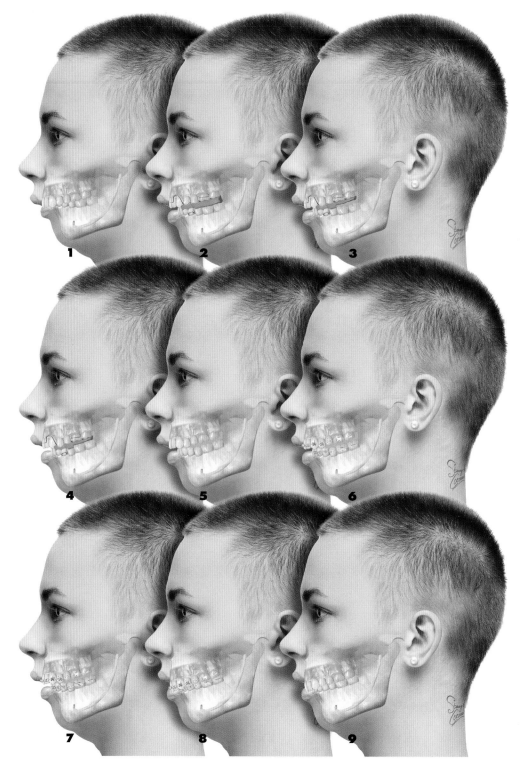

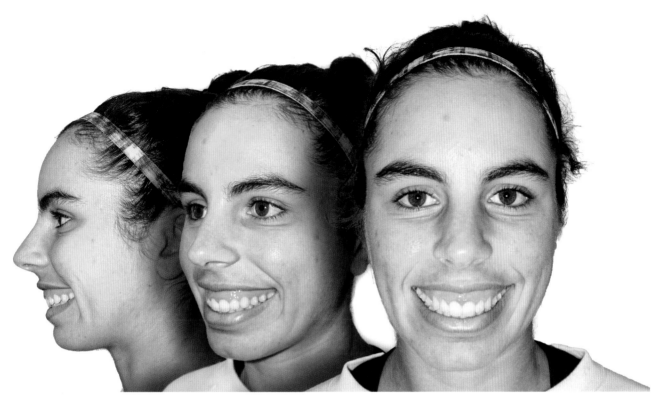

FIG 12-5 This 19-year-old patient underwent a course of camouflage orthodontics in adolescence involving maxillary jaw expansion and 4 years of nonextraction orthodontics to reduce her original prominent dental incisor overjet. While her Class II, division 1 malocclusion was successfully converted into a Class I state, her third molars are impacted, she holds her jaw forward, she snores at night, and she has chronic open mouth breathing due to lip incompetence. Therefore, she independently sought remedial BIMAX surgery to reverse the effects of her clockwise orthodontic camouflage treatment as well as to increase her mandibular length and reduce her vertical facial height. Clockwise orthodontic camouflage, particularly when not associated with premolar extractions, typically generates a greatly increased lower vertical facial length, prominent gummy smile (now called *vertical maxillary excess*), and general lip incompetence. Here the patient is smiling not because she is happy, but because I asked her to in order to show her gummy smile and the steepness of her bite. She is currently undergoing mild presurgical Invisalign therapy, which will continue once remedial BIMAX surgery is completed.

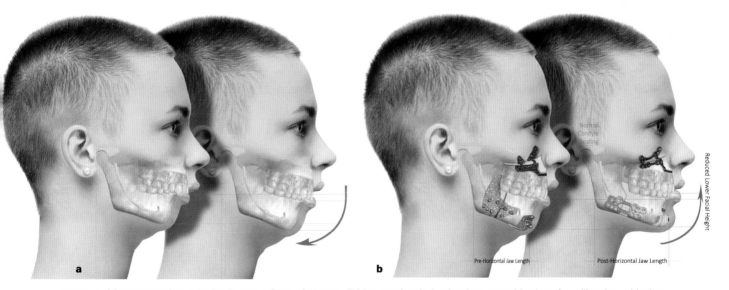

FIG 12-6 *(a)* Nonextraction orthodontic camouflage of Class II, division 1 malocclusion involves a combination of maxillary jaw widening and clockwise rotation of the dentoalveolus. Facing east, this lengthens the face, rotates the jaws downward (clockwise), and produces a gummy smile and lip incompetence. *(b)* The classic remedial BIMAX is an opposite, counterclockwise rotation of the jaws to normally seat the condyles, reducing vertical facial height and providing lip competence while also increasing horizontal jaw length. There is a physical limit to the amount the mandible can be advanced and the distance of the "gap" that can be held by a plate, which is about 10 mm. Using digital design and understanding custom titanium is the key to predictable corrective jaw surgery. The bigger the bilateral sagittal split osteotomy (BSSO) distance, the bigger the plate, the more unstable the pull-back forces, and the greater the chance of postoperative infection and poor healing.

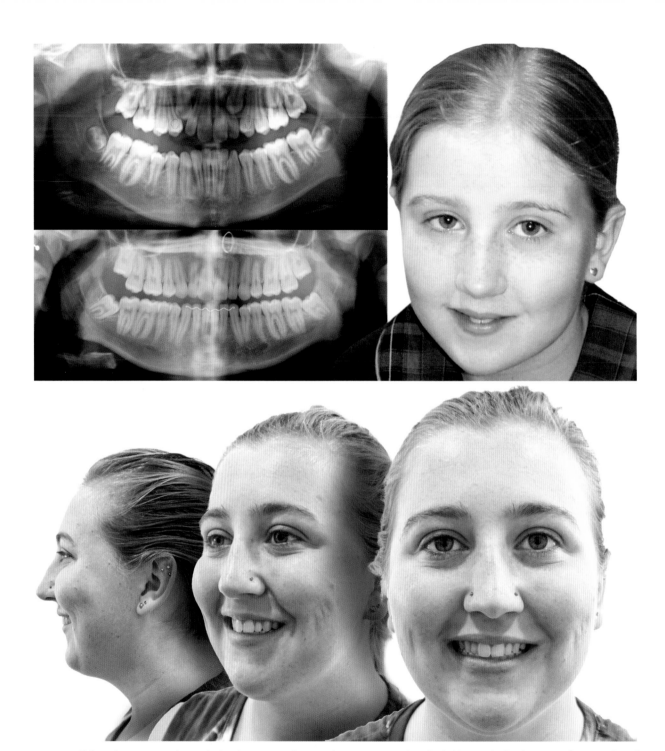

FIG 12-7 This patient was seen by me in October 2005 at the age of 12 years, 6 months. She held an orthodontic request for extraction of the maxillary first premolars, after which she had a course of camouflage orthodontics to relieve her impacted canines (see Fig 12-8). She was classified as orthodontic Class I crowding—but is better described as orthognathic Class D. When she was 20, she again held a request form for extraction of four third molars. At 27 years old, she returned again, this time asking me to perform a remedial BIMAX to fix her snoring and clinically confirmed OSA. She also asked why she needed six teeth extracted, her tonsils removed, and 3 years of adolescent orthodontics all to avoid this surgery she now needed anyway. Retrospectively, the orthodontist, surgeon, parent, and now adult patient were all upset at the series of opportunities lost to us. The IMDO protocol would have been an ideal treatment for her at age 12 years, but in October 2005 it was yet to be developed.

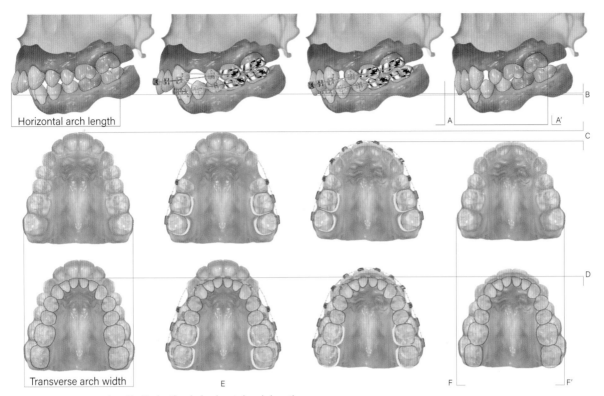

A + A' - Reduction in horizontal arch length
B - Increase in vertical incisal height
C - Retraction of maxillary incisal edge backward
D - Proclincation of mandibular incisal edge forward
E - Expansion of midline suture
F + F' - No increase in transverse arch width. Should be the same as pretreatment state.

FIG 12-8 Camouflage orthodontics with maxillary premolar extractions for treatment of prominent or crowded anterior teeth, like the patient in Fig 12-7 underwent. The extraction of maxillary premolars has a long tradition in orthodontics and is a simple and community-accepted treatment sequence. Extracting "excessive" teeth to cosmetically reduce the prominence of crowded anterior teeth appears to be benign, cheap, nonsurgical, and inconsequential for a child. But the overall facial cosmetic effect, especially of a collapsed upper lip and narrow smile, can be devastating for the adult. This methodology of treatment severely reduces dental mass and does not result in any potential to gain a natural or normal occlusion.

condition, the subsequent surgical treatment of that condition becomes more and more difficult. Because patients are knocking on orthodontists' doors and not surgeons' doors, it is clear that parents are looking to avoid surgery in favor of orthodontics. However, considering the future adult that the child patient will eventually become means that the mature clinician should offer a mature consideration of the primacy and reality of corrective jaw surgery from the start.

After all, the vast majority of my patients presenting for BIMAX surgery are remedial cases to address previous treatment failures with camouflage orthodontics.

Over the course of my career, I've noticed three major complaint sets among my patients presenting for remedial BIMAX. The first major complaint set involves primary symptomatic issues of jaw joint pain or joint dysfunction (Fig 12-10), or more widely of face or jaw or

After all, the vast majority of my patients presenting for BIMAX surgery are remedial cases to address previous treatment failures with camouflage orthodontics.

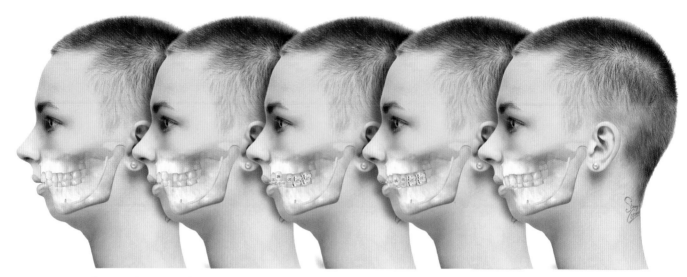

FIG 12-9A The normal sequence of extraction-based camouflage orthodontics used to treat severe dental crowding. This model of orthodontic care requires premolar extractions first and often eventual removal of the impacted third molars later. Losing a total of eight teeth out of a full complement of 32 represents a dental mass reduction of approximately 35%. This style of orthodontics preserves temporomandibular joint (TMJ) position and long-term jaw joint health but results in maintenance of the original small jaw (AMHypo) and the cosmetic sense of dewlap, a collapsed upper lip, and prominence of the nose. There is also persistence of the future risk of OSA development from the original glossoptotic condition. The final profile with the sense of a small jaw and narrow, collapsed smile is an enormous driver for an adult to later seek facial cosmetic change.

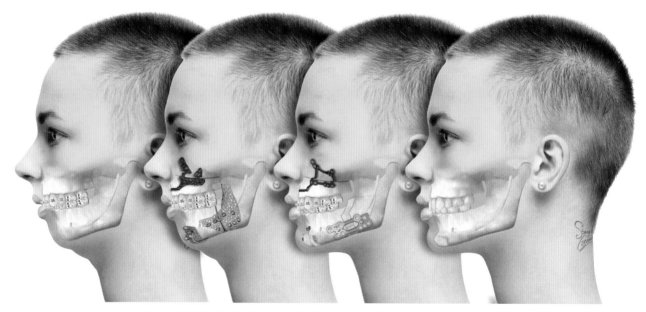

FIG 12-9B The sequence of remedial BIMAX following extraction-based camouflage orthodontics involves custom design and custom titanium and often repeat full fixed orthodontic appliances. To the orthodontist, the aim is to preserve or gain a Class I occlusion. To the patient, the aim is to correct the facial proportional imbalance and to relieve snoring or CPAP dependency. The surgeon's primary aims are entirely for medical therapeutic reasons and are defined by the medical remediation of the original AMHypo and associated glossoptosis. Preserving or improving the orthodontically acquired occlusion, or creating a normalized facial proportionality, are secondary aims but obviously no less important. Nothing, however, exists to enable replacement of missing teeth, to reverse secondary camouflage cosmetic procedures, to overcome any long-term issues impacting TMJ health, or to reverse the systemic medical secondary effects of established OSA.

general headache. These patients commonly complain of grinding their teeth while asleep, and their teeth often have objective signs of excessive wear. They have joint issues such as click, or crepitation, or lack of normal gliding motion. They have features of muscle tenderness, or what we call "tension" headache, or earache or just general "ache." They progress to many dental appointments, usually involving many dental experts

FIG 12-10 The forward jaw joint displacement associated with chronic forward jaw posture training is therapeutically represented as "unlocking the trapped condyle" and is well known to be associated with "condylar remodeling". Such chronic jaw posturing completely reverses every night when the individual enters nontone (or deep) sleep, when the jaw simply falls backward to allow for open mouth breathing. To remain in toned light sleep (and therefore with the jaw postured forward) relieves any associated nocturnal glossoptosis but is often associated with complaints of grinding or clenching behavior, general muscle ache or cranial "tension," or jaw joint symptoms such as clicking and ache. These features of chronic jaw posturing, associated joint remodeling and symptoms, and nighttime clenching and grinding habits complicate subsequent remedial BIMAX surgery.

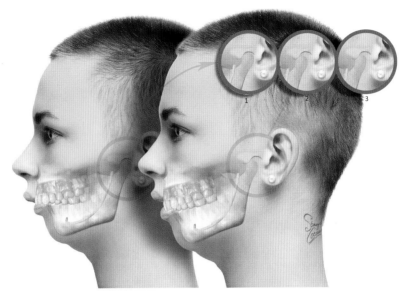

FIG 12-11 At first sight, there is little obvious connection that links the adolescent experience of extraction-based orthodontics and adult use of therapeutic jaw advancement splints for relief of snoring. Jaw advancement splints are an effective therapy to help enable sleep. By pulling the mandible forward using a splint that is locked to the maxilla, the tongue is also pulled forward. These appliances have significant negative consequences on long-term jaw joint health and can also permanently alter the occlusion. Splints are not recommended preceding BIMAX surgery due to these TMJ- and occlusion-altering effects.

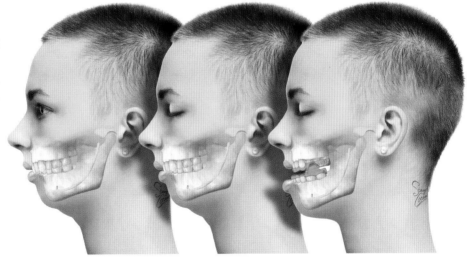

and dental bite splints (Fig 12-11), maybe the removal of redundant or impacted third molars, and maybe also repeat orthodontics.

In a secondary complaint set, adults at different ages and at different stages of life and wellness are experiencing the previously unknown airway consequences that come from having small jaws (see Fig 12-7). The dominance of OSA becomes more prominent in later age groups but is usually predated by ever-worsening snoring or a decreased tolerance for aerobic exercise. These postorthodontic camouflage adult patients visit the dentist and start wearing snoring splints (Fig 12-12), which are not unlike the bite splints used

for TMJ problems, except now these splints can worsen TMJ health. Or they visit the physician and start using a CPAP.

A third complaint set relates to esthetics—diminutive jawline, neck lines, big noses, thin lips, and the general loss of the thin veneer of youth. These problems, society tells us, are easily solved with cosmetic procedures.

While the scientific evidence abundantly shows that adolescent orthodontics does not *cause* any of these complaint sets, it certainly does not prevent them either. All these things—camouflage orthodontics, removing impacted third molars or extracting crowded ones, tonsillectomy, nasal reduction surgery, jaw splints, CPAPs—they are all Band-Aids on bullet holes. The small jaw is still there.

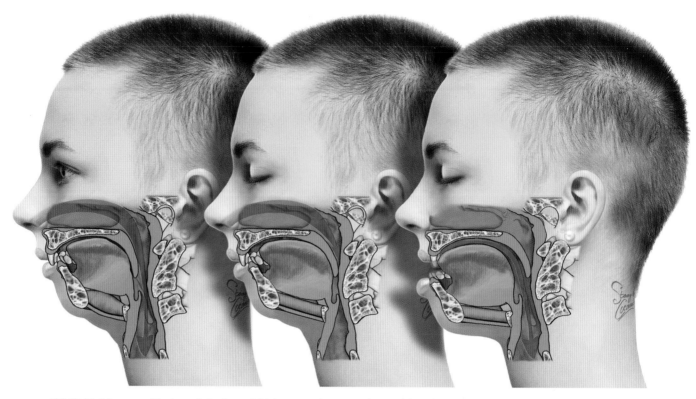

FIG 12-12 A jaw-repositioning splint relieves OSA by converting an awake nasal-based breathing state to a supine, asleep, open mouth, forward jaw position breathing state. The therapeutic retroglossal effect of the jaw splint (also called a *mandibular advancement device*) is to bring the relaxed tongue mass forward and to splint the airway open during sleep. The anatomical basis for tongue collapse is dependent only upon the degree of contraction or stretch of the geniohyoid muscle needed to open or close the collapsed airway. As sleep transitions from light to deep, general muscle tone relaxes. This means that the tongue also relaxes and thus collapses the airway.

The only thing in this context that can fix the real problem in the end is surgical correction—through BIMAX surgery.

THE BIMAX OPERATION

BIMAX involves a LeFort 1, a bilateral sagittal split osteotomy (BSSO), and a modified genioplasty called Genio-Paully. Sometimes the LeFort 1 is combined with subtle expansion (called SARME [surgically assisted rapid maxillary expansion]), and occasionally the mandible also needs to be divided in order to create width and symmetry and levelness to the actual bite planes. Orthodontics in the form of classical brackets and wires or Invisalign then follow to perfect the bite. Orthodontics certainly does not need to be in place for surgery.

If the remedial BIMAX is planned properly and executed precisely using custom titanium technology, we tick three major boxes:

1. A symmetric, wide, and Class I occlusion that is amenable to postsurgical orthodontic settling through ongoing (or new) orthodontics and with symmetric and balanced TMJ seating
2. A maximally advanced chin point in order to maximize geniohyoid pull and thus maximally tent the retroglossal airway, simultaneously maintaining or enhancing the nasal airway and bilateral nasal patency
3. Proportional and symmetric facial balance matched to the femininity or masculinity and smile of the patient, without gumminess

Figures 12-13 to 12-19 give examples of the surgical planning and execution of remedial BIMAX in seven different patients with various presenting conditions, all of whom previously underwent camouflage orthodontics in adolescence.

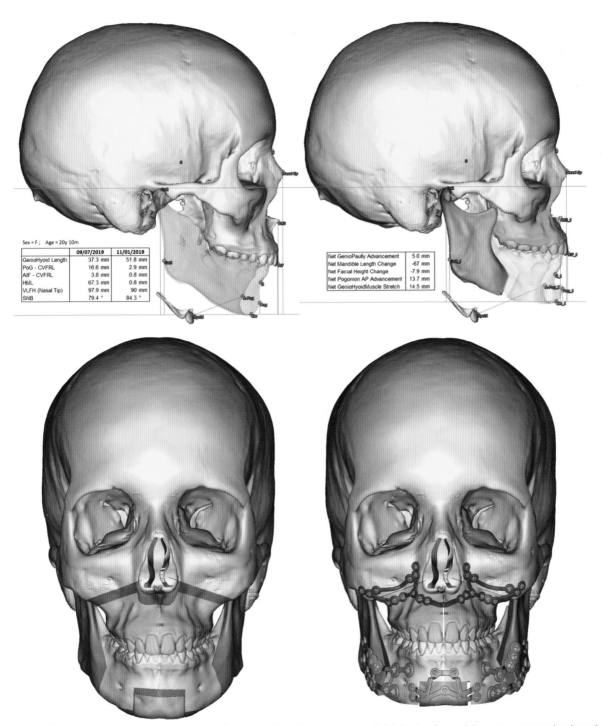

Sex = F ; Age = 20y 10m		
	09/07/2019	11/01/2019
GenioHyoid Length	37.3 mm	51.8 mm
PoG - CVFRL	16.6 mm	2.9 mm
AIF - CVFRL	3.8 mm	0.8 mm
HML	67.3 mm	0.8 mm
VLFH (Nasal Tip)	97.9 mm	90 mm
SNB	79.4 °	84.3 °

Net GenioPaully Advancement	5.0 mm
Net Mandible Length Change	-67 mm
Net Facial Height Change	-7.9 mm
Net Pogonion AP Advancement	13.7 mm
Net GenioHyoidMuscle Stretch	14.5 mm

FIG 12-13 This 20-year-old patient presented wanting a reduction of her "gummy smile" following from adolescent nonextraction-based camouflage orthodontics. She still has a significant dental overjet remaining and wears an occlusal splint to help relieve her from nighttime grinding. Counterclockwise advancement BIMAX (11-piece) allows for the creation of a wider, level smile without rolling of the maxillary occlusion. The GenioPaully in combination with a maxillary impaction (shown in red) reduces facial height by 8 mm and restores natural lip competence. Overall mandible length increases by 13.7 mm (20%) for a net therapeutic geniohyoid stretch of 39%. Pre- and postsurgical orthodontics surrounding surgery is with Invisalign only via a general dentist followed by cosmetic incisal veneers using Digital Smile Design technology. For this patient, the primary driver for therapy was for the functional therapeutic effect that comes with formal surgical care. Success is thus primarily measured in the subjective relief of snoring, improved sleep, and improvement in daytime alertness, cognition, and general happiness. Her before and after photographs are shown in Fig 3-12.

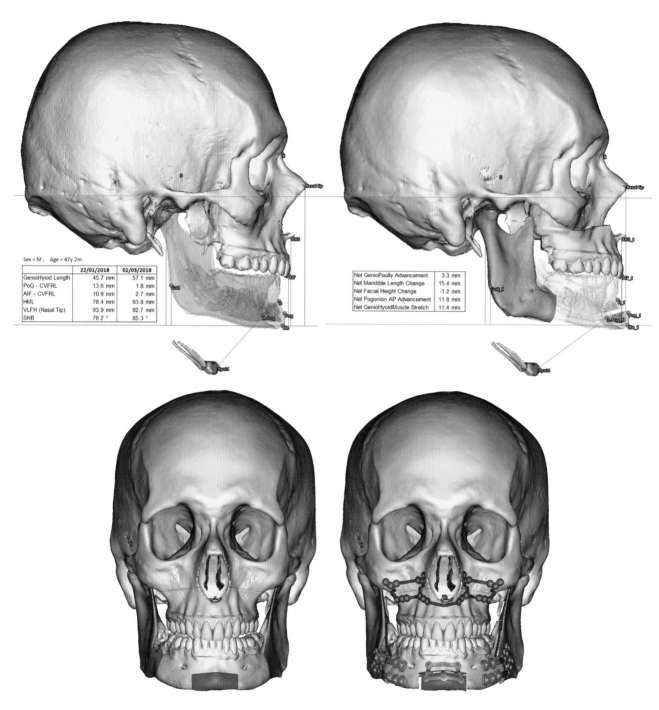

	22/01/2018	02/03/2018
GenioHyoid Length	45.7 mm	57.1 mm
PoG - CVFRL	13.6 mm	1.8 mm
AIF - CVFRL	10.9 mm	2.7 mm
HML	78.4 mm	93.8 mm
VLFH (Nasal Tip)	93.9 mm	92.7 mm
SNB	78.2 °	85.3 °

Sex = M ;   Age = 47y 2m

Net GenioPaully Advancement	3.3 mm
Net Mandible Length Change	15.4 mm
Net Facial Height Change	-1.2 mm
Net Pogonion AP Advancement	11.8 mm
Net GenioHyoidMuscle Stretch	11.4 mm

FIG 12-14 This patient is a 48-year-old craniofacial surgeon with primary OSA. He is intolerant of CPAP or mandibular advancement splint therapy. He had nonextraction camouflage orthodontics as an adolescent with mild maxillary arch widening and maxillary incisor retroclination to reduce his initial dental incisor prominence. A simple BIMAX counterclockwise advancement maximizes the geniohyoid stretch to fully reverse his apnea-hypopnea index score from about 6 to 0. To correct his latent mandible asymmetry, BSSO extension was at the maximum limit for extension at 13 mm (on the left side), while maintaining a sliver of medial vertical ramus bone contact for healing. Widening of the jaw across the vertical rami is possible by small rotation movements of the condylar heads. After surgery, Invisalign is used to further procline the maxillary anterior teeth toward the esthetic vertical line limit, thus reversing his adolescent camouflage orthodontics. This case shows that surgeons can also suffer the same conditions as their patients.

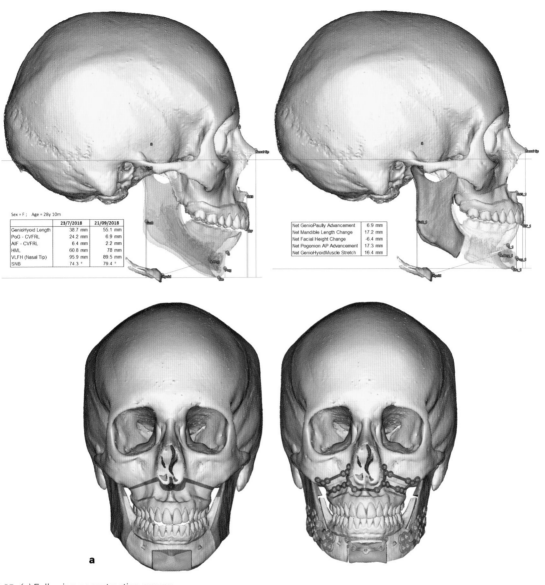

	23/7/2018	21/09/2018
GenioHyoid Length	38.7 mm	55.1 mm
PoG - CVFRL	24.2 mm	6.9 mm
AIF - CVFRL	6.4 mm	2.2 mm
HML	60.8 mm	78 mm
VLFH (Nasal Tip)	95.9 mm	89.5 mm
SNB	74.3 °	79.4 °

Sex = F ;   Age = 28y 10m

Net GenioPaully Advancement	6.9 mm
Net Mandible Length Change	17.2 mm
Net Facial Height Change	-6.4 mm
Net Pogonion AP Advancement	17.3 mm
Net GenioHyoidMuscle Stretch	16.4 mm

a

FIG 12-15 *(a)* Following nonextraction camouflage orthodontics in her teens, this patient is now 27 years old and chronically postures her mandible forward to achieve occlusal interdigitation, and she has condylar remodeling from this, which medically is better described as early osteoarthritis. With forward jaw posturing, she appears as a "perfect" Class I occlusion. Lying supine, her jaw position relaxes backward, leading to an anterior open bite, posterior molar prematurity, and a significant dental overjet. She wakes each morning with chronic jaw ache and daytime tiredness, and her partner says she snores. Her remedial BIMAX is a counterclockwise rotation, with vertical maxillary impaction (represented in red) to reduce her gummy smile. Note that vertical maxillary impaction requires formal imaging of the nasal mucosa. GenioPaully improves lip competence as well as further stretching of the geniohyoid. Overall mandible length has increased by 17.2 mm (28%), and the geniohyoid length has increased by 42% to eliminate snoring completely. *(b)* Facial views before and after BIMAX.

b

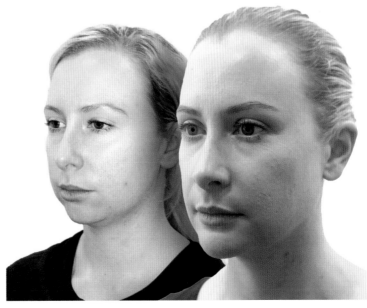

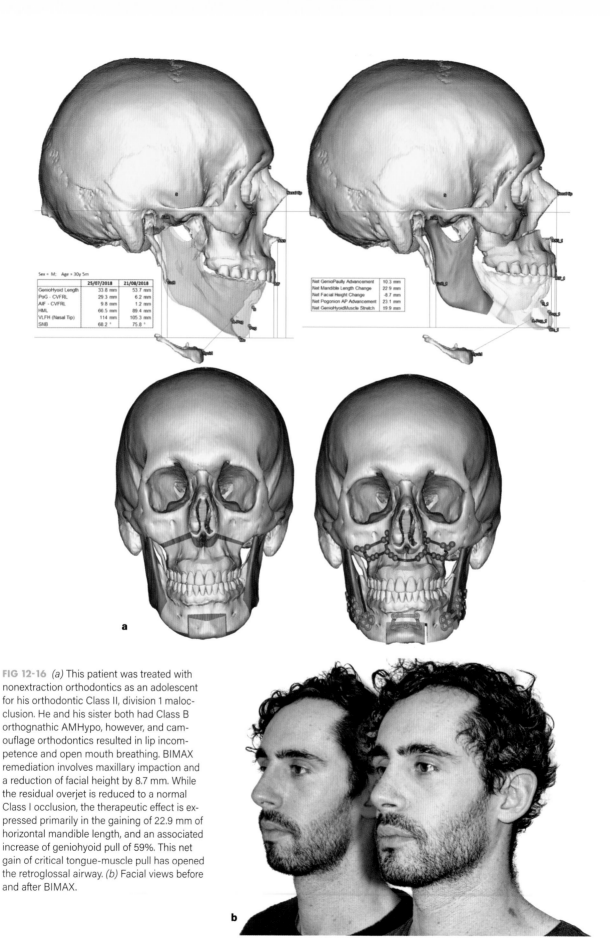

Sex = M; Age = 30y 5m		
	25/07/2018	21/08/2018
GenioHyoid Length	33.8 mm	53.7 mm
PoG - CVFRL	29.3 mm	6.2 mm
AIF - CVFRL	9.8 mm	1.2 mm
HML	66.5 mm	89.4 mm
VLFH (Nasal Tip)	114 mm	105.3 mm
SNB	68.2 °	75.8 °

Net GenioPaully Advancement	10.3 mm
Net Mandible Length Change	22.9 mm
Net Facial Height Change	-8.7 mm
Net Pogonion AP Advancement	23.1 mm
Net GenioHyoidMuscle Stretch	19.9 mm

FIG 12-16 *(a)* This patient was treated with nonextraction orthodontics as an adolescent for his orthodontic Class II, division 1 malocclusion. He and his sister both had Class B orthognathic AMHypo, however, and camouflage orthodontics resulted in lip incompetence and open mouth breathing. BIMAX remediation involves maxillary impaction and a reduction of facial height by 8.7 mm. While the residual overjet is reduced to a normal Class I occlusion, the therapeutic effect is expressed primarily in the gaining of 22.9 mm of horizontal mandible length, and an associated increase of geniohyoid pull of 59%. This net gain of critical tongue-muscle pull has opened the retroglossal airway. *(b)* Facial views before and after BIMAX.

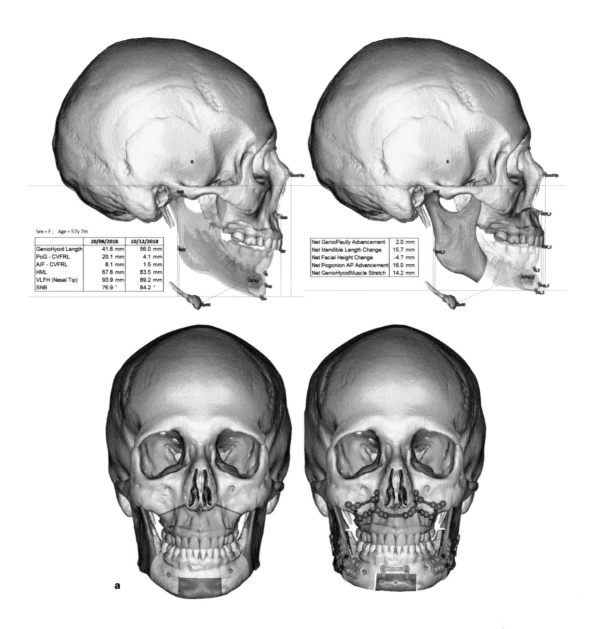

Sex = F ; Age = 57y 7m		
	20/08/2018	10/12/2018
GenioHyoid Length	41.8 mm	56.0 mm
PoG - CVFRL	20.1 mm	4.1 mm
AIF - CVFRL	8.1 mm	1.5 mm
HML	67.8 mm	83.5 mm
VLFH (Nasal Tip)	93.9 mm	89.2 mm
SNB	76.9 °	84.2 °

Net GenioPaully Advancement	2.0 mm
Net Mandible Length Change	15.7 mm
Net Facial Height Change	-4.7 mm
Net Pogonion AP Advancement	16.0 mm
Net GenioHyoidMuscle Stretch	14.2 mm

a

FIG 12-17 *(a)* At 56 years old, this patient requires an 11-piece remedial BIMAX of her 24-tooth occlusion (premolars and third molars were removed during adolescence alongside camouflage orthodontics). Finding a neutrally passive, bilateral jaw joint position leaves her with an anterior open bite, molar premature contacts, and significant dental overjet. Counterclockwise rotation increases mandible length by 16.7 mm (25%) and increases the geniohyoid length by 34%, therapeutically eliminating her CPAP dependence and curing her of OSA. Achieving a perfectly level maxillary dental arch, with slight posterior widening, can only be achieved by "dividing" the maxilla jaw into two halves. The maxillary custom plate then acts as a precise 3D torque and repositioning device, which is only possible through this bespoke digital custom design process. *(b)* Facial views before and after BIMAX.

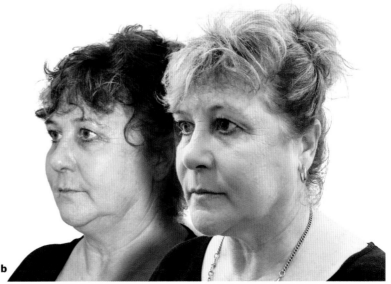

b

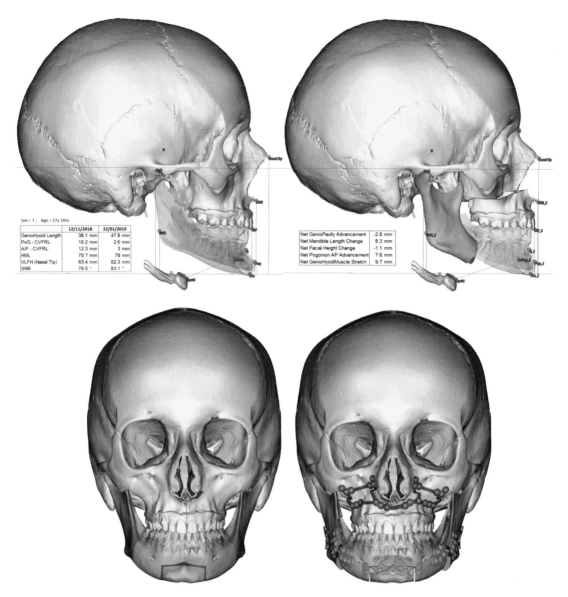

	12/11/2018	22/01/2019
GenioHyoid Length	38.1 mm	47.8 mm
PoG - CVFRL	10.2 mm	2.6 mm
AIF - CVFRL	12.3 mm	3 mm
HML	70.7 mm	79 mm
VLFH (Nasal Tip)	83.4 mm	82.3 mm
SNB	76.5 °	83.1 °

Sex = F ; Age = 27y 10m

Net GenioPaully Advancement	-2.8 mm
Net Mandible Length Change	8.3 mm
Net Facial Height Change	-1.1 mm
Net Pogonion AP Advancement	7.6 mm
Net GenioHyoidMuscle Stretch	9.7 mm

FIG 12-18 This patient, shown in Fig 12-1, already had orthodontic retroclination of the mandibular anterior teeth for Class III malocclusion, which pushed the mandibular anterior roots outside the surrounding alveolar bone. The remedial seven-piece advancement BIMAX includes a rare GenioPaully set back to femininely soften the sense of a strong chin. The geniohyoid is still stretched a therapeutic 25% distance. The etiologic basis for almost the entirety of Class III malocclusion is a small mandible, not a large one (orthognathic Class F AMHypo). The sense of a strong chin is from a relatively smaller maxilla, which is pneumatically small from chronic open mouth breathing (due to the small genetic mandible or AMHypo).

A BETTER WAY

Remedial BIMAX follows on and remediates the clinical failures of the past, but orthognathic surgery was never meant to be a back-door fix to the failure of classical orthodontics or cosmetic surgery or CPAP therapy. Corrective jaw surgery is meant to be *first*. By correcting the actual problem, the potential and actual symptoms of that problem will disappear entirely. It is common and easy for orthodontists, ENT surgeons, and cosmetic surgeons to demonize corrective jaw surgery as too invasive or too extreme—instead offering patients "easier" procedures that are easy to access and simple to perform but really only act as semipermanent makeup. All the while the real culprit behind all the artificially separated problems—the small mandible—is still there. Comprehensive digital

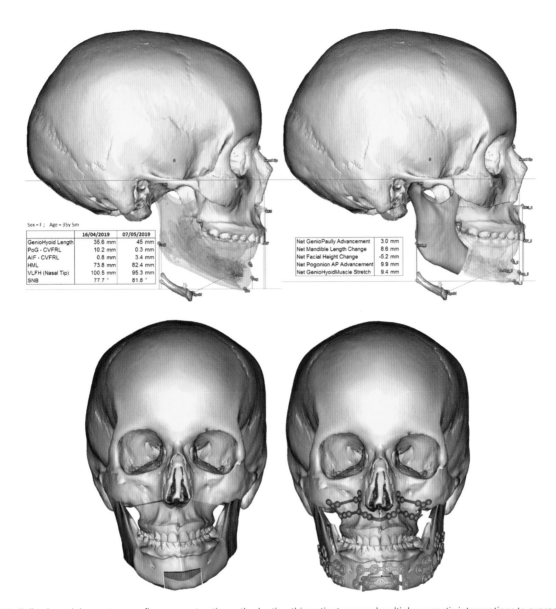

Sex = F ; Age = 35y 5m		
	16/04/2019	07/05/2019
GenioHyoid Length	35.6 mm	45 mm
PoG - CVFRL	10.2 mm	0.3 mm
AIF - CVFRL	0.8 mm	3.4 mm
HML	73.8 mm	82.4 mm
VLFH (Nasal Tip)	100.5 mm	95.3 mm
SNB	77.7 °	81.8 °

Net GenioPaully Advancement	3.0 mm
Net Mandible Length Change	8.6 mm
Net Facial Height Change	-5.2 mm
Net Pogonion AP Advancement	9.9 mm
Net GenioHyoidMuscle Stretch	9.4 mm

FIG 12-19 Following adolescent camouflage nonextraction orthodontics, this patient pursued multiple cosmetic interventions to overcome the facial cosmetic effects of camouflage orthodontics and the original asymmetric AMHypo (aggravated by mild hemifacial microsomia). These secondary surgical interactions included cosmetic nasal hump reduction, silicone cheek implants, and permanent subdermal fillers, all of which complicate remedial BIMAX correction in treating her for CPAP dependency. Overall, advancing past the vertical esthetic line (where the nasal bone tip has been surgically reduced by prior cosmetic rhinoplasty) risks creation of a saddle deformity to the nasal bridge. Therapeutic geniohyoid stretch is seen as increased from 35.6 to 45 mm (only a 26% change), which may be subtherapeutic and fall short of the minimum distensible need required to overcome OSA. The osteotomization needed to level the bite relative to the eyeline and to coordinate anterior and posterior symmetrification and centralization of the face and occlusion involves 13 different segments, 4 custom guides, 4 custom plates, and 57 screws. All orthodontics is coordinated through Invisalign technology, without intermaxillary fixation or splints, and the orthodontic practitioner is a general dentist accredited for this purpose.

orthognathic surgery that complements adult (or adolescent) orthodontics or cosmetic surgery should instead *start* with the corrective jaw surgeon. Through IMDO, the corrective jaw surgeon can eliminate the gun, saving the patient a world of trouble in the future. The custom remedial BIMAX is the complex treatment that peels away all the Band-Aids after the genetic bullet was first fired.

Corrective jaw surgery is meant to be first.

13

THE SUPERBIMAX

THE FOURTH WAY

WHY DO WE FEAR CORRECTIVE JAW SURGERY?

A question I often ask myself is why parents and patients are okay with surgical removal of third molars but not okay with interventional jaw surgery to prevent third molar impaction in the first place. Is any jaw surgery operation really that different from another? Is the "invasiveness" of losing two or four or eight teeth during or after orthodontics any less or more invasive than the invasiveness of corrective jaw surgery before, during, or after orthodontics?

It seems any patient or parent staring down a jaw surgery that can potentially be avoided by an alternative "conservative treatment" will naturally choose conservatism. But is removing teeth more natural or easier or healthier than fixing the fundamental problem and keeping all the teeth through corrective jaw surgery?

CREATING THE NORMAL ADULT JAW

Some people simply have super small jaws. When we are faced with assessing just how far things need to come forward in these patients in order to normalize this smallness to match the dimensions and functional demands of the rest of the face and body, the question arises: Just how far away is normal? Once this question is answered and we see the distances and the volumes needed, we may be frightened because it's too hard, too far, too invasive—or just too much.

Intermolar mandibular distraction osteogenesis (IMDO) has a fantastic ability to create real volume in a jaw, but it

If we need a massive change in order to overcome snoring or to get to the maximum esthetic limit or the minimum distensible need, we may need distances that exceed the ability of any one operation.

was designed for adolescents and for people with jaws that are expected to "grow" more. That being said, IMDO can still be used in fully grown adults. However, we are limited by how far the IMDO distractors can work. They have a certain "maximum" distance, and at 14 mm in an adolescent, this might represent as much as a 25% increase in jaw length. But for an adult, the same 14 mm might only mean a 15% increase. For an adolescent who is still expected to grow after IMDO, 14 mm of advancement may be all that is needed to overcome snoring. But for a large adult male, 14 mm may still fall far short of our imaginary yet very real line.

Likewise, the bilateral sagittal split osteotomy (BSSO), even in combination with custom BIMAX, may not be enough to overcome the total distance needed to gain this "normal." If we need a massive change in order to overcome snoring or to get to the maximum esthetic limit or the minimum distensible need, we may need distances that exceed the ability of any one operation.

So what if we do both? Is it possible to perform IMDO and surgically assisted rapid maxillary expansion (SARME) first, then perform custom BIMAX later? By combining our operations, is it possible to obtain the distances and volumes we need to gain a perfect bite, decrowd the teeth,

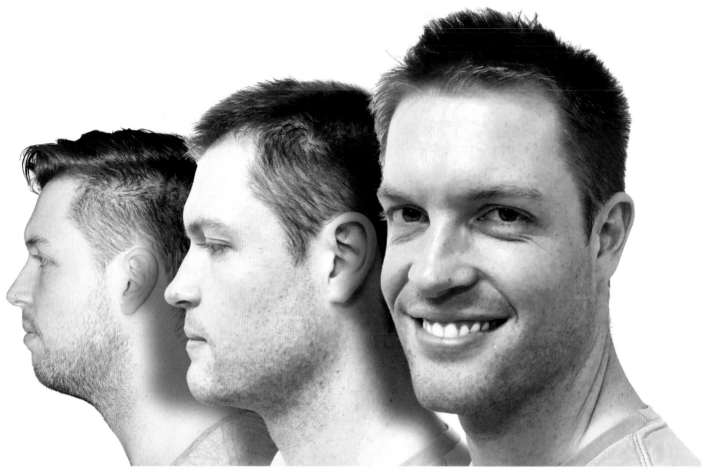

FIG 13-1 Profile views and smile view of a 24-year-old man before and after SuperBIMAX.

overcome snoring, and obtain the full esthetics of a normalized jaw size? The answer is yes, and that process is called the SuperBIMAX.

WHAT CAN THE SUPERBIMAX DO?

Figure 13-1 shows a 24-year-old man who presented with this detailed brief: "I snore. I want a wider smile. And, can you make my jaw as big as possible?" The only way to accomplish all this was to combine everything in my toolbox: IMDO, SARME, BIMAX, and GenioPaully. I needed it all—the SuperBIMAX. Treatment was completed over 24 months and involved four independent surgical procedures as well as cotreatment with Invisalign. By combining all four procedures, I was able to achieve a 27% increase in mandible length and 11% increase in mandible width (Fig 13-2).

The only way to accomplish all this was to combine everything in my toolbox: IMDO, SARME, BIMAX, and GenioPaully.

Figures 13-3 to 13-5 illustrate three more case examples in which SuperBIMAX was used to dramatically advance the jaws and overcome airway and esthetic problems. These cases show that pulling the mandible forward while advancing the maxilla can radically alter the facial profile (Fig 13-6). With the SuperBIMAX, care is taken to obtain maximum airway pull matched to idealizing the facial balance (Fig 13-7).

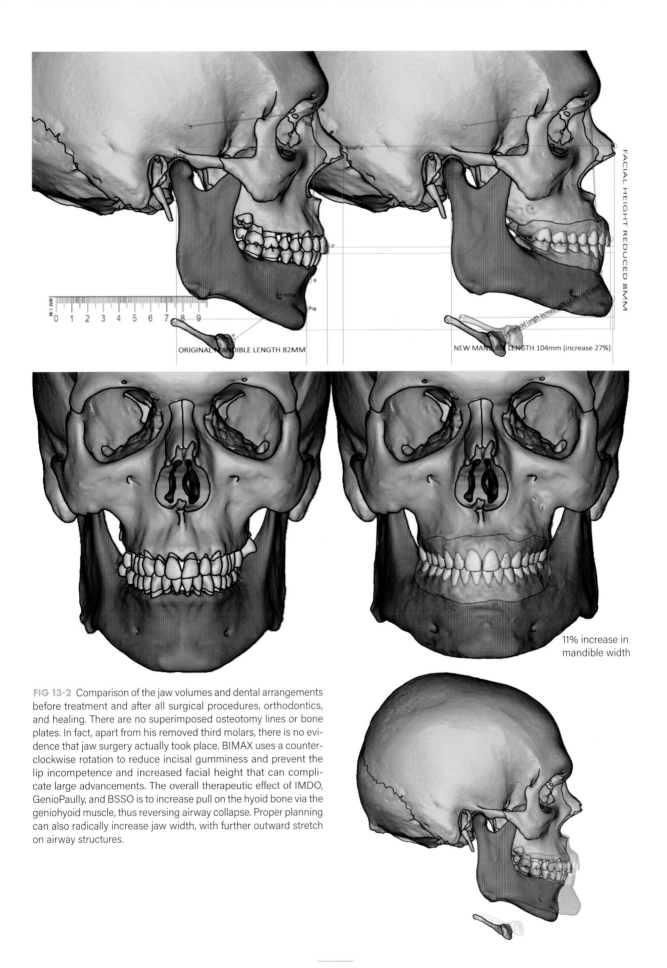

FIG 13-2 Comparison of the jaw volumes and dental arrangements before treatment and after all surgical procedures, orthodontics, and healing. There are no superimposed osteotomy lines or bone plates. In fact, apart from his removed third molars, there is no evidence that jaw surgery actually took place. BIMAX uses a counterclockwise rotation to reduce incisal gumminess and prevent the lip incompetence and increased facial height that can complicate large advancements. The overall therapeutic effect of IMDO, GenioPaully, and BSSO is to increase pull on the hyoid bone via the geniohyoid muscle, thus reversing airway collapse. Proper planning can also radically increase jaw width, with further outward stretch on airway structures.

11% increase in mandible width

ORIGINAL MANDIBLE LENGTH 82MM

NEW MANDIBLE LENGTH 104mm (increase 27%)

FACIAL HEIGHT REDUCED 8MM

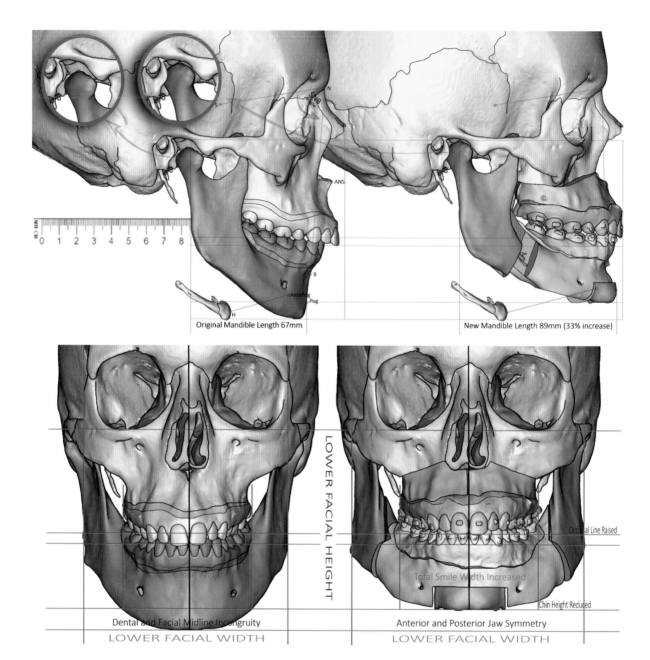

Original Mandible Length 67mm

New Mandible Length 89mm (33% increase)

LOWER FACIAL HEIGHT

Occlusal Line Raised

Total Smile Width Increased

Chin Height Reduced

Dental and Facial Midline Incongruity

Anterior and Posterior Jaw Symmetry

LOWER FACIAL WIDTH

LOWER FACIAL WIDTH

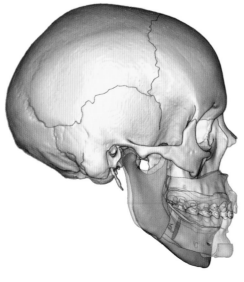

FIG 13-3 At age 14 years, this patient had had four premolars removed and her prominent maxillary anterior teeth orthodontically pulled backward. Such camouflage orthodontics produces a "clockwise" orthodontic movement, and for this patient in particular, it produced an exceptionally gummy smile and unnaturally lengthened her lower face. It also proclined the mandibular anterior teeth forward. Fast forward to age 29 years, and this patient now snored and slept with an open mouth, and her lips could not naturally meet. She chronically held her jaw and neck forward in order to breathe, which affected precise cephalometric comparisons. The adaptive postures also exacerbated her tension headaches, and she had jaw joint pain. When she first saw me, the plan was to perform a posterior SARME and widen the upper smile and nasal airway. Simultaneously, a 13-mm IMDO advancement would obtain an initial degree of mandible lengthening. Invisalign was used to align the dentition, and a final BIMAX with GenioPaully completed the picture. No single operation could achieve everything, but piecemeal and with planning, it was possible to eventually achieve everything—lip competence, a normal bite, a normal facial volume, and normal breathing—with each procedure performed as one small bunny hop in series. Retrospectively, the ideal treatment would have been for adolescent IMDO alone, which was not then available for this patient. At age 31 years, she finally achieved what she had wanted at age 7—a normal smile.

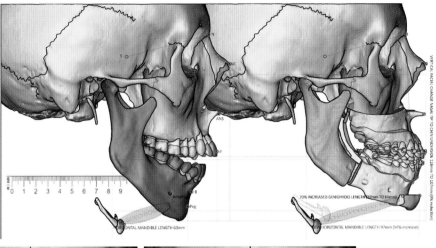

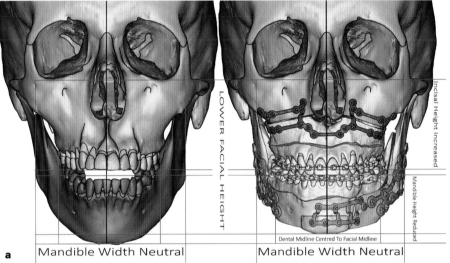

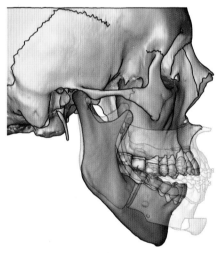

a

FIG 13-4 Anterior open bite is extremely difficult to treat with orthodontics alone. Surgically, the aim is to normalize the jaw volume, and that in itself is also difficult. Anterior open bite has a complex etiology. It is always dominated by an extreme form of the small mandible (usually caused by anterior mandibular hypoplasia [AMHypo]). The intrinsic glossoptosis leads to chronic open mouth breathing from birth. The child can spontaneously discover thumb sucking as a means for adaptive nasal breathing. As the child ages, the habit can be difficult to socially break and can also lead to dentoalveolar molding. As the permanent dentition develops, the posterior teeth often overerupt, aggravating the chronic "open bite" look. IMDO and SARME improve the dental arch space, allowing for orthodontic decrowding. Final BIMAX settles the bite, usually with a posterior LeFort impaction. In this patient's case, he was treated throughout adolescence with camouflage orthodontics to attempt to extrude the teeth into a functional bite and avoid surgery. Dental extrusion causes serious periodontal disease that would follow this patient throughout his life. It also leads to high rates of orthodontic "relapse," as the anterior open bite reverts to its original state. Later repeat orthodontics to help coordinate remedial SuperBIMAX takes care not to extrude the teeth any further and may involve intrusion mechanics with temporary anchorage devices. Getting to "the line" to overcome snoring and close the lips and bite and normalize the profile is challenging. As each successive surgical step occurs, skin and

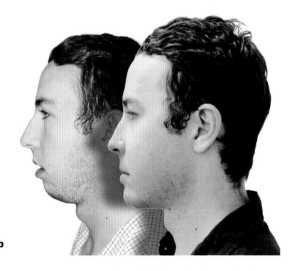

b

tongue muscles do not elastically stretch easily to help overcome the often severe glossoptosis. *(a)* Jaw volumes before and after SuperBIMAX surgical procedures. Note the astounding 54% increase in mandible length and 70% increase in geniohyoid stretch to permanently overcome snoring and reinstate natural nasal breathing. This is the most advancement I've ever achieved so far. *(b)* Facial profiles before and after surgery. Note the forward head posture and open mouth breathing in the before photograph. By contrast, in the after photograph the profile is straight, and the dewlap has been completely eliminated. More importantly, this patient will likely no longer face a lifetime of snoring, the effects of tooth and masticatory loss, or the once very real risk of developing obstructive sleep apnea (OSA).

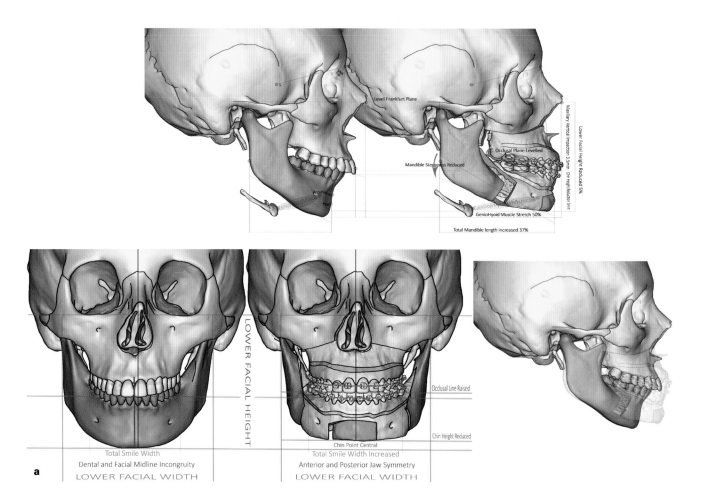

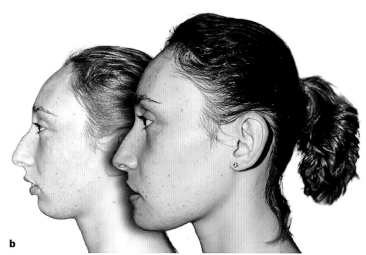

FIG 13-5 Prolonged retraction-style orthodontics to reduce prominent anterior teeth will work only while the midface is growing. The typical feature of retraction-style orthodontics is a nasal dorsal hump, incisal gummy display, and lip incompetence, with a vertically long face. At age 19 years, this patient retained a dental overjet and gummy smile despite 5 years of camouflage orthodontic therapy. Her original Class II malocclusion was just a little "less" Class II. Her orthodontist, unfamiliar with the practicalities of orthognathic surgery, requested that her surgeon "please bring the upper jaw backward" to help close the remaining incisor overjet. We had a different surgical plan. *(a)* First, SARME widened the upper smile, and then a combination of IMDO, BIMAX, and GenioPaully advancement followed. There was dramatic increase in mandible length (total increase of 37%) and geniohyoid stretch (50%). It is hard to explain in cases of an existing large incisor overjet that the equation of surgical therapy requires an even greater increase in forward maxillary incisor movement, magnified by mandibular incisor retraction (using the IMDO intermolar space). Fortunately, a necessary maxillary advancement forward can be overcome by massive mandibular movement combining IMDO, custom BSSO, and GenioPaully. Maxillary advancement also raises and advances the nasal tip, thus reducing the dorsal nasal hump (see part *b*). At 14 years old, this patient was never going to avoid jaw surgery. By engaging camouflage orthodontics, her jaw surgery needs changed from a par 3 to a par 8. *(b)* Profile views before and after SuperBIMAX. The combination of procedures produced a massive change to her profile, airway patency, and self-confidence.

FIG 13-6 Drawings representing the profile before and after SuperBIMAX. The after drawing deliberately shows the profile "over" advanced to demonstrate the facial effect of the big advancement.

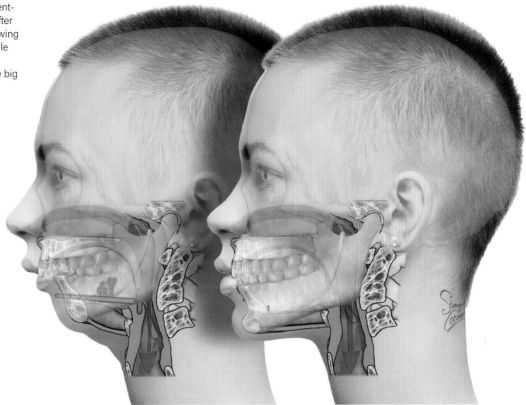

FIG 13-7 The effects of SuperBIMAX in this 20-year-old young woman. She had camouflage orthodontics between the ages of 12 and 15 years old and retrospectively would have been far more easily managed by adolescent IMDO. At 20 years old, she presented with an anterior open bite, and she had chronic open mouth breathing and a chronically small retroglossal airway. Figure 6-8 shows the presurgical cervical and airway state.

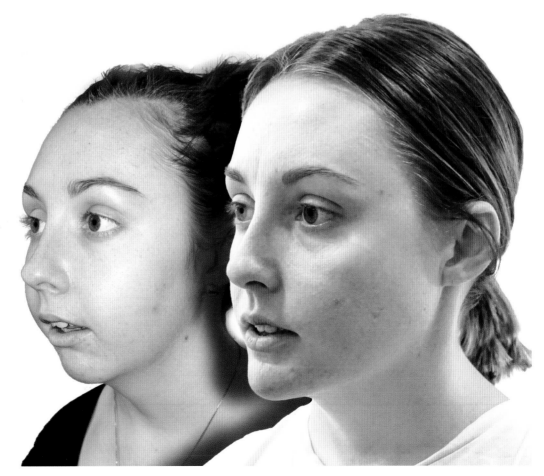

Figures 13-8 to 13-11 illustrate the airway, skeletal, and facial effects of the various stages of SuperBIMAX. For many adults, IMDO or BIMAX alone is not enough to overcome snoring or the risk of developing OSA. Only a combination of IMDO, SARME, BIMAX, and GenioPaully—the SuperBIMAX—will lead to sufficient advancement in these cases.

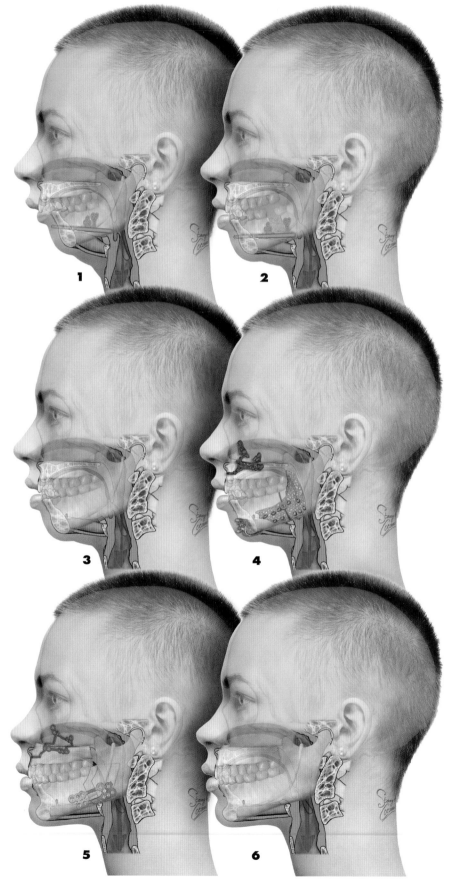

FIG 13-8 The airway effects of the various stages of SuperBIMAX are shown to demonstrate comparative possibilities. *(1)* Original AMHypo and hypogenia (orthognathic Class B) with IMDO distractors in place. The geniohyoid muscle, when the patient is awake, is extremely contracted and cosmetically contributes to the dewlap. *(2)* IMDO distraction extended 14 mm (maximum 16.5 mm). IMDO alone has a substantial but incomplete reversal of glossoptosis. In the adult, IMDO alone is unlikely to overcome snoring. *(3)* Healing and occlusion settling. Dewlap, lip incompetence, a vertically long chin, and hypogenia remain. *(4)* BIMAX and GenioPaully planning and custom titanium guide planning is by sophisticated 3D analysis software, where there is simultaneous imaging of airway structures. Performing BIMAX after IMDO is only applicable to adults. *(5)* BIMAX straight-line advancement to maximum BSSO distance of 10 mm, LeFort 8 mm, and GenioPaully 8 mm. The soft tissue distortion and stretch is maximized at these combined distances. Considerable structural design of custom titanium printed plates is required to overcome glossoptosis. There is substantial movement, or "relapse" of big movements, where retention is by small hand-bent "off-the-shelf" surgical plates. *(6)* After plate removal and bone grafting to osseous defects. After 6 to 12 months, plates and screws are removed to take away stress shielding and maximize natural healing.

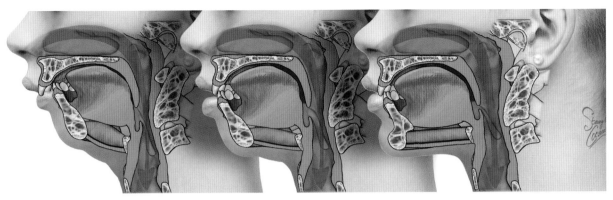

FIG 13-9 Comparing the airway effects from AMHypo to post-IMDO to SuperBIMAX. There is an overwhelming stretch of the muscles attaching the back of the chin to the hyoid. This tension brings the hyoid forward and thus tents open the retroglossal airway. The greater the geniohyoid "stretch," the less likelihood there is for supine collapse of the airway during relaxed sleep. The entire aim of surgical advancement of the jaws is to overcome snoring and OSA risk.

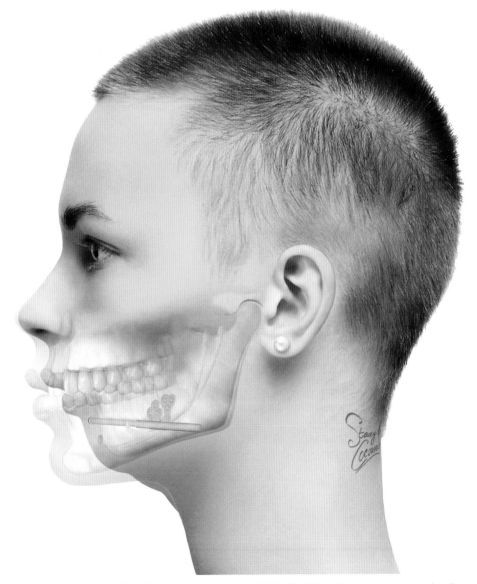

FIG 13-10 Direct overlay comparison showing maximum extensible limit of bimaxillary advancement using the combination of IMDO, BIMAX, and GenioPaully.

FIG 13-11 Pure skeletal and profile views demonstrating skeletal and facial effects of the various steps involved in the SuperBIMAX sequence. *(1)* Original profile of AMHypo with hypogenia and IMDO distractors in place. Dewlap, lip incompetence, incisor prominence, and a diminutive chin projection are all features. There is no other way to gain substantial interdental space for orthodontic arch decrowding other than by dental extractions or interdental enamel stripping. *(2)* IMDO distraction extended 14 mm (maximum 16.5 mm). IMDO is combined with SARME to the maxilla, all to gain interdental space to help dental decrowding. In adults, IMDO has a much longer healing time compared to in adolescents. *(3)* Healing and occlusion settling occurs over several months and with the assistance of Class I orthodontics. Bone healing and dental movement is much slower in adults than in adolescents. *(4)* BIMAX and GenioPaully planning and titanium custom guides. Planning for further custom BIMAX utilizes sophisticated 3D planning software. Guides are printed in titanium. *(5)* BIMAX straight-line advancement to maximum BSSO distance of 10 to 13 mm, LeFort 8 mm, and GenioPaully 8 mm. At these distances, large custom-made titanium plates are used, which must be eventually removed. *(6)* After plate removal and bone grafting to osteotomy defects. Retaining the plate limits the bone to naturally heal and adapt to chewing forces.

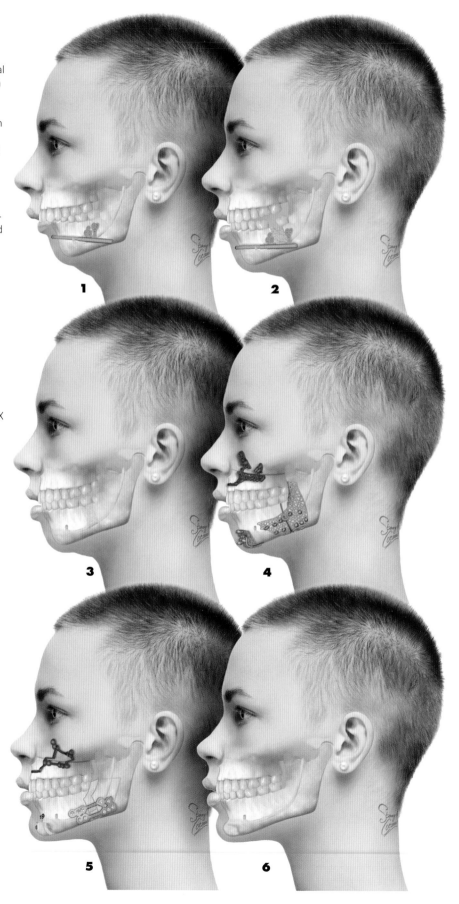

14

WHAT PATIENTS CAN EXPECT WITH BIMAX

BIMAX surgery is the biggest operation a corrective jaw surgeon will routinely perform. It involves two jaw operations coordinated together: maxillary LeFort 1 surgery and mandibular bilateral sagittal split osteotomy (and often with a chin). These combined surgical procedures can still be coordinated with orthodontics, but it is increasingly rare. Even rarer is the traditional use of heavy archwires and placement of surgical hooks, whose role has changed with the development of custom plate solutions. The fitting and use of a surgical splint is something belonging to another era.

What BIMAX surgery has NOT entirely eliminated is the need for postsurgical orthodontic bite alignment and settling using orthodontic brackets or Invisalign. The surgical planning session with the patient will have importantly determined this need.

It is important to note that 100% perfection 100% of the time in 100% of people is not possible with orthognathic surgery. In the weeks and months following surgery, habitual jaw positions, relapse of orthodontic tooth movements, and unpredicted abnormal healing may lead to a treatment outcome that is not ideal, especially when it comes to the bite. Secondary operations may become necessary to adjust bone plates or make minor "tweaks" to idealize the surgical outcome. Reoperation rates are close to 30% in cases of normal BIMAX and as low as 1% to 5% in custom BIMAX. With digital planning, these risks and unknowns are reduced to as close to zero as possible, but it is never and will never be a perfect rate.

> With digital planning, these risks and unknowns are reduced to as close to zero as possible, but it is never a perfect rate.

IMMEDIATE POSTOPERATIVE PERIOD

In the immediate postoperative period, patients should expect the following:

- Moderate discomfort in the upper and lower face
- Swelling in the lower face and midface, as well as in the lips and into the upper neck
- Some nasal or postnasal blood clotting
- General facial numbness, with perhaps the sense of a "floating" jaw (particularly with surgically assisted rapid maxillary expansion [SARME])
- Sutures along the inside of the upper lip, above the teeth, and at the back of the jawline below the lower cheek
- Inability to open the jaws normally

These immediate effects of surgery are normal and temporary, lasting only a few weeks. Patients should not be alarmed by this.

Nasal care

Immediately after surgery, the patient will wake with nasal tampons inserted into the nose (Fig 14-1). These are left in

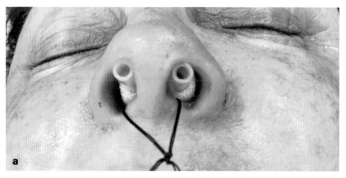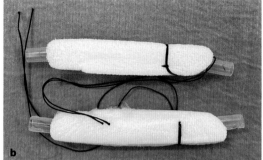

FIG 14-1 *(a and b)* Nasal tampons in the nose immediately following BIMAX surgery.

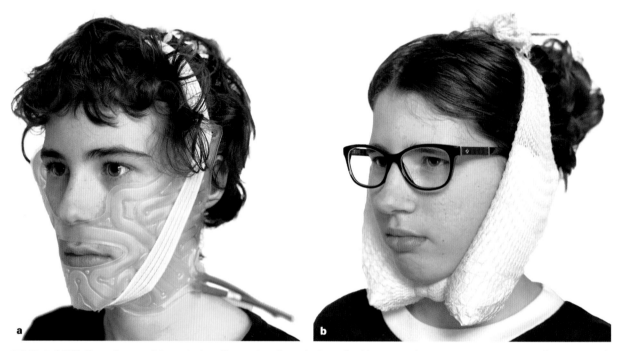

FIG 14-2 *(a)* Hilotherm face mask to control swelling and soothe pain. A small refrigerator unit pumps a constant stream of water through the mask, reducing surface skin temperature to between 15°C and 19°C. Used over 3 days, this reduces swelling from surgery and provides pain relief to the patient. *(b)* Barrel sock bandage. Using a simple stocking with a knot tied in the middle, ice packs can be introduced to each side and tied over the top of the head. This can produce an intense cold that in short bursts can prevent deep bruising and larger swelling resulting from jaw surgery.

place for 24 hours, which can make the first night in the hospital comfortably difficult for the patient. Afterward, a hilotherm face mask is worn to manage swelling and pain; this can be quite soothing for the patient (Fig 14-2a). These can be replaced with normal barrel bandages using ice (Fig 14-2b).

After the first 24 hours, nasal sprays are used for nasal decongestion. By 10 days after surgery, 80% of the swelling will have dissipated. Bruising can travel lightly down the neck and will most likely disappear by 14 days.

While the sutures are still in place (up to 15 days after surgery), patients should NOT blow their nose.

> While the sutures are still in place (up to 15 days after surgery), patients should NOT blow their nose.

If any nasal bleeding occurs, the oxymetazoline nasal spray provided by the hospital can be used to stop it. If mouth or nasal bleeding persists, crushed ice can be applied to the roof of the mouth, or—the more enjoyable alternative—the patient can eat an ice slushy. The "brain freeze" caused by this ice block is usually effective to stop nasal bleeding.

Nausea, pain, and oral care

Nausea is not uncommon in the immediate postoperative period due to the anesthesia. A good vomit is often relieving for patients and should not be seen as something to actively prevent.

The teeth can be brushed carefully with a baby toothbrush and toothpaste, but nothing should be rinsed in the mouth while the sutures are in place, and of course any stitches should be avoided while brushing. It is important that patients not rinse the mouth at all.

About 24 hours after surgery, mouth soaks using hot salt water laced with numbing anesthetic (dispensed by a pharmacist), and chlorhexidine 0.2% aqueous solution, are introduced to clean the teeth and soothe the inside of the lips and mouth. Again, the solutions should NOT be rinsed.

Once home (usually following a 3-day stay in the hospital), the patient must completely rest for 2 days and avoid all active exercise for 12 days. No smoking is permitted, and the patient should actively avoid people who do smoke. All prescribed medications must be taken (see section below), and all dairy should be avoided while the sutures are in place.

No need for banding

The patient will wake with their mouth able to open normally; the mouth will not be banded shut. A combination of presurgical design and the use of custom bone plates and screws maximizes the chance of long-term stability of the final surgical repositioning without the usual need for bite splints or elastics.

> The patient will wake with their mouth able to open normally; the mouth will not be banded shut.

When moving jaws, we are stretching tissues, and stretched tissues will resist the bodily movements that have been applied. Until these stretched tissues have relaxed and accommodated the new positions (ie, until healing is complete), the neck and jaw skin and tongue may feel stretched, which some describe as a burning sensation. Until these tissues have completely healed and become used to their new positions, normal range of movement, normal eating, and normal talking will be affected.

Diet

In the immediate postoperative period, the patient's diet is restricted to liquids and purées and vitamin supplements that do not require any chewing.

Appropriate nondairy foods include puréed fruits and vegetables, beef broth, soups, overcooked pasta and rice, and scrambled eggs. For the first few weeks following BIMAX surgery, it is important that the patient only ingest cold or warm foods that do not require biting, nibbling, or chewing. Overhot foods can stimulate bleeding, and scalding may occur if the mouth and lips remain numb.

A narrow syringe can be provided to patients for squirting food directly down the back of the throat or for introduction through the spaces down the side and behind the back of the teeth. This should only be used if the patient feels they cannot open the mouth sufficiently to insert a spoon between the open front teeth.

> It is extremely important not to bathe mouth oral wounds in ingested milk by directly drinking through a glass.

Dairy products should be avoided while the sutures are in place. If a dairy-free diet cannot be tolerated, milkshakes can be ingested via a feeding syringe and introduced directly down the back of the throat. It is extremely important not to bathe mouth oral wounds in ingested milk by directly drinking through a glass.

Patients will often ask, "When can I eat normally?" Our answer is always given by clinical consideration of the doctor on a week-to-week basis. Normal eating depends on many factors, including the stability or fragility of the surgery performed, whether any reoperations are required, the state of wound healing intraorally, the patient's recovery, and of course the patient's general medical state.

A soft diet, including milk products, is usually achieved in about 10 days, but most people will dramatically lose between 10 and 20 pounds during this time, depending on their initial weight. Most patients should have a normal diet by 10 weeks after surgery. Everything in between is a gradual self-titrated process.

Most people undergoing jaw surgery will be wanting weight loss to occur, especially as they are seeking relief from their obstructive sleep apnea (OSA). As weight loss is a cofactor with therapeutic OSA management, dietary control is extremely important and can be suggested by the doctor's office to also incorporate dietician and general practitioner input. It is here that dedicated weight loss programs can have significant advantage from the immediate anorexic effects of BIMAX recovery.

MEDICATION USE

It is important for patients to take all prescribed medications following BIMAX surgery.

Antibiotics to prevent infection

With big surgeries like custom BIMAX, where significant hardware is placed into living tissue, there is a high risk for plate infection, hence the need for short periods of postsurgical antibiotics (and eventual plate removal). Repeat infections should have repeat antibiotics started early and often. This is always under the treating surgeon's direct supervision.

> With big surgeries like custom BIMAX, where significant hardware is placed into living tissue, there is a high risk for plate infection, hence the need for short periods of postsurgical antibiotics (and eventual plate removal).

As with IMDO therapy, amoxicillin and clavulanate is the standard antibiotic provided to all patients after surgery to prevent postsurgical infection. For penicillin-allergic patients, clindamycin may be used instead.

NSAID to control swelling

A nonsteroidal anti-inflammatory drug (NSAID) such as piroxicam is provided after surgery to reduce swelling and pain in the 10 days following surgery. It is important to take the course for 10 days to control postoperative swelling. Following BIMAX, this NSAID is designed to be dissolved in 50 mL of water and drunk.

Pain reliever

For the first 24 hours following surgery, two tablets of acetaminophen (500 mg with codeine 30 mg) should be taken every 6 hours to relieve postoperative pain. The first dose should be taken before the local anesthetic wears off. After

the first 24 hours, it can be taken as needed, not to exceed eight tablets in 24 hours.

Mouth and wound care

Anesthetic mouth salts containing benzocaine (100 mg in a 20-g mixture of plain salt and bicarbonate of soda) can be used in a ratio of 1 small teaspoon to half a glass of hot water to soak wounds (see Fig 14-4). This salt compound is dispensed by a compounding pharmacy. It is safe to use this solution as regularly as the patient desires, but three times daily is the recommended protocol. This solution can be used starting 24 hours after surgery. This is to be used as a soak, not a rinse, and it should NOT be swallowed.

> All solutions should NOT be rinsed, as this may open up fresh wounds, may cause bleeding, or may accidentally be swallowed.

Oral surgery mouth soaks containing aqueous 0.2% solution of chlorhexidine in a 200-mL bottle are also used three times a day (morning, noon, and night) to clean the wounds (see Fig 14-4). This solution prevents bacterial colonization of wounds and sutures. The anesthetic mouth salts should be used prior to this soak because chlorhexidine solutions may contain minimal alcohol and can sting otherwise. All solutions should NOT be rinsed, as this may open up fresh wounds, may cause bleeding, or may accidentally be swallowed.

Anesthetic throat lozenges or spray

Sore throat is a common postoperative side effect of jaw surgery. Anesthetic lozenges including benzocaine (8.2 mg/lozenge) or lidocaine (10 mg/lozenge) may be used to control this unpleasant side effect. Benzydamine throat sprays can also be used to treat sore throat or any oral ulcers that may have developed as a result of surgery.

Antiemetic drugs

Vomiting up unsettling stomach contents is both normal and relieving for the patient. When nausea persists, when we need the patient to keep down necessary medications or food, or when there is the rare use of jaw elastics, antiemetic drugs may be prescribed to control the nausea.

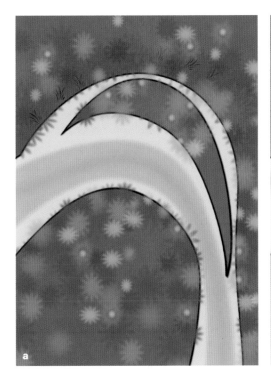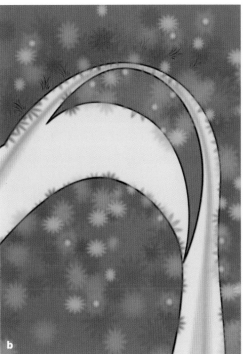

FIG 14-3 Opening the mouth creates a natural high-flow, low-resistance system that makes nasal airflow impossible. People who open their mouth to breathe at night do so because the closed small jaw potentiates airway blockage behind the tongue. Chronically opening the mouth to breathe makes the nasal airway passages more likely to become smaller, further developing the dependence upon open mouth breathing. Diverting a river (high-flow, low-resistance system, *a*) so that water flows through a branch canal (low-flow, high-resistance system, *b*) requires the creation of a dam. Unless the canal has normal flow, the waters will remain stagnant, the canal banks will develop weeds, and eventually the canal will fill with sediment and debris. Similarly, establishing normal nasal airflow requires a closed mouth. With normal nasal airflow, the nasal mucosa will not collect stagnant mucus and collected debris. Chronically inflamed nasal mucosa is a feature of stagnant airflow and is prone to irritation and further airflow blockage by increased thickness and polyp development. Keeping the nose clean with regular irrigation will help clear stagnant mucus, help relieve nasal membrane irritation, and help improve natural nasal airflow.

SINUS CARE FOLLOWING JAW SURGERY

Irritable nasal disease affects a large segment of the community, and for patients undergoing jaw surgery, nasal disease and a small upper jaw go hand in hand (Fig 14-3). This nasal disease may have affected the growth of the nasal passages and of the midface in general, and ongoing irritable nasal disease may also modify recovery from jaw surgery, BIMAX in particular.

Acquired nasal disease is usually supported by a history of nasal blockage, postnasal drip, nasal itchiness, nosebleeds, watery reactive eyes, an admission to active or passive smoking, repetitive sneezing, mouth breathing, and purulent (foul) breath and loss of smell. Patients often report a history of asthma or eczema, formal

Nasal care is an important part of overall maxillary surgical management, and one that should be continued over a lifetime.

allergy testing, long-term use of CPAP, or high rates of viral colds or bacterial airway infection.

Following surgical procedures to the maxilla like BIMAX, oral mucosal healing is only successful if the mucosa of the maxillary sinus lining is also healthy and the person is able to normally breathe through both nostrils 24 hours a day. As such, nasal care is an important part of overall maxillary surgical management, and one that should be continued over a lifetime.

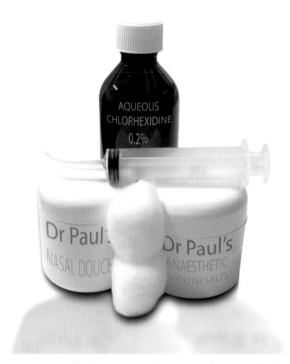

FIG 14-4 Prescribed medicaments for oral and sinus care following BIMAX surgery. Aqueous chlorhexidine 0.2% is used as a mouth soak over oral wounds using cotton balls. Anesthetic mouth salts containing benzocaine, salt, and bicarbonate are also used to bathe oral wounds after being mixed into a half glass of coffee-hot water. Both are used three times daily. Dr Paul's Nasal Douche contains salt, sugar, eucalyptus, and bicarbonate and is introduced via the nose as a light solution and snorted twice daily.

Two weeks after surgery (NOT before), nasal washing should commence with special nasal douche salts. This preparation, called Dr Paul's Nasal Douche in Australia, is made at a compounding pharmacy and from a pharmaceutically prepared batch of pharmaceutical-grade salt (75%) 500 g, sucrose (9%) 60 g, bicarbonate (15%) 100 g, and eucalyptus 5 mL (1%) and distributed in 66.5-g jars (Fig 14-4).

When prepared as a solution, small 0.5-g amounts of the prepared salts are combined with plain water and inhaled by use of a tapered syringe (Fig 14-5). This is the most effective and cheapest way to maintain nasal cleanliness. The douche is to be used initially morning and night, and we advise using it in the shower. The solution is designed to be snorted into each nostril to physically clean and whet the nose. This lavage of the nose expels dry crust, blood, and tenacious secretions, which may also contain irritating allergens.

The solution is a self-prepared one. The aim is to obtain a solution at about 38°C to 40°C, with a salt content slightly stronger than that of natural nasal secretions. If the patient cannot taste the salt, then they have not added enough. If it is too strong, it will feel like being dunked in a wave at the beach. The approximate amount of salt is a small scoop on the inner ¼ of the plunger end of the syringe (see Fig 14-5a), with the volume of the syringe to be filled with warm water taken from the shower head. A small squirt should be "sniffed" into each nostril and expectorated, until the syringe is empty. One syringe morning and evening is usually enough to last the day and night. The syringe should be cleaned with flushing after each use.

After a few weeks, the patient should notice a difference in their nasal health. This nasal douching should become a regular part of the patient's self-care routine for the rest of their life.

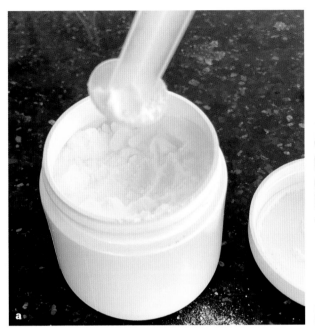 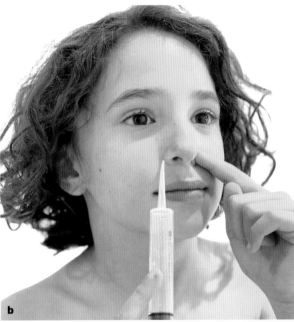

FIG 14-5 Dr Paul's Nasal Douche regimen. *(a)* Use ¼ of the syringe plunger to collect a small amount of salts. Pour the salts into the syringe barrel, and fill the rest of the syringe with warm water. *(b)* Squirt and "sniff" a small amount of the solution into each nostril while holding the other nostril closed and expectorate, until the syringe is empty. Perform this in the shower once or twice daily.

AFTER THE BIMAX

Healing takes time. Swelling will rise and fall and is variable among people.

The patient will typically want to reenter society as soon as possible, and they will be keen to show off their new face. It is very important to understand that everything that has been done is a collection of extremely subtle and intercoordinated movements and that biologic processes are still ongoing. It will take some time for these natural processes to complete. However, fundamentally the patient's new smile and face may have been acquired so gradually and subtly that an old photograph is all they will have to remind them of the journey.

Braces and/or Invisalign is a final step in the remediation puzzle. Moving teeth through surgery is like moving house. The movers only move the boxes into the house; the homeowner still needs to unpack and arrange the plates on the shelves and hang the paintings.

Getting a perfect bite can take considerable time. The bite may feel off or unsettled for a long period, and expensive and laborious processes are needed as each tooth is individually moved and settled into its new arch position by the orthodontist.

Eventually the surgical plates need to be removed too—and small bone nooks filled in and bumps smoothed over. The patient may also want to eventually seek cosmetic interventions to enhance their symmetry or to reduce self-perceived facial defects as they advance toward their own esthetic desires.

The therapeutic relationship between the surgeon and patient will eventually reach its natural end. Bariatric surgeons, dieticians, general practitioners, the family dentist, the orthodontist, and cosmetic surgeons can follow, but they do not normally need to interact with the maxillofacial surgeon. Hopefully any need for a sleep physician and interventional ENT surgeon has been eliminated. By this stage, there should be little if any evidence that corrective jaw surgery has occurred at all.

15

CREATING THE IDEAL MAXILLA
THE FIFTH WAY

To achieve ideals in smile and facial esthetics, and to normalize airways and a bite that is common to both jaws, the consideration of a small lower jaw naturally has to include a discussion of the maxilla as well. Almost all people with a small mandible also have a small maxilla. Mandibular dental crowding and maxillary dental crowding often go hand in hand. The coupling of a retruded mandible and a narrow maxilla is extremely common. An asymmetric mandible means an asymmetric maxilla also.

In a global assessment of a face, it is rare that a single growth problem does not also have a negative effect on another adjacent part that would have otherwise been normal. This assessment must consider not only the primary condition but also the secondary effects of that condition as well. The small mandible has many effects that magnify as the child's face and adolescent face grow

But the single biggest effect of the small mandible is that it causes the otherwise normal maxilla to become a little— or a lot—smaller too.

into the final adult face. If these problems can be identified early on, some of these secondary effects can be avoided or even easily reversed without a direct need for surgery. If they have already occurred, then there are things we need to surgically coordinate and correct so that the whole adult face is normal and balanced (Fig 15-1).

But the single biggest effect of the small mandible and by a variety of means is that it causes the otherwise normal maxilla to become a little—or a lot—smaller too.

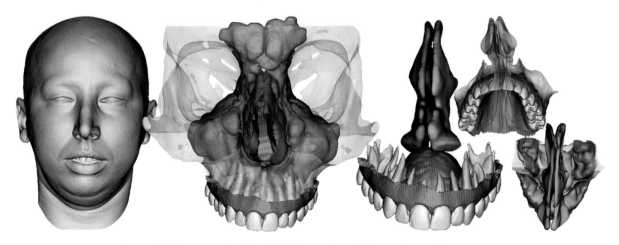

FIG 15-1 How we assess the maxilla has as much to do with looking at the smile line and overall face, as well as the nose, sinuses, and dual nasal airway passages. The LeFort 1 is a workhorse for the orthognathic surgeon, and this chapter explains how we manage the ideal volume, dimensions, and spatial position of the maxilla to coordinate maxillary esthetics, bite, and airflow.

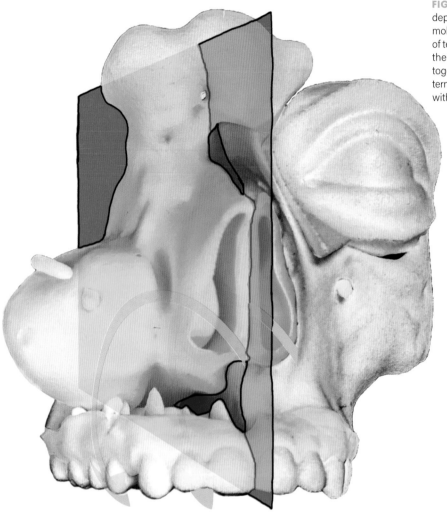

FIG 15-2 Normal sinus inflation is dependent on natural airflow, tongue molding of the palate, and the number of teeth, all of which contribute to how the cheekbone and maxilla develop together as a one-sided unit and determine how well it pairs symmetrically with the other side.

HOW THE NORMAL MAXILLA DEVELOPS IN CHILDHOOD AND ADOLESCENCE

The normal maxilla develops from three separate natural processes:

1. **Teeth:** There needs to be a normal compliment of primary and then permanent teeth. Having fewer naturally developed teeth or fewer teeth as a result of extraction will reduce the bony volume of the dentoalveolus.

2. **Tongue dome:** The tongue dome (the top of the tongue) must naturally be present to shape the palatal vault (the arch or shape of the palate). A small tongue, or a tongue that sits naturally backward or is chronically held away from the roof of the mouth, will cause the palatal vault and dental arch to underwiden and underexpand. Chronic mouth breathing is the most common cause of a high arched palate or a narrow maxillary dental arch.

3. **Maxillary sinuses:** The inside of the maxilla is filled with two large air sacs, the maxillary sinuses. Normal inflation and pneumatization of these air sacs is the single biggest influence on normal maxilla development. These sacs lie on either side of the maxillary airway and naturally expand (like balloons) with nasal breathing. Like papier mâché, the overall shape of the maxillary bone (which includes the dentoalveolus, connecting palate, and developing teeth) occurs in the hard bony crust that develops and surrounds these softly inflating air sacs (Fig 15-2). Anything that affects regular nasal breathing, or natural nasal air passage, will cause underinflation of these air sacs and will lead to a small maxilla.

FIG 15-3A The maxillary sinuses lie on either side of the nasal airway. Having equal nasal airflow is important to gain symmetric inflation of the maxillary air sinuses. Just like playing with papier mâché in kindergarten, the membranous bone of the cheekbone and maxilla concretes onto the surfaces of the developing nasal mucosa, palate, and maxillary sinus balloons. Underinflation of the sinus balloons leads to asymmetric effects on eyeball position, developing teeth, and normal facial shape. ⟶

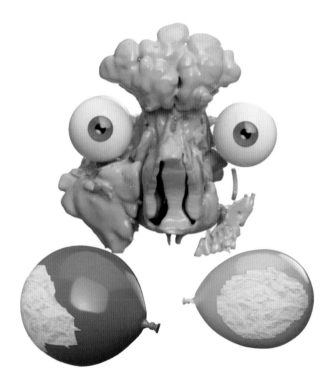

The biggest cause of a small maxilla is underinflation of the maxillary sinuses and secondary downward displacement of the tongue dome.

Maxillary jaw volume, the number of maxillary teeth and their alignment, normal palatal width, and normal natural nasal air passage are therefore all interrelated.

The biggest cause of a small maxilla is underinflation of the maxillary sinuses and secondary downward displacement of the tongue dome. Both are the result of chronic open mouth breathing, which is caused not by chronic nasal blockage but as an adaptation to relieve the glossoptosis, mainly at night and during sleep, that is consequent to the small mandible (see Fig 1-17).

Chronic nasal blockage, underdevelopment of the maxilla, and maxillary dental crowding are inherently and primarily due to this small mandible.

WHAT IS SILENT SINUS SYNDROME?

Maxillary sinuses inflate. They inflate by steady, normal, symmetric breathing—back and forth—through the nose and on each side. Breathing occurs at an approximate resting adult rate of 14 times a minute. This means there are 28 air movements 60 times an hour. Over a full 24 hours, this is a total of 40,320 individual micropressure events each and every day and on both sides of the mandible.

If there is anything that prevents normal natural nasal airway breathing, then there is a reduction in the number of these natural air movements. If a person is a chronic mouth breather at night and when asleep, then up to a third of all natural nasal air movements do not occur. Over the developmental period of that person's face, this reduced proportion of natural nasal air movements will have a significant effect on natural sinus health, development, and normal inflation.

Because the maxillary sinus is the major contributor to how the midface forms, small underinflated maxillary sinuses lead to the appearance of a small maxilla and cheekbones. Normally this underinflation occurs on both sides of the face, but occasionally underdevelopment of the maxillary sinus is more prominent on one side (Fig 15-3a). This leads to an asymmetric maxilla and therefore

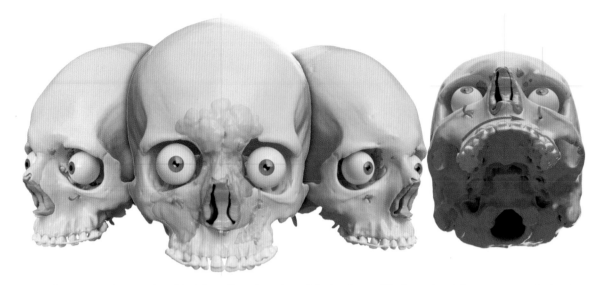

FIG 15-3B Nonpneumatic expansion of the left maxillary sinus, due to left chronic nasal blockage since infancy, causes underdevelopment of the left zygomatic (cheek) bone. This in turn leads to rearward and downward drop of the eyeball and a twist of the maxilla and dental arch to that side. Restoring the lost zygomatic volume requires a combination of LeFort 1 repositioning surgery as well as custom polyetheretherketone (PEEK) implants (see chapter 16) involving restoration of globe position as well as orbital rim symmetry. The maxillary dental arch has been expanded with a rapid palatal expander to gain both normal nasal bilateral airflow and increased dental arch circumference to accommodate the previously crowded maxillary teeth.

an asymmetric level of the eyes (Fig 15-3b). Doctors refer to this asymmetric inflationary effect as silent sinus syndrome (SSS).

Asymmetry does not mean that only one nasal air passage is affected. Both maxillary sinuses may still be underinflated, and reduced nasal air passage usually occurs on both sides but is relatively worse on the smaller side. However, the end point of developmental underinflation and its negative effect on midfacial development is significantly greater on one side than the other.

The most important dental feature of SSS is the associated asymmetry of the dental arch and smile. There is significant movement of the facial midline from the central dental midline toward the smaller side. There is developmental distortion of the relatively bigger side toward the relatively smaller side. This distortion exacerbates the asymmetry.

PLANNING FOR IDEAL MAXILLARY SHAPE AND POSITION

Setting the position and shape of the maxilla is the single key feature to creating the rest of the face around it. How we obtain CT data and how we segmentalize and create 3D imagery that combines mucosa and bone and maxillary teeth is explained in chapter 4. Our first segmentation process enables us to formalize a diagnosis of why the

maxilla has developed as it has. It also serves as a basis to plan how to correct it. This segmentalization process enables the surgeon to visualize many complex structures that all interlink with each other—bone, dental roots, occlusion, smile lines, eyes, face, and air passages.

> Setting the position and shape of the maxilla is the single key feature to creating the rest of the face around it.

The most important thing we segment is the nasal and sinus mucosa. Without visualizing the septum, valves, conchae, and air sacs, it is virtually impossible to blindly correct or improve the nasal air passages through our LeFort surgery (Fig 15-4). And it is only by accurately correcting the ideal position and dimensions of the maxilla that the surgeon can then plan to correct the ideal position and dimensions of the mandible through either intermolar mandibular distraction osteogenesis (IMDO) or bilateral sagittal split osteotomy (BSSO) surgery.

The maxilla is always the first thing we look at fixing—either through expert pre-IMDO orthodontics, through surgically assisted rapid maxillary expansion (SARME) and then preparatory orthodontics, or through formal correctional LeFort surgery. The mandible comes second.

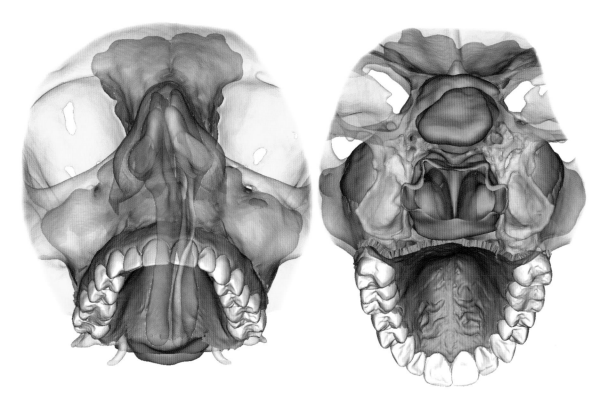

FIG 15-4 The nasal mucosa is extremely important to visualize with computed tomography (CT) imaging, because success or failure of our surgical procedures can ignore, aggravate, or improve nasal airway passages. The nasal airway begins at the nasal valves. Anything that increases the anterior dental arch width will increase airway through the nasal valves. The nasal airway ends at the conchae, which lie above the soft palate. Anything that increases the dental arch across the back of the palate will increase airway before it enters the space above the soft palate.

THERAPEUTIC MAXILLARY EXPANSION

When the maxillary teeth are crowded, when nasal breathing is difficult, when nasal breathing with a closed mouth during sleep is impossible, and when there is complaint of chronic nasal blockage, the maxilla must be assumed to be small.

There are two classical clinical ways to look at the abnormal smallness of the maxilla. Dentists can look in the mouth and see it as a case of dental crowding, or malocclusion, or of impacted teeth or a constricted palate. Or doctors can look in the nose and see it as a case of chronic nasal blockage, narrow nostrils, copious mucus, nasal allergy or chronic irritation or nasal stuffiness, large polyps or inflamed membranes, or a deviated septum, prominent adenoids, and big turbinates. Either way, upstairs or downstairs, most clinicians will see only one story or the other in this two-floor house. And most clinicians can only see that there is too much furniture. Either there are too many teeth and a small mouth in the lower floor, or there are too many

adenoids and turbinates and a blocked nose in the upper floor. As dentists and doctors we fall into a habit of being household removalists. By only seeing crowded furniture, the danger is that we ignore the need to become builders instead and to make the whole house bigger—and keep all the furniture.

HYRAX expansion and MARME

From the dental perspective, the palatal expander or HYRAX can be affixed to the teeth to gain an expanded dental arch and to help decrowd maxillary teeth, hopefully allowing the clinician to keep all of them. It is commonly used in camouflage orthodontics (see Fig 12-3). Used slowly (maybe only 0.33 mm per week), the effect is mostly on the dental arch and dentoalveolus rather than by expansion of the palate. In adults, this means that HYRAX devices can easily push teeth beyond their natural bone boundaries, leading to effects such as orthodontic relapse, loose teeth, or later periodontal disease. This outward dental tipping effect is an adverse outcome that most dental practitioners want to avoid.

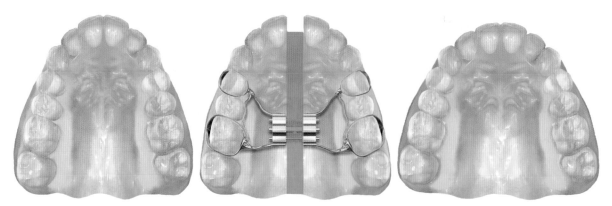

FIG 15-5 The "hygienic rapid expander" or HYRAX was developed by William Biederman in 1968. This is a tooth-borne device. Used slowly, it will only tip out the teeth. Used rapidly at 1/3 mm per day, it will spread the unfused sutures of the midface.

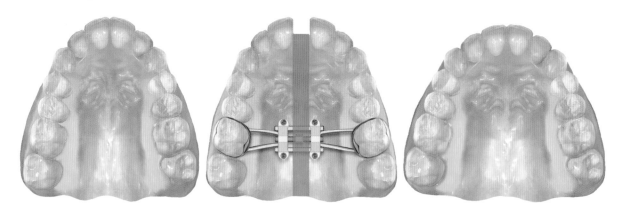

FIG 15-6 MARME. Both systems expand the maxilla and the entire nasal cavity outward but rely upon a nonfused set of sutures contained throughout the midface, particularly the palatal suture. Both systems are very successful in adolescents, but after age 17 years (and up to possibly 25), only MARME is effective. Beyond this age, or where expansion does not occur in the young adult, formal LeFort 1 surgery must be performed to aid expansion (ie, SARME). The frontal effects are illustrated and explained in Figs 15-7d and 15-7e.

In adolescents (girls up to age 15 years and boys up to age 17 years), rapid expansion with the HYRAX (around 1/3 mm per day or every other day) achieves dental arch widening primarily by separation of the central palatal suture (Fig 15-5). Because of the rapidity, there is little orthodontic tooth movement. Like opening the midline base of a pyramid, the palatal suture expands by also spreading all other interconnected natural bone sutures throughout the entire midface. Experienced and informed dental clinicians will therefore use a HYRAX for midfacial orthopedic purposes to expand the midfacial airway volumes, massively increasing nasal airway patency and reducing chronic nasal blockage.

To further magnify this midfacial sutural opening but reduce the chance that teeth are simply tipping outward,

SARME is a workhorse for the orthognathic surgeon.

dentists have come up with ingenious ways to maximize forces applied more specifically to the midfacial bones themselves. One way is via mini-implant assisted rapid maxillary expansion (MARME), and its effect is to separate all the sutures of the face and thus minimize outward dental tipping movements (Fig 15-6).

There are many types of MARME devices, the most popular being the mixed dental-skeletal devices based on the HYRAX designed by Professor Won Moon or Professor Benedict Wilmes. These devices have obvious widening benefits on the midline nasal airway passages and can

FIG 15-7 Almost everyone is asymmetric, and expanding the maxilla *(d)* almost certainly requires secondary LeFort surgery to accurately position the maxilla centrally and proportionally with the rest of the face. *(a)* Mommaerts SARME expanding only the posterior maxilla requires a binding plate under the nasal spine and four loose plates to hold the LeFort up while expansion occurs, as it does with *b*, where full anteroposterior SARME widening is needed with use of a HYRAX. *(c)* An anterior SARME only needs two loose anterior hitching plates and a Mommaerts device, as there is no "posterior dysjunction" through the pterygoid fissures. Overall, expansion of the nasal airways only occurs very low—along the nasal base—whereas when using the Moon-Wilmes device in young adults or a normal HYRAX in adolescents as in *e*, there is expansion of the entire nasal airway—high and low—with profound airway relief. It is with dubious claims that a Moon-Wilmes device will expand a truly adult maxilla without requiring formal SARME surgery. *(f)* Removing a deviating nasal spine (green) and anterior wedge (purple) can impact *g*, a slanting maxilla, and reduce a gummy smile, and this can be held up with four small plates with screws *(h)*. To do this freehand is brave, because it is challenging to get positionally correct—and difficult to understand how inadvertently crushing an already small nasal airway can be avoided. *(i and j)* SARME and midline miniplates used with LeFort surgery.

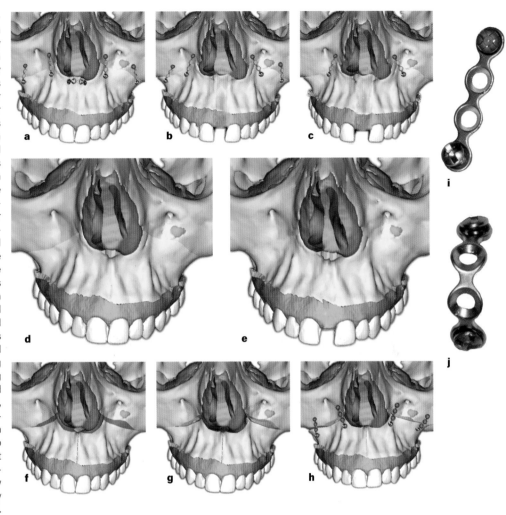

also dramatically improve the maxillary dental arch width and circumference to help orthodontically relieve maxillary dental crowding. Both HYRAX and MARME devices also widen the cheekbones, broaden the smile, and stretch and widen the hard and soft palate.

The major problem with using both HYRAX and MARME devices is that they are dentally fixed, and when used in adolescents, they are being placed into growing faces. Prolonged use beyond the period of actual expansion can actually bind teeth and indirectly prevent vertical and forward natural expansion of the maxilla. This binding effect obviously negates any advantage of the effect on improved maxillary expansion through the establishment of widened nasal airflow. It is also difficult to simultaneously use normal orthodontic appliances to straighten teeth while these dentally fixed expanders are in place.

SARME

The age to which we can absolutely predictably stretch the midfacial sutures ends at about 17 years. Beyond this age (particularly past 25 years) and under increasing forces and increasing potential discomfort, there is an accumulative chance that facial sutures are simply too bound or too fixed to be so easily expanded. The experiment of natural expansion can be performed, but if there is a failed trial or if the patient is simply too mature for natural expansion, the only means of expanding the maxilla is through the surgical creation of expandable sutures—ie, surgically assisted rapid maxillary expansion (SARME).

SARME is a workhorse for the orthognathic surgeon. The bone-borne palatal Mommaerts device is the key instrument, together with suitably placed miniplates to help guide the direction and form of expansion (Fig 15-7). Used properly, and with careful planning, there can be deliberate

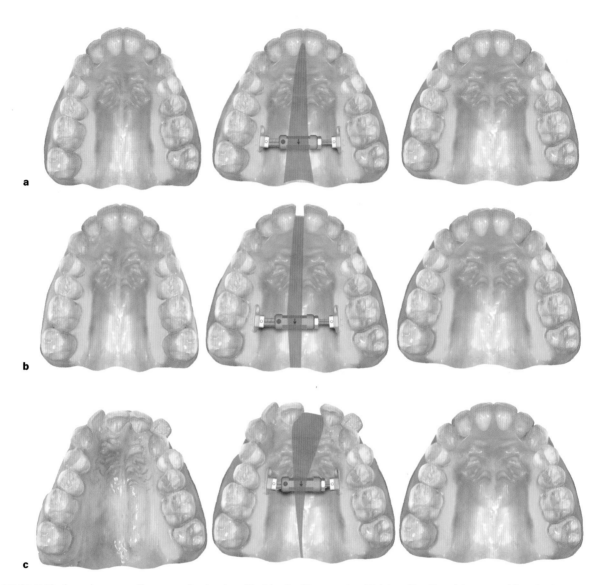

FIG 15-8 The bone-borne maxillary expander developed by Maurice Mommaerts of Belgium. Used in adolescents without LeFort surgery, it is both highly predictable and more comfortable than a HYRAX or MARME device, and unlike those devices, it does not attach to teeth, leaving them free to independently decrowd or receive orthodontic appliances. For late adolescents and adults of all ages, the Mommaerts is a workhorse device that can predictably expand the maxilla at strategic areas, such as posteriorly *(a)*, anteroposteriorly *(b)*, or anteriorly *(c)*. To gain differential expansion either forward or backward requires the use of miniplates affixed across the lines of the LeFort and midline suture.

expansion of surgically created sutures, achieving differential expansion based on its location in the palate (Fig 15-8). The Mommaerts device does not bind the maxilla or interfere with normal orthodontic straightening appliances, but it is both tricky and uncomfortable to accurately place, and it is notoriously prone to unwinding itself, unless the patient strictly follows directions on the use of the locking screw.

SARME is based on the LeFort 1 operation, where artificial bone sutures (created by the surgeon) allow for expansion

of the maxilla across the palatal midline. The midline suture in the palate is called a *midline split*, and SARME will only expand the maxilla across this split; it will NOT also expand all the midfacial sutures of the face. But SARME is *almost* as effective as MARME or HYRAX appliances at widening the nasal airway and in being able to stretch the soft palate and achieve widening of the maxillary dental arch.

FIG 15-9 *(a)* How the maxilla is repositioned anteroposteriorly, vertically, and frontally affects smile fullness, gumminess, and symmetry and has profound effects on the nasal airway. Knowing how far to impact a maxilla requires a knowledge of how much bone from the piriform rim and nasal floor also needs to be removed in order to not compress the nasal mucosa. *(b)* Finally, after the mandible has also been moved, we can make an analysis of the critical changes that combine to increase nasal airway and retroglossal airway with combined custom BIMAX surgery.

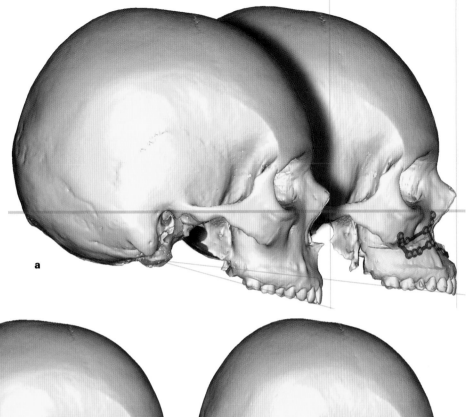

a

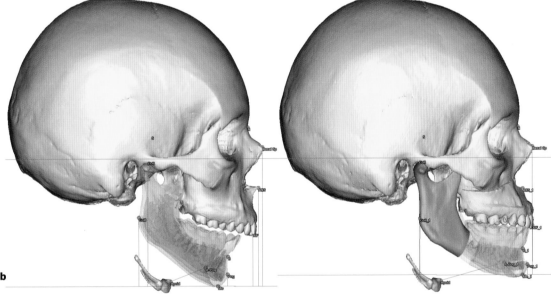

b

The problem with expansion

The overriding problem with widening a small maxilla, no matter which device or modality is chosen, is that palatal expansion will only widen left to right or right to left. There is no guarantee that widening will be symmetric or level (see Fig 15-11). Used alone, the procedure will not guarantee centrality, evenness, or even completeness. Most importantly, as small jaws are three dimensionally small, simple widening will not increase vertical maxillary height or forward projection or affect the spatial qualities of abnormal yaw, pitch, or roll. Secondary LeFort surgery is often required to accurately position the maxilla centrally and proportionally with the rest of the face (Fig 15-9).

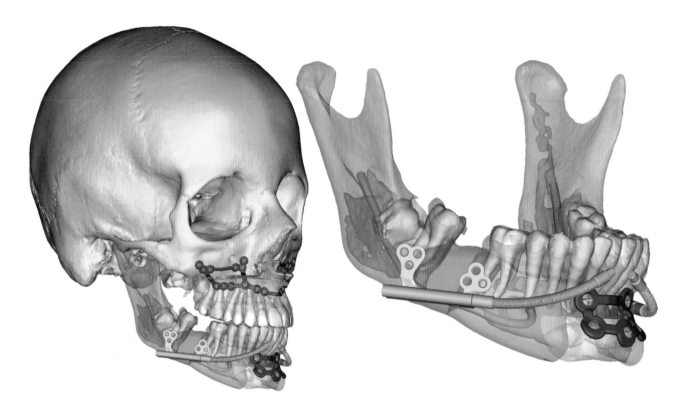

FIG 15-10 Integrating LeFort 1 advancement using custom titanium corrects the secondary developmental smallness of the maxilla that arises because of the genetically small mandible. LeFort advancement also enables an increase in the available capacity for the IMDO distractors to be maximally advanced in order to normalize the very small mandible. Adding GenioPaully provides further maximal support to stretch the geniohyoid forward in order to overcome nighttime upper airway obstruction.

LEFORT ADVANCEMENT

LeFort advancement takes advantage of the principle of en bloc movement of teeth—in this case surgical 3D repositioning of an entire jaw, the maxilla. In this way, corrective jaw surgeons can correct nasal airways, enhance lip and soft tissue fullness, and of course give fundamental correction to smiles and bites (see Fig 15-9).

The LeFort operation is an amazingly versatile procedure. It is safe to conduct (in experienced hands), and with custom titanium it is extremely predictable, infinitely designable, and very stable. What's better is that the LeFort can be used safely to move the maxilla in precise 3D directions—up and down, side to side, and forward. Angulations can also be changed, affecting pitch, yaw, and roll. And it can be split in two, allowing perfect symmetrification (see Fig 15-11).

Integrating expansion and LeFort advancement with IMDO

To meet the vertical esthetic line, surgeons can advance the maxilla into an ideal forward position at the same time as applying IMDO distractors (Fig 15-10). LeFort advancement increases the dental overjet, and any orthodontic distance can then be closed by the massive mandibular growth achieved with IMDO. In young adults and late adolescents, IMDO can be combined with SARME as well, using the Mommaerts device in place of the orthodontically placed HYRAX.

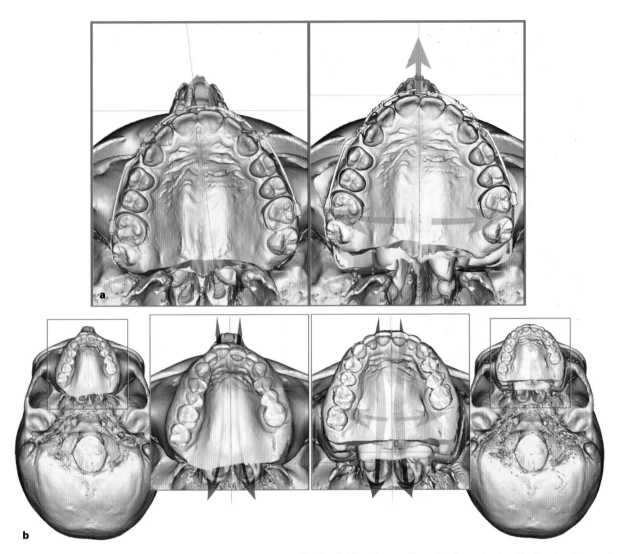

FIG 15-11 *(a)* Absolute correction of yaw, pitch, and roll is magnified by dividing the maxilla and independently widening, leveling, and advancing each side. Posterior expansion is to a maximum of 4 mm when combined with overall LeFort bodily movement. Beyond this, an independent primary SARME procedure must be performed. *(b)* A narrow dental arch that is also set back requires initial broad expansion through SARME, then later advancement using custom titanium. Splitting the maxilla at the time of secondary BIMAX allows it to be treated in two halves to enable leveling of the dental arch and maximal occlusal interdigitation. Posterior expansion at the same time as LeFort 1 advancement is extended to a maximum of 4 mm and overall produces a significantly symmetric dental arch, a wide broad smile, and profound airflow improvement to both sides of the nasal cavity from nasal valves to conchae. The soft palate is also pulled forward, eliminating the soft palatal flap and the distinct nasal snore.

Integrating LeFort surgery with "midline split" to gain perfectly shaped maxillas

The most important technical advancement that has happened in custom LeFort surgery is the discovery that by splitting the maxilla, each half of the dental arch can be precisely controlled independently and relative to one another. Division of the maxilla into two digital halves enables us to gain perfect arch symmetry, perfect levelness, and ideal width (Fig 15-11). In combination with midline mandibular halving and the BIMAX operation, occlusions can be far more predictable and precise (see Fig 12-19).

The most important technical advancement that has happened in custom LeFort surgery is the discovery that by splitting the maxilla, each half of the dental arch can be precisely controlled independently and relative to one another.

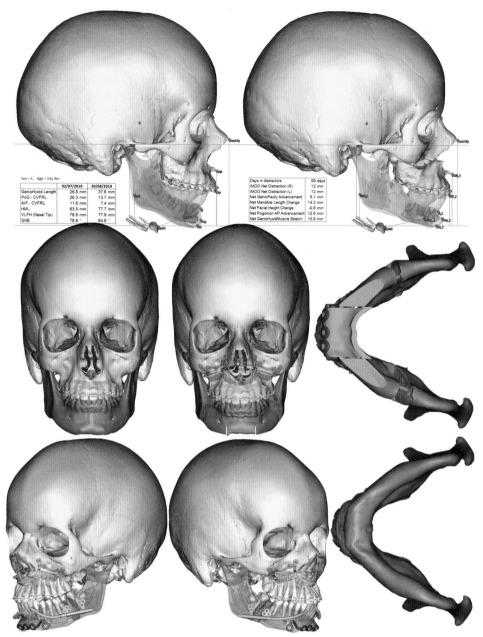

	02/07/2019	30/08/2019
GenioHyoid Length	26.8 mm	37.6 mm
PoG - CVFRL	26.3 mm	13.7 mm
AiF - CVFRL	11.6 mm	7.4 mm
HML	63.5 mm	77.7 mm
VLFH (Nasal Tip)	78.5 mm	77.9 mm
SNB	78.9 °	84.8 °

Sex = F; Age = 14y 4m

Days in distractors	59 days
IMDO Net Distraction (R)	12 mm
IMDO Net Distraction (L)	12 mm
Net GenioPaully Advancement	5.1 mm
Net Mandible Length Change	14.2 mm
Net Facial Height Change	-0.6 mm
Net Pogonion AP Advancement	12.6 mm
Net GenioHyoidMuscle Stretch	10.8 mm

FIG 15-12 This 14-year-old adolescent girl had the yaw of her maxilla corrected so that the maxillary dental midline fell on the facial midline. Overall there was a significant relative advancement of the right maxilla (10 mm) compared to the left (2 mm), in part due to right silent sinus syndrome and chronic right nasal airflow blockage. The increased overjet enabled a greater gain with IMDO and the ability to grow the mandible forward symmetrically, thereby enabling the development of a symmetric bite. An advancement GenioPaully further enhanced geniohyoid pull and created normal lip competence. Overall there was a normalization of both nasal and retroglossal airflows through a combined LeFort-IMDO.

IMPORTANCE OF DESIGN

Design is a major component of how clinical jaw surgery is practiced. Without some form of initial design pathway, it is impossible to coordinate the complex orthodontic, dental, facial cosmetic, and functional airway needs of the patient. And without design it is impossible to maximize the potential of individual jaw operations and the predictability of the final outcome (Figs 15-12 to 15-15). Design is paramount. If it begins early, the whole roadmap is revealed, and the journey's start and ending are known from the beginning.

> Design is paramount. If it begins early, the whole roadmap is revealed, and the journey's start and ending are known from the beginning.

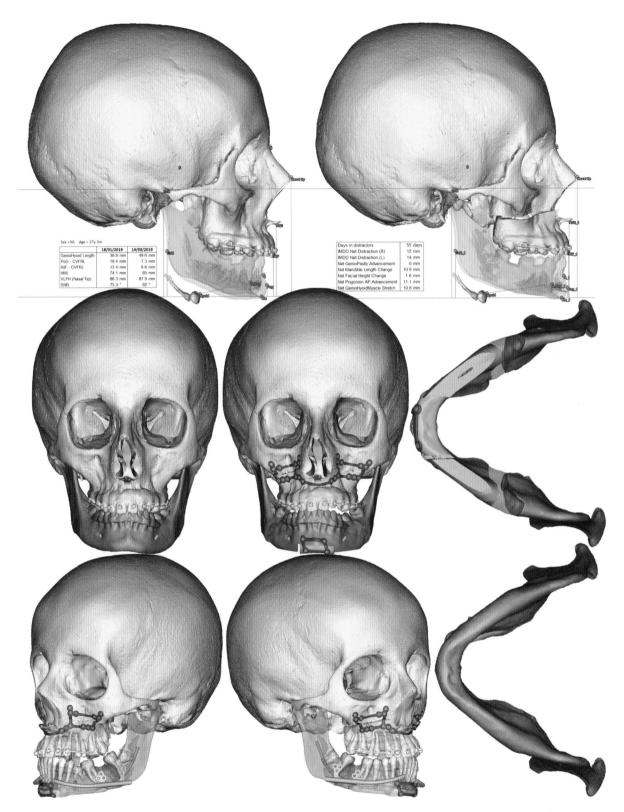

Sex = M; Age = 17y 3m	18/01/2019	14/03/2019
GenioHyoid Length	38.8 mm	49.6 mm
PoG - CVFRL	18.4 mm	7.3 mm
AIF - CVFRL	13.4 mm	6.6 mm
HML	74.1 mm	85 mm
VLFH (Nasal Tip)	86.3 mm	87.9 mm
SNB	75.3 °	82 °

Days in distractors	55 days
IMDO Net Distraction (R)	12 mm
IMDO Net Distraction (L)	14 mm
Net GenioPaully Advancement	0 mm
Net Mandible Length Change	10.9 mm
Net Facial Height Change	1.6 mm
Net Pogonion AP Advancement	11.1 mm
Net GenioHyoidMuscle Stretch	10.8 mm

FIG 15-13 This 17-year-old adolescent girl is severely hypoplastic (small) in the maxilla as a result of chronic open mouth breathing, originally derived because of her innately small mandible. To effectively overcome her fundamentally severe glossoptosis requires a significant IMDO distance, which is maximized by also advancing the maxilla about 6 mm with custom LeFort 1 surgery. The pattern of this procedure is performed over three operations. The first is to advance the maxilla and place the IMDO distractors. The second is to remove the IMDO distractors and perform the GenioPaully procedure. The third is to remove both the GenioPaully and LeFort plates. Creating a symmetric face enables the natural eruption of teeth into a normal bite before application of further Class I orthodontic mechanics.

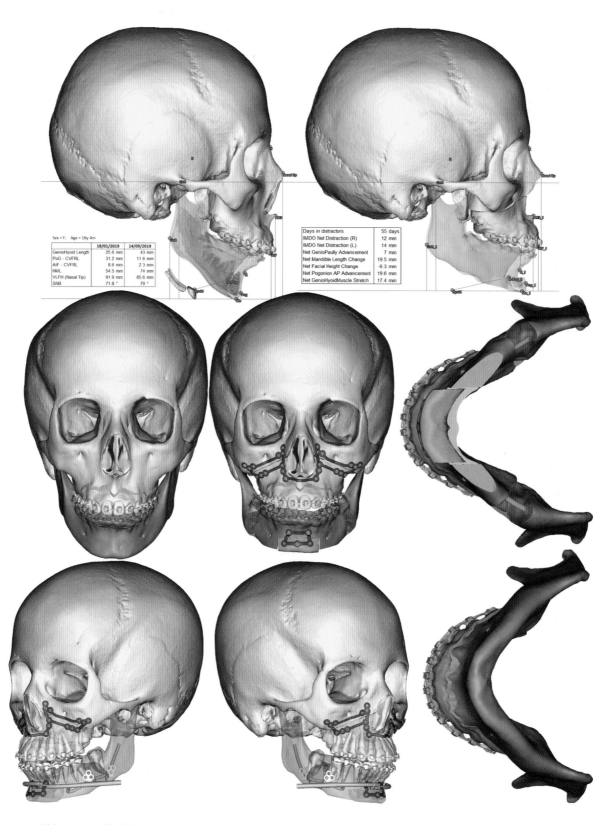

	18/01/2019	14/03/2019
GenioHyoid Length	25.6 mm	43 mm
PoG - CVFRL	31.2 mm	11.6 mm
AIF - CVFRL	8.6 mm	2.3 mm
HML	54.5 mm	74 mm
VLFH (Nasal Tip)	91.9 mm	85.6 mm
SNB	71.8 °	79 °

Sex = F;   Age = 16y 4m

Days in distractors	55 days
IMDO Net Distraction (R)	12 mm
IMDO Net Distraction (L)	14 mm
Net GenioPaully Advancement	7 mm
Net Mandible Length Change	19.5 mm
Net Facial Height Change	-6.3 mm
Net Pogonion AP Advancement	19.6 mm
Net GenioHyoidMuscle Stretch	17.4 mm

FIG 15-14 This 16-year-old adolescent girl was in orthodontics since she was 12 years old, and the attempt to close the dental overjet from her original Class II, division 1 malocclusion created a significantly vertical and asymmetric maxilla and mandible. It can be very hard to convince the orthodontist that these secondary maxillary effects from prolonged orthodontics occur, and there is little that can be surgically offered apart from an impaction-advancement-symmetrifying LeFort to accompany the referred-for IMDO—and thus maximize the mandibular lengthening that is needed to overcome the very small mandible, which started everything.

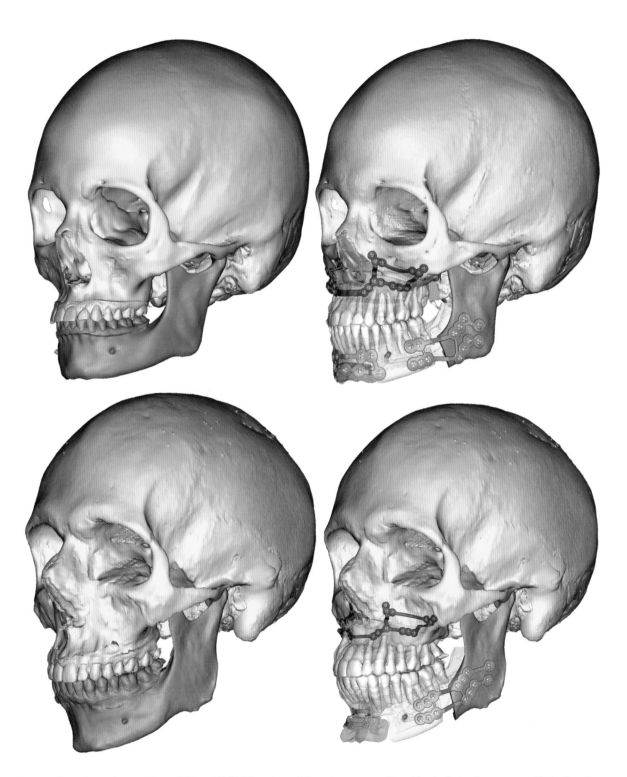

FIG 15-15 Once the patient reaches adulthood, IMDO is not possible, unless we are attempting to first gain some mandibular length as part of a SuperBIMAX series. Custom titanium allows for enormous advancement, but it is always to remediate a previous attempt at camouflage orthodontics, which has essentially shrunk and distorted the maxilla. Like IMDO, the BSSO also requires hardware removal. Unlike IMDO, the BSSO does not physically grow bone volume, which requires further bone grafting. If there is no prior orthodontics and things are allowed to develop naturally, then remediation is simply widening the maxilla and lengthening the jaw through IMDO with GenioPaully. The terminal two holes of the mandibular ramus plate are designed by the writer as a rescue extension, to be used only in case of a bad split—a rare complication of the BSSO.

16

INTRODUCING PEEK IMPLANTS
THE SIXTH WAY

n this book, I have elaborated on the beautiful interplay of GenioPaully, remedial BIMAX, IMDO, LeFort-SARME, and SuperBIMAX in being able to restore the bite and airways and jaws of the undergrown face. The final cherry on top of this five-tiered cake is the jawline polyetheretherketone (PEEK) implant (Fig 16-1).

In discussing PEEK implants, we must be careful not to introduce an idea that cosmetics is the underlying driver for their placement. For silent sinus syndrome, for condylar resorption, and for hemifacial microsomia in particular, reconstruction using PEEK is fundamentally functional in that it restores primary teratologic abnormality.

PEEK-Optima implants (Invibio), made using patented polyetheretherketone polymerization technology, come as Class IIB CE approved, medical-grade CNC-machinable polymer blocks. The final milled implants, performed under ISO13485 standards, replicate the digital design provided by the biologic reconstruction engineer together with perfect retention-screw placement. From the start, PEEK implants are designed to be practically insertable and easily secured by the surgeon.

PEEK implants are steam-sterilizable, nonporous, and nonbiologically degradable, and unlike titanium or other metals, they are radiolucent and do not scatter or reflect

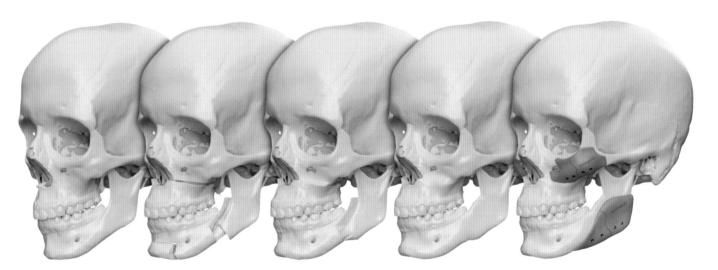

FIG 16-1 The sequence of jaw surgery begins with a decision to create volume. BIMAX advancement is an operation for adults, and for a number of functional reasons—including improvement to the bite and airway—BIMAX is an extraordinary and life-changing operation. However, the commitment to such dramatic facial change can exacerbate or disclose other problems that BIMAX cannot correct. Fortunately, we have custom PEEK design and manufacturing technology to fully restore us.

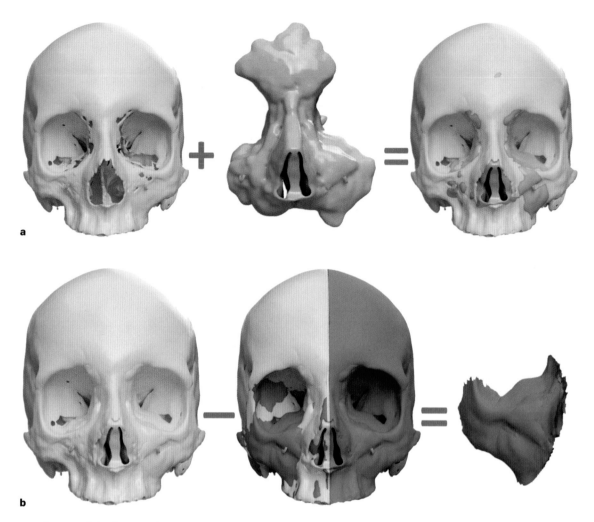

FIG 16-2 Segmentalizing bone produces many pseudoforamina, or holes, as well as areas of inaccurate bone thickness in areas where midfacial bone is particularly thin, such as the lamina papyracea. Segmentation is more capable of assuming the thickness and aerated volumes of the sinuses and nasal mucosa, and on the right there is significant reduction of the maxillary air sinus, such that the overlying right zygomatic bone is also "underinflated" and small (a). Merging the midface and mucosa allows us to see the drop in both the right orbital floor (leading to a drop in eye level) and decreased prominence and size of the orbital rim (eye socket) and the zygomatic bone itself. (b) Boolean uniting of the mucosa and calvarium produces a composite midface free of pseudoforamina. Mirroring the normal left side (blue) over the right side (bone color) allows us to subtract the original composite. The difference leaves the volume deficit, against which the engineer can digitally reconstruct the right orbital floor and hypoplastic zygomatic bone.

or absorb x-ray photons. PEEK implants also resist creep and fracture fatigue and have flexion properties similar to natural bone, enabling natural bone healing and local tissue biocompatability.

There are essentially six types of reconstructive PEEK implants for the jaws:

1. The combined orbital floor and cheekbone implant to restore silent sinus syndrome (Fig 16-2)
2. The jaw angle implant to restore ramus asymmetry in the mandible (see Figs 16-8 and 16-9)

3. The chin implant to centralize and project the central chin button in those who do not want GenioPaully (see Fig 16-5)
4. The cheekbone implant to restore cheekbone projection and symmetry after BIMAX advancement surgery (see Figs 16-9 and 16-10)
5. The posterior mandible implant to achieve absolute symmetry and increase volume of the bilateral posterior mandible following bilateral sagittal split osteotomy (BSSO) or IMDO surgery (see Fig 16-11)
6. Lateral nasal implant to support the nasal base, nasal valves, and underlying columella base (see Fig 16-11)

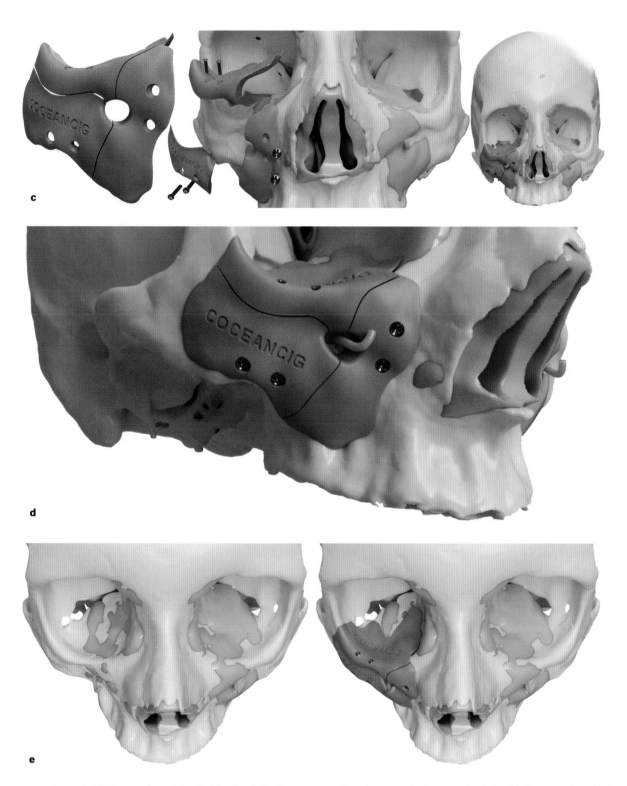

FIG 16-2 (CONT) *(c)* The creation of the final implant is in three parts, and each surrounds the emerging infraorbital nerve. The orbital implant, including the new rim, is inserted by a subconjunctival or infraorbital incision, which aims to safely lift the depressed eye globe. The remaining two implants are inserted via the mouth, through the superior sulcus and under the cheek skin. *(d)* The final implant reconstructs the normal orbital and cheekbone contours perfectly—and gives relief to sensory nerves that provide sensation to the cheek. Retention is through normal maxillofacial bone screws. *(e)* Seen from above, the new orbital and zygomatic implant reconstructs the volume and projection of the orbital rim, restores symmetric orbital volume, and levels globe support.

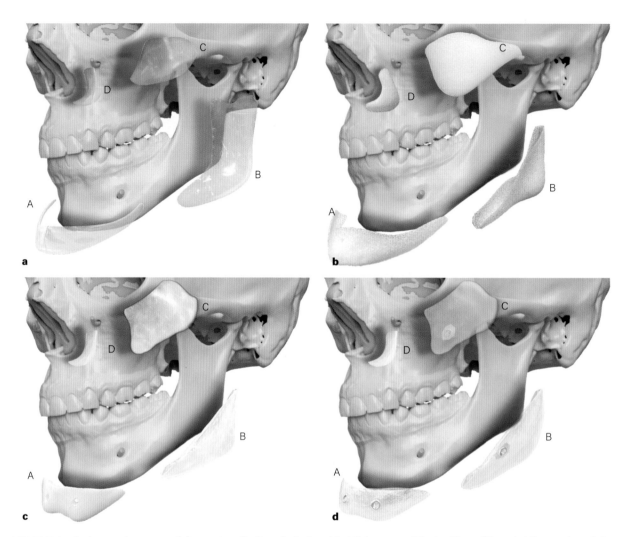

FIG 16-3 Implants come in a range of sizes and applications, including chin (A), jaw ramus (B), cheekbone (C), and piriform or lateral alae (D). *(a)* Silastic implants come in a range of off-the-shelf sizes, and while flexible, they are notorious for being very hard to accurately locate and hard to stably fixate. They also resorb away underlying bone in a process called *embedding erosion*. *(b)* Expanded or porous polyethylene is extremely stiff and difficult to resize and accurately fit. A kind of hard fibrotic tissue invades the porous surface, making overlying skin and muscle extremely hard and removal almost impossible. With 3D printing of the patient's jaws, wax buildups can be made in a maxillofacial prosthetic laboratory. *(c)* The wax can be optically scanned, and zirconia pucks can be accurately milled in five-axis CNC mills. *(d)* Alternatively, the wax can be converted to polymethyl methacrylate (PMMA) through the lost-wax technique common to established denture manufacturing. Both zirconia and PMMA implants are extremely tissue inert, and potentially zirconia can integrate with bone. Only zirconia is extremely radiopaque, while the other materials cannot be seen on plain radiographic film. When comparing all of these implants, only the combination of remedial BIMAX with custom PEEK implants gives the potential to maximally combine full reconstruction with the long-term benefits of radiolucency and maximal tissue compatibility.

OTHER TYPES OF FACIAL IMPLANTS

I have a steady stream of people who ask me about having a silastic implant placed in their chin or cheekbones (Fig 16-3). I have never once in my professional career placed one, but I do remove quite a few.

There are many reasons why I avoid silastic implants, and principally it is because I am not a cosmetic surgeon. I am very firmly a functional surgeon. While I understand

the argument that facial esthetic issues can lead to functional psychologic problems for a patient, alone this argument does not override my assessment of the imbalances, disproportions, and asymmetries of the underlying structure, nor my understanding of the compounding effects of anatomical disturbances upon chewing and biting, and of course breathing.

The moment a patient asks me for a specific cosmetic thing—like a facial silastic implant—I know that I am seeing

FIG 16-4 If a patient's sole and only issue is agenia (no chin button) in orthognathic Class A, then the option of a standalone chin implant seems an attractive option. If there is one advantage of custom PEEK implants *(right)* over off-the-shelf silastic *(left)*, it is that there is bespoke design and the security of a perfect fit. Neither form of implant imparts any functional benefit in a patient's airway patency.

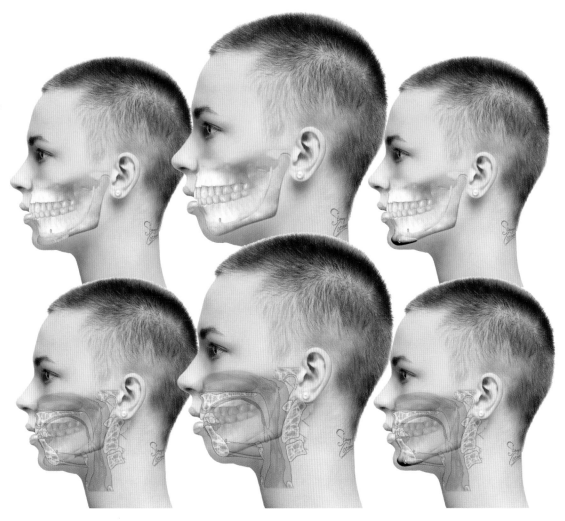

I have never once in my professional career placed a silastic implant, but I do remove quite a few.

a patient who will never be truly internally or fundamentally or psychologically satisfied. The ever-present danger is that by fundamentally correcting or deleting one focus of attention, another *more* fundamental cosmetic anomaly is revealed that pushes the patient closer toward an unknown psychiatrically abnormal boundary. This trajectory can easily lead to a full-blown and expressed psychiatric disease if the patient is enabled down this road by the surgeon. Therefore, in patients seeking facial implants alone, it is best to proceed compassionately but cautiously.

The functional uselessness of the standalone chin implant

The decision to proceed with a chin implant is one that belongs entirely to the patient. Advancing a chin through GenioPaully is to therapeutically gain two things: lower lip competence and fundamental advancement of the back of the tongue. The chin implant, on the other hand, does neither of these two things.

There are two broad groups of chin implant. The first are off the shelf, coming in a range of different sizes, and include silastic and porous polyethylene (see Fig 16-3). The second type are custom made and include polymethyl methacrylate (PMMA), titanium, zirconia, and finally PEEK. Of these choices, the PEEK implant is best, based on assessment of biologic compatibility, design predictability, and the long-term hope of lasting patient cosmetic satisfaction (Fig 16-4).

FIG 16-5 When considering standalone custom PEEK implants to augment a small mandible affected by AMHypo or PMHypo (anterior or posterior hypoplasia) or both, the choice becomes a consideration of fundamental remedial change (using the jaw surgery procedures described in this book) or a consideration of implants alone. Far greater volumes and far more therapeutic change can only occur by remedial surgery.

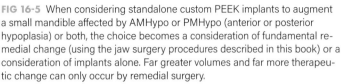
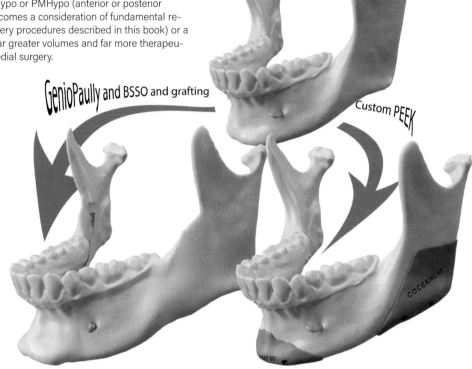

Once the bone contours are set and healing is complete, we can start looking at PEEK implants to fix those things that custom BIMAX could not.

The PEEK chin implant can be combined with PEEK angle implants, but nothing beats doing a fundamental jaw correction procedure for all the therapeutic benefits it brings (Fig 16-5).

BONE GRAFTING AFTER BIMAX ADVANCEMENT SURGERY

A major purpose of BIMAX surgery is to restore or recreate volume. After the advancement of the jaws, however, there are still a few steps to undergo as we progress toward full normalization.

Both the LeFort and BSSO procedures require a period of healing. The large plates that are intrinsic to digital design and large advancements eventually require removal, but not before the individual bone movements have healed in their new relationships. This first round of healing can take between 3 and 6 months, and with it some bony infill naturally occurs in the osteotomy gaps.

Once healing is complete, I like to remove all the plates and screws that we put in. If left in place too long, they completely fuse, making removal extremely difficult, not to mention expensive. There are a number of reasons why

removal is necessary, but mostly it has to do with leaving evidence behind. The devices we use are titanium, and because of the extreme tissue stretching that has to occur with successful and therapeutic BIMAX advancement, these titanium devices are made to be very large. This large size means that they are obvious on radiographs and can potentially hide underlying dental disease. For the patients themselves, the plates add unnecessary bulk and a feeling of lumpiness under the skin or local tenderness. Their very size, which is even bigger with larger jaw advancements, is also associated with high rates of local infection.

Removing plates and screws also allows me to recontour and bone graft some of the remaining osteotomy defects (Fig 16-6a). This is done with collagen sheets, powdered hydroxyapatite, and stiffer collagen-hydroxyapatite microsponges, all of which populate easily with the patient's own circulating and local stem cells to create new and natural bone (Fig 16-6b). A new round of healing then follows for another 6 months (Fig 16-6c).

Once the bone contours are set and healing is complete, we can start looking at PEEK implants to fix those things that custom BIMAX could not—primarily the cheekbones that were left behind and the jaw angles that may remain asymmetric (Fig 16-7).

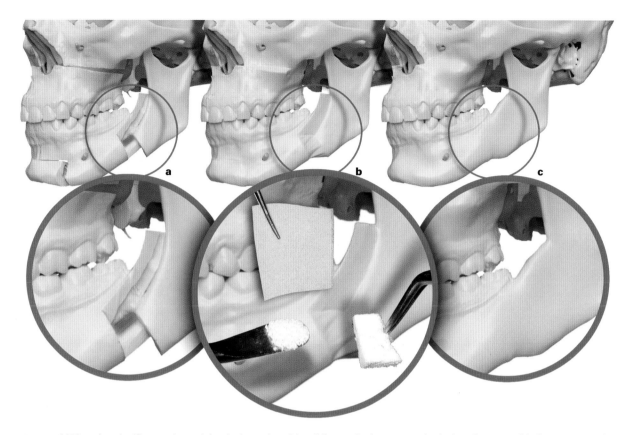

FIG 16-6 *(a)* There is a significant volume defect in the region of the sliding sagittal osteotomy, intrinsic to the BSSO. *(b)* After 3 to 6 months, the bone plates are removed, and while some bone infill has occurred, a combination of powdered hydroxyapatite, collagen sheeting, and collagen hydroxyapatite sponges is used to help create normal volume and contours. *(c)* Another 6 months of healing is required before we can assess how much normal bone formation has successfully occurred.

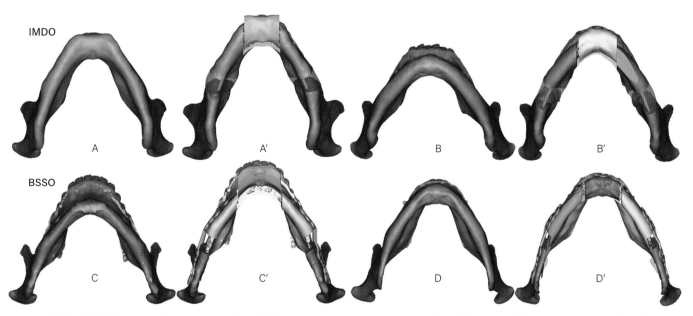

FIG 16-7 IMDO intrinsically grows bone. The BSSO cuts and pastes, creating a significant thinning that fills in with a combination of natural healing and further bone grafting. PEEK gives further enhancement to either the post-IMDO or post-BSSO grafted mandible only at the jaw angles.

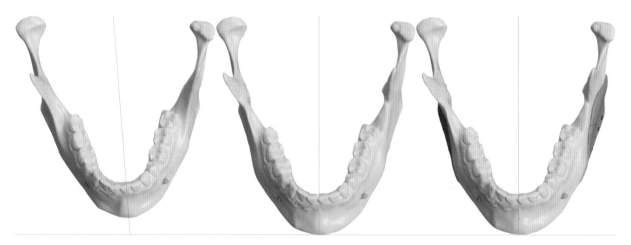

FIG 16-8 These 1:1 overviews demonstrate that custom BIMAX together with GenioPaully can achieve central anterior symmetry but not posterior symmetry. Custom PEEK implants restore the jaw angles in order to achieve posterior symmetry. The left implant is significantly larger than the right.

RESTITUTION OF JAW ANGLE SYMMETRY AFTER BSSO OR IMDO

After advancement BSSO has restored central symmetry to the mandible, what remains to be addressed is what BSSO and IMDO can never truly fix—posterior asymmetry (Fig 16-8).

Asymmetric jaws are very common. They can result from congenital conditions such as hemifacial microsomia, where one side of the face is underdeveloped (Fig 16-9a), or from acquired conditions that affect how the jaw joint develops (eg, juvenile rheumatoid arthritis). No matter the cause, we use the remedial BIMAX to correct central asymmetry and the changes in the bite plane that occur because of smaller joints. While the BSSO and GenioPaully are very good at being able to level the mandibular dental arch and centralize the chin button and the mandibular dental midline, they cannot fix the vertical shortness of the back of the jaw caused by the small jaw joint. After corrective jaw surgery, plate removal, and osteotomy defect grafting, the jawline and jaw angles can remain distinctly and obviously asymmetric (Fig 16-9b). For women in particular, it is the normal side that appears bigger. For men, the smaller side appears smaller. PEEK angle implants allow us to symmetrify these asymmetric areas (Fig 16-9c). Remodeling and 3D-printing of post-BIMAX jaws can enable a rational discussion between surgeon and patient of where jawlines can be trimmed or carved back.

Even if a person didn't notice the fundamental reasons for their jaw asymmetry before their surgery, it can be that their new facial focus highlights the last thing remaining: the residual asymmetry of the jawline. They no longer notice the uneven cant of their smile, or their gumminess, or the sense of midline asymmetry, or their dewlap, or lack of chin, or their snoring, or their bad bite, or whatever it was that drove them to seek surgery in the first place. They have a new facial focus—the thing that the BSSO cannot fix. Even if I clean the rest of the room perfectly and make everything tidy, patients will always notice the one thing I left behind—the sock in the middle of the floor. PEEK implants are my last surgical tool left in the box.

RESTITUTION OF CHEEKBONE PROJECTION AND SYMMETRY AFTER BIMAX

Particularly in the case of hemifacial microsomia, cheekbone asymmetry following BIMAX is common. The obvious cheek flatness is a result of the original complex deformity, but it becomes more apparent as a one-sided smallness of the cheekbones (Fig 16-10). Large advancements of the small maxilla can also leave the cheekbones behind. When I remove the large custom LeFort 1 plate, the step that was created has filled in a little, but grafting also helps smooth these contours.

Repeating the CT about 6 months after plate removal allows me to reprint facial models and use silastic lab putty to guide the conversations between my patient and myself. The same models, with marking pen, can also help with a discussion of trimming oversized areas too. Each cheek implant is rarely more than 2 cm³, but with them we can

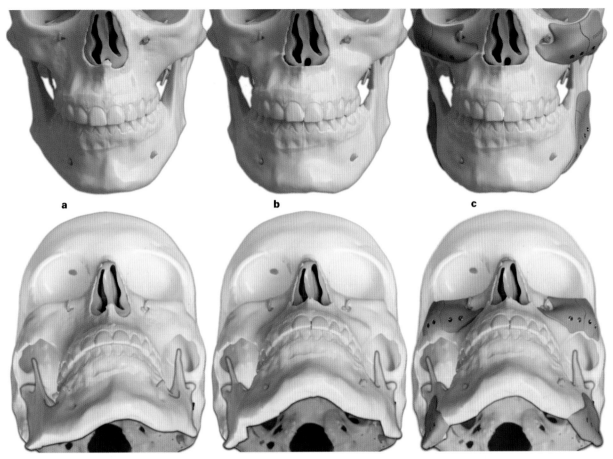

FIG 16-9 Hemifacial microsomia is notoriously hard to perfectly correct, particularly in the area of the smaller jaw angle. *(a)* Note the considerable distortion that occurs with Pruzansky Type 1 hemifacial microsomia. *(b)* Bimaxillary advancement and bone grafting centralizes and projects the lower facial skeleton, achieving central skeletal symmetry. *(c)* Combination of cheekbone and jaw angle implants to restore lateral facial volume and posterior symmetry of the jawline.

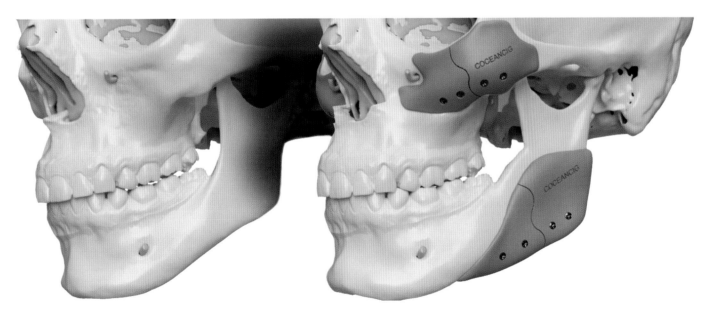

FIG 16-10 The full restoration of the deficient left jaw angle and the deficient left cheekbone following initial BIMAX is intrinsic to the ultimate correction of hemifacial microsomia (in this case, the reduced side is the left). These images are in exact 1:1 proportion and in precise orientation for direct comparison.

imagine how much more bony volume we need—usually laterally, but sometimes frontally—to restore balance and cheekbone symmetry (Fig 16-11).

Cheekbone implants are very subjective and very much dependent on user experience. The surgeon is not only determining whether they can be physically placed through the intraoral incisions we make, but also we want to try and predict their soft tissue bulking effects. In the end, less is always more.

My only advice is to not oversize anything, in women or men. Making the outer cheekbone edge at least meet the vertical edge of the jaw angles gives visual balance. Once the general design is settled, the silastic putty examples can be sent to the engineer as a guide to his or her own digital workflow.

Insertion is again under general anesthesia. If eventually the patient wants larger implants, then the process is repeated. PEEK is advantaged by its tissue neutrality, radiolucency, and ease of removal and replacement.

THE FINAL WORD: THE PIRIFORM IMPLANT

The deep nasolabial folds that extend from the base of each nostril and run to either side of our mouths really do tell people something of our age. The recessive maxilla, the collapsed upper lip, and the prominent nose accentuate these lines.

Once I have lifted the maxilla and reshaped and centralized the nasal spine, I can try and trim and symmetrify the piriform rims too. To a significant degree I am trying to give a new and symmetrified support to the squishy soft tissue lump and two holes we call a nose. But it is very unpredictable how it is handled. I can use PEEK implants to help fill in these areas to get as much digitally predictive symmetry and fullness as possible (see Fig 16-11).

But before anyone goes to the cosmetic rhinoplasty surgeon or to have their nasal septum "straightened," they should let me do the job I explained in these pages first.

In the end, less is always more.

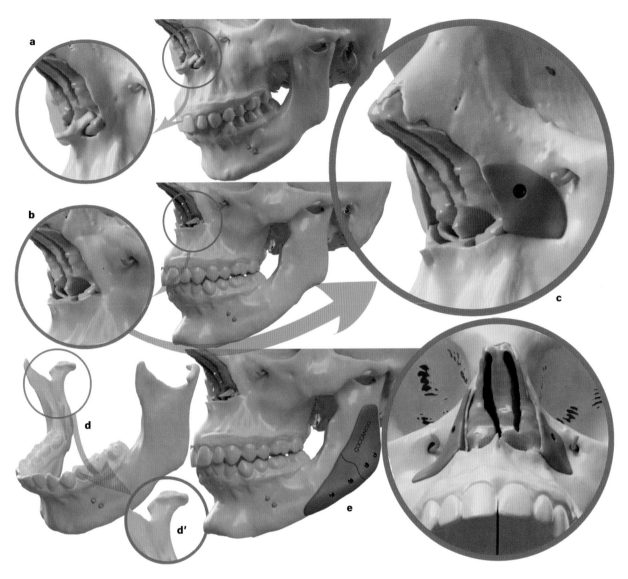

FIG 16-11 *(a and b)* A small counterclockwise rotation to anteriorly impact and advance a small maxilla can require some nasal spine resection, some anterior septal straightening, and reshaping too of the piriform rim, so as to enable some symmetric nostril creation. After the maxillary plate is removed and the grafting has been allowed to heal, small lateral piriform steps can occur on either side of the nostril (alae) base, which can deepen the nasolabial crease. *(c)* This can be lifted by symmetrically designed lateral piriform PEEK implants, each fixated with a screw. *(d–d')* The deformity of bilateral juvenile rheumatoid arthritis, which has destroyed the condylar heads, leads to vertical shortening of the vertical ramus. Rather than commit to joint replacement surgery of what is effectively a functional though small joint, the small mandible is managed by BSSO and GenioPaully and grafting as part of the overall counterclockwise remedial BIMAX. *(e)* Later, custom angle implants are manufactured alongside the piriform implants as well.

17
THE NEGATIVES OF CORRECTIVE JAW SURGERY

In surgery, we are trained to think adversely. To always think of negatives. The surgeon is always looking for what will fail. And we're always looking for an escape route too. To help make decisions in surgery, surgeons apply game theory. Instead of looking at the chance to win, we look at the chance to lose. Surgeons assimilate the negatives of each side and choose the side with fewer. And then we work on deleting each remaining negative, one by one.

> In my mind, the biggest risk surrounding corrective surgery is being convinced NOT to have corrective surgery.

In game theory, you always lose if you only bet on the long shot, or hope on a miracle, play the short game, or rely on anecdote, magic, or rumor. Hoping it will be okay just doesn't work in surgery. In game theory, the surgeon always wins at the horse race if he bets on the favorite and shoots the other horses.

In my mind, the biggest risk surrounding corrective surgery is being convinced NOT to have corrective surgery. So rather than talk of risks, I want to talk of negatives: the negatives that arise in the practice of corrective jaw surgery that may sway a person away from the treatment they should really have.

GENERAL ANESTHESIA NEGATIVES

There is a false and enduring community belief that general anesthesia is bad for you. But it isn't. It is perfectly safe.

My own anesthesiologist is a highly trained medical specialist, and in over 20 years we have never had an anesthetic negative event involving corrective jaw surgery. We treat by specific and established protocols, in standardized world-class medical hospitals, using state-of the-art anesthesia machines and medicines, with access to full level 3 trauma hospitals.

In Australia, where we have about 3 million general anesthesia events per annum, the numbers of mortal outcomes under routine, elective general anesthesia is literally counted in single digits over decades. The same experience of modern anesthesia exists in most every modern developed country. Maxillofacial surgeons are representative of the most highly trained and qualified surgeons you will find from any of the 11 surgical specialties.

General anesthesia is painless. It is safe. It is totally dependable. There is no "good luck" with anesthesia or with surgery. There is only supremely excellent planning and complete medical professionalism in the execution.

ESTHETIC NEGATIVES

If you point to a photograph of a child's knee, he will say, "That's my knee." If you point to an elbow, he will say, "That's my elbow." But if you point to a child's face in a photograph, he will say, "That is me."

Inwardly, we see our outward beauty very differently to how others esthetically perceive us, and our entire self-perception is through our face and by what we see in the mirror. We give our identity to it, and our personality, and our sense of self.

But the majority of us are also inherently, thoughtlessly, reflexively, and callously cruel to the facially flawed. And yet it's those same observers—us—who view the facially flawed as simplistic, naïve, insecure, or vain in seeking remedial relief for those flaws.

It is a wonderful thing to treat young people, especially those with simple problems like buck teeth or little chins, through the dramatic immediacy and simplicity of IMDO. Children breathe better. They sleep better. They run better. They eat better. But they also look better. And these shy little children, who cannot even talk to me because of their inner fears and schoolyard taunts, emerge like beautiful butterflies from their chrysalislike entombment in poor self-esteem. People simply interact with them differently. They are more popular at school or in social settings. And suddenly they are "normal."

In every emotional and rational sense, the notion of operating on a child for esthetic reasons is inherently wrong. Yet parents bring their children to orthodontists to cosmetically reduce a dental overbite or to cosmetically remove excessively crooked teeth. Adolescents are brought to me to cosmetically advance a diminutive jaw. Adolescents are brought to an ear, nose, and throat (ENT) surgeon to cosmetically reduce a prominent nose. Children are brought to a dermatologist to cosmetically remove a prominent birthmark, or to cosmetically cure adolescent facial acne.

All clinical professional interactions involving the face of a child or adolescent are inherently initiated by esthetics. Yet a direct conversation about a child's facial esthetics is extremely hard to engage. Parents have an inherent need to protect their children from narcissistic harm. Some parents will even ask that the entire conversation regarding esthetics not be engaged. But does this request absolutely negate the doctor's direct therapeutic obligation to the child—a child who eventually will become an adult—to deny a discussion on the inherent lifetime esthetic effects of adolescent corrective jaw surgery?

In part to avoid the socially negative connotations of such a conversation taking place, my passive trick is to give a series of before and after photographs that parents can casually glance through. This usually avoids the subliminal question or doubt or degree of what positive cosmetic change is possible.

All that a corrective jaw surgeon can offer is symmetry, centrality, proportionality, and balance in the skeleton.

To a surgeon, our analysis of facial beauty isn't an analysis of beauty at all. What we are doing is giving an objective measurement of the proportionality and symmetry and levelness of the facial skeleton and teeth alone. But to the layperson, beauty is the entirety of their analysis on a self-known scale from ugliness to handsomeness.

I often say to patients that in operating I am not changing the person's self-perception of their own beauty. Instead I am changing the opinions of seven billion strangers. The conversations revolving around this idea of physical appearance are difficult. After all, treating a child through the opinions of a love-blind parent is impossible. And treating an adult through the expectations of their social peers is also impossible. As a surgeon, I cannot promise beauty. I cannot promise social benefit. I cannot promise a better job, or a better wage, or better self-esteem. I cannot promise an amazing face, or even a normal face. All I can promise is that your face will remain your face. And no one else's.

All that a corrective jaw surgeon can offer is symmetry, centrality, proportionality, and balance in the skeleton. In constructing a face, we are defined first by surgical safety, then functional benefit. Esthetics runs dead last. If a patient wants maximal esthetics, then it is best to move in small steps, not leaps, and to build each advancement incrementally and steadily in one direction. It is hard to get a hole in one.

PSYCHOLOGIC NEGATIVES

General

Most surgeons don't want to talk about a patient's psychiatric wellness. It is an unusually sensitive topic to ask people about depression, anxiety, obsessive thoughts, or recreational drug use. It can be an uncomfortable conversation and is safely and reasonably avoided in 99% of most surgical visits. In the context of corrective jaw surgery, however, these topics become more relevant. There is, much more intrinsically involved concerning a person's mood state and anxiety level when considering facial surgery.

Emotion and normal anxiety

Children and parents who are made to wait for surgery over a long period of time can become more anxious as time passes. Once the surgery is performed, there can be an almost cathartic release of emotions that can appear as the extremes of anger or fundamental happiness. For young adolescents forced to wait for pre-IMDO orthodontics or for parents to make a difficult decision or for insurance waiting periods to expire, real psychologic harm is a possibility.

For adults involved in surgery, there is an increased likelihood of an underlying mood or anxiety disorder that can magnify these basic emotional reactions to surgery. The emergence or magnification of frank psychiatric disease can obviously affect postsurgical compliance and personal care. A parent may refuse to turn distractors in their child due to overwhelming anxiety. A patient's underlying ruminations and depression may transform to crippling cataplexy or anorexia or withdrawal from care.

In my surgical experience, even people with some form of psychiatric illness are in perfect and rational need of the corrective facial operations they seek. Given normal general physician or specialist psychiatric or general psychologic support, corrective jaw surgery is very mental-health safe. The need for discussion of one's psychiatric state doesn't really exist. If the patient is psychiatrically well enough to visit, they are psychiatrically well enough to be treated as well.

But be attentive to children. The ways we innocently discuss things as adults are not interpreted the same way by them.

Body dysmorphic disorder

There is, however, one specific psychiatric disorder that has the reputation of causing great harm to those pursuing facial surgery. Body dysmorphic disorder (BDD) is formally an anxiety disease, characterized as constant thinking, ruminating, and obsessing over perceived flaws in one's appearance. Individuals with BDD become anxious, depressed, and absolutely driven to delete what they see as wrong or deformed or broken.

About 99% of the time, those who seek a series of remedial operations to correct a complex facial deformity do NOT have BDD. These people are in every way psychiatrically normal. There is nothing unusual about wanting to fix the jaws or face or broad esthetic.

In my entire jaw surgery career, I have only ever met four people with BDD. I deliberately elected to treat one. I deliberately did not treat the other three. All of them had already had multiple previous jaw surgery correction–oriented operations. None of these operations had worked to the satisfaction of the patients concerned. The one that I did treat had a legitimate objective jaw deformity, about which he ruminated and thought about constantly, and for which there was high likelihood of surgical remediation by a single operation. Despite successful surgery, his BDD did not allow alleviation of his anxiety, and he went off to seek further surgical opinion and interaction.

This notion in the public mind that the person who seeks multiple facial surgical operations has BDD is frankly wrong. BDD is exceedingly rare. The false accusation that people seeking facial surgery are vain, or self-loving, or narcissistic are terrible social labels to place. The vast majority, almost the overwhelming entirety of people seeking corrective facial surgery, are psychiatrically normal people. It is completely normal to want to have the combination of functionality and esthetic balance.

Pathologic narcissism

What is NOT normal is another tiny subset of people who suffer from a formal and specific and fundamentally destructive persona, and which also drives cosmetic surgical seeking, called *narcissistic personality disorder* (NPD).

In my practice, we try to detect these people as early as possible. We do not want to treat them at all. NPD is not a psychiatric condition. It is not treatable by medications or talking or group therapy. It is immutably formed from the basic temperament and being of the person. It belongs to a cluster of similar personality disorders that we also want to avoid—both socially and professionally—including antisocial, borderline, and histrionic personality disorders. Unfortunately, all jaw surgery correction practices uniquely and specifically attract people with NPD.

Those with NPD seek jaw surgery not for functional remediation but for the cosmetic effects of jaw surgery and for the promise of professional attention. They are normally exceedingly polite and deliberately engaging in superficial and initial interaction, but they are entirely without empathy for others and histrionically volatile and aggressive and dangerous when denied surgical service. They will falsely represent the need for jaw surgery in terms of a functional reason they have researched but is entirely without objective support. They will perpetuate the claim of a functional complaint only until their inner cosmetic or self-serving drive for attention is expunged. There is no professional satisfaction or promise of a therapeutic end.

Inner drives vs external influencers

The final psychologic negative lies in a discussion of drive. Of motivation. Of who wants what. It is a discussion of the psychologic differences separating the primary patient and the secondary supporter.

Orthognathic surgery is intrinsically associated with the changing of a face. For a surgeon, these changes relieve the patient of a structural abnormality, thereby providing a better way to eat or breathe. To a patient, though, these fundamentally structural changes also represent how they may see and identify with themselves in a mirror.

For there to be a fundamental and intrinsic acceptance in the "my face looks better" quality of facial surgery, it has to be matched to a fundamental acceptance that "my face works better." For that happy intellectual link to happen, the primary driver for all facial surgery has to be a consensus agreement between two objective patient and surgeon assessments of the functional deficiencies of the face.

Much like I never want to treat people who are seeking only esthetic change with surgery, I also do not want to treat people whose parents or partners are the ones pushing the surgery onto the patient. Instead the ideal jaw correction patient is the patient who knows that their face is broken somehow, and that no other solution exists. They are those people who do not suffer from BDD, and who do not have NPD, but are still intrinsically, inwardly, and normally driven.

For all of these psychologic reasons, 99% of all people who present for jaw correction surgery have normal inner-driven motivations that are a combination of everything in their normal lives that we call social, cosmetic, or functional. These 99% are the best patients for corrective jaw surgery. It is the other 1% that are to be avoided at all costs.

THE NEGATIVE OF WORKING WITH MULTIPLE PRACTITIONERS FIXING A COMPLEX INTERWOVEN SYSTEM

Jaw surgery is naturally very complicated by the need to have multiple people, often from divergent professional backgrounds, working together and in a coordinated way.

For instance, orthodontists are not medical doctors, and maxillofacial surgeons are not practicing dentists, and on many fundamental levels they have the potential to hold opposite points of view on how things should be started, coordinated, delivered, or led.

Using corrective jaw surgery to fix obstructive sleep apnea (OSA) naturally comes into philosophical conflict with other competing treatment groups. ENT surgeons offer ENT operations to relieve or diminish OSA effects. Respiratory physicians use sleep studies and continuous positive airway pressure (CPAP) devices to establish and reduce apnea-hypopnea index (AHI) scores. Sleep dentists use snoring splints for the same purpose.

Likewise, using jaw surgery for fixing a small jaw potentially comes into conflict with orthodontists who believe they can use jaw splints to grow small jaws and fix overbites and thus avoid corrective jaw surgery.

The three major themes of corrective jaw surgery are bite, airway, and facial balance, and all three can be achieved when the treating professionals—dentist, orthodontist, and surgeon—work together for the overall benefit of the patient and come to the table with the same philosophy about care. Any infighting will only lead to confusion and uncoordinated (and thus subpar) care for the patient. At worst, these arguments and fear-mongering can frighten the patient away from the very treatment they need. And it is unethical too.

THE THEME OF TRUST

In any therapeutic relationship between a surgeon and their patient, there comes a fundamental point where intellectually the client has to give in to an inherent social trust. There has to be trust that the surgeon knows what the problem is that needs to be fixed. There has to be trust in seeing that it will be fixed. There has to be trust that the patient will not be fundamentally hurt or harmed. There has to be trust that if a random unanticipated technical negative occurs, that it can be recognized and resolved. There has to be trust in the deliverance of compassion. There has to be trust in the perseverance of the therapeutic relationship no matter what.

Trust is a complex thing. Like the acceptance of a surgeon to treat a patient, and the acceptance of that patient to be treated by that surgeon, the establishment of trust goes both ways. All normal relationships between two people are founded on an intermutual social trust between them. However, unlike normal human relationships, the patient-doctor relationship is a professional and therapeutic one. There is an absolute need for both to retain an emotional and social distance from each other. And yet within this professional union, there is still this very intrinsic, very human, very socially based need for trust.

Once this social trust is broken, there is rarely any recovery. Perhaps the patient loses trust in the surgeon because they feel they were not told the entire truth about a given procedure, or perhaps the surgeon loses trust in the patient when they choose a coincident or side treatment that goes against the surgeon's philosophy of care. No matter the cause, the loss of social trust is a death knell.

The only cure for this great complication—the loss of social trust—is prevention. To retain trust, and to retain the fantastic benefit of an intact therapeutic relationship, both parties have to respect the gift of it, the fragility of it, and the risks of losing it. The therapeutic relationship is above all the one thing neither party wants to lose. Ever.

> The therapeutic relationship is above all
> the one thing neither party
> wants to lose. Ever.

Preventing its loss is by constant, open, and honest communication by both parties. There can never be accusations of negativity either way. There is only ever just two people—a surgeon and a patient working personably and together to fix a common problem. Communication means access to each other. And the major tools are given in the form of time, open doors, a phone call, and the fundamental intersocial means of polite conversation.

THE NEGATIVES OF TREATMENT ECONOMICS

Globally there are three broad areas of health care. Within those divisions are associated known health economics that surrounds the broad funding of health care that either directly or indirectly deals with the health effects of small jaws.

The first area is dentistry, which in the context of small jaws is dominated by camouflage orthodontics for dental crowding and malocclusion, sleep dentistry for mandibular advancement splints to help with OSA and snoring, and oral surgery for things like removal of impacted teeth (especially third molars) or routine orthodontic extractions for dental crowding relief.

The second area is medicine, which includes many fields that indirectly deal with the secondary medical and surgical effects of small jaws. The first medical arm includes physician care for OSA and its medical effects (ie, obesity, diabetes, and hypertension). And the other medical arm is surgical care mostly for upper airway surgical procedures that can help relieve either nasal or retroglossal airway obstruction, such as nasal or sinus or septal surgery or soft palate, tonsillar, tongue, or upper throat surgery. In this medical-surgical group too are maxillofacial procedures, such as for remedial BIMAX (for all the reasons already detailed in chapter 12) as well as consideration for bariatric surgery or surgical obesity management.

The third area is cosmetic surgery. This includes cosmetic dentistry, for instance in providing for full dentures or cosmetic veneers or even orthodontics that enable correction of abnormal bites and smiles that are intrinsic to jaw size problems. But most people consider "cosmetic" to include formally medical cosmetic procedures oriented to surgical or semisurgical procedures, such as dermal filler injections, silastic chin or jaw angle implants, underchin liposuction (for dewlap) or neck or facial "lifts," or cosmetic rhinoplasties.

Without recognition of the broad effect of small jaws, and because of the disconnect of many of the clinical groups that independently practice in this region, it is hard to actually quantify what total health care costs actually apply to an individual having one treatment over another—all as consequences of the small jaw—but which are spread out over a lifetime.

In this book, I hope that I have demonstrated that when you are considering the natural life of an individual, there are two broad methods by which a child and eventually an adult with a small mandible can be treated. By directly comparing them, it's possible to consider the serial treatments involved, then the broad economics of either pathway, and finally the total health economic cost in terms of overall health, well-being, and general effect on lifespan.

The classical ENT, orthodontic, and oral surgery cost pathway

By 12 years old, the adult teeth—a total of 28—should have emerged, and the final pattern of the face and how it will mature will essentially be known. The remaining four third molars are universally considered redundant, and 95% of all people will have these prophylactically or symptomatically removed in most Western societies. Twelve is also the age at which most children will first present to an orthodontist for the commencement of orthodontic treatment for crooked teeth and the associated bad bite, which in all cases is associated with small jaws, be it Class I, II, or III or anterior open bite. At this age, all initiated orthodontics will be aligned with some form of camouflage pathway—being that treatment by an orthodontist cannot possibly make jaws bigger but can only move and shuffle and align the teeth and visual smile. These dental treatments have a routine and defined cost, but added to them are the costs of time and of the visits themselves. And at the end, third molars are almost always also inevitably removed, possibly also with premolar extractions, which carry treatment costs.

> Treatment by an orthodontist cannot possibly make jaws bigger but can only move and shuffle and align the teeth and visual smile.

Associated within this broad age group are the phenomenon of enlarged tonsils, inflamed adenoids, and middle ear obstructions.

In early adulthood comes the emerging focus on cosmetic medicine. There is a cost for reduction rhinoplasty, submental liposuction, septal deviation correction and turbinate reduction, and the silastic chin implant, alongside lip or dermal fillers, as well as for cosmetic dentistry to improve the smile built upon the previous camouflage orthodontics.

At the other age-end is the middle-aged person and beyond—no longer with an overbite, with fewer natural teeth, and with the memory of orthodontics or pediatric ENT or cosmetic surgery long gone. In these patients, a sedentary lifestyle and high-calorie intake combine to thicken the neck and potentiate the OSA expression from the persistent small jaw and innate glossoptosis. Sleep studies and CPAP machines and snoring splints follow, as well as medical management for insulin resistance, hypertension, and other obesity effects.

ENT procedures may follow, with uvulopalatopharyngoplasty (UPPP) or frank glossectomy or indirect hyoid suspensions.

Of course the fundamental treatment is the remedial BIMAX, which could have been employed at any point following the initial camouflage orthodontics.

All of these multiple and seemingly unconnected clinical care costs are associated with the small jaw. But apart from remedial BIMAX, no treatment outside of maxillofacial surgery is directed to the fundamentality of that condition. Everything else—dental, orthodontic, ENT, oral surgical, or cosmetic—is instead considered as independent and isolated and unconnected diseases.

The cost pathway for IMDO

IMDO considers that the single fundamental disease is the commonality of the small mandible, which I call anterior mandibular hypoplasia (AMHypo), and that everything else is a secondary sign or consequence of that single and primary condition.

There is no room for camouflage orthodontics in the IMDO model. The moment camouflage orthodontics has been undertaken, there is either the LeFort-IMDO procedure in late adolescence or remedial BIMAX in adulthood.

For IMDO to work, orthodontics is included but limited to pre-IMDO maxillary expansion, which also relieves nasal airway obstruction and thus replaces nasal-ENT as an airway intervention, and post-IMDO orthodontics, which is usually far simpler and far quicker than alternative camouflage orthodontic mechanics.

> The moment camouflage orthodontics has been undertaken, there is either the LeFort-IMDO procedure in late adolescence or remedial BIMAX in adulthood.

The IMDO operation combined with the GenioPaully procedure is also far cheaper than any other classical orthognathic surgical procedure, and IMDO distractors are relatively cheap as well, especially in comparison to the custom titanium material manufacturing costs associated with remedial BIMAX.

Added to those fundamental cost benefits, IMDO is also fundamentally curative of glossoptosis, thus removing any snoring and OSA risk. By correcting the fundamental volume of the jaws, it dentally deletes the requirement for premolar extractions and gives the maximum preventive potential for third molar impactions, thus eliminating the need for their surgical removal down the line after camouflage orthodontics. By widening the nasal airway and pulling the tongue forward, adenoids and tonsils are naturally deobstructed, Eustachian tubes are cleared, and the turbinates no longer block the nose. All this deletes the upper airway intervention of adolescent or adult ENT airway opening procedures.

Cosmetically there is great advantage too. The nose size is normal, being that it is now proportional to the lower face, and the potential for cosmetic rhinoplasty as well as cosmetic jawline or chin enhancement or dewlap correction or lip filler procedures is deleted also.

Despite these clear comparisons, the economic choice between the two options is difficult to reconcile for the classical orthodontic pathway. First, orthodontics does not acknowledge any codependency upon either oral surgery or ENT procedures, and secondly it does not consider or compete against alternative models of care such as IMDO.

Specifically, the classical treatment model does not consider the commonality of the small jaw to all three classical clinical care disciplines. Instead, orthodontics considers dental crowding as common, alongside the redundancy of tonsils and third molars, all of which are irrationally considered a consequence of modern or recent

> To a parent, however, and eventually also to the child when they become the adult, all these procedures and all the diseases they treat are obviously linked within the individual.

human evolution—and the devolution of the modern need for these anatomical structures by the epigenetics of soft diets.

Thus by separating the specialty disciplines into orthodontics, ENT, and oral surgery, there is no classical health economic model, and almost no professional costs incentive that can causally link all of them as fundamentally treating the same condition.

To a parent, however, and eventually also to the child when they become the adult, all these procedures and all the diseases they treat are obviously linked within the individual. And over the lifetime of the person, the economic costs of both disease and treatment pathway, within either model, eventually become fully and inevitably realized.

Considering the divisions still alive in clinical care today, my only advice to the parent of a child with a large dental overjet or crooked teeth or with enlarged tonsils or with clear difficulty in nasal breathing is to choose early—and to choose wisely. The ramifications of that early choice stretch over a lifetime.

EPILOGUE

The gods give us all a road, but they don't give a map. As long as we travel it without pride and hubris, they leave us alone along our journeys of discovery. I had no idea where my road was to lead me. I just drove it. I was given a good brain. A good heart. Energy. Empathy. Ethic. All just unknown unappreciated gifts for a good life. The special people I met along the way, they were diamonds in my asphalt.

My father, Bruno, and my mother, Roslyn, were my initial drivers. My wife and children and brother have been my most recent passengers. In Australia, we are a nation of immigrants, and the intercontinental experiences of billions are concentrated here in a polyglot that is the entirety of the human horizon. A most excellent panorama for driving along a good and unique road.

I hope all readers of this book have their own equally excellent journey. I've loved the random discovery of this hill and that river. I'm sorry that I have given you some clues as to the roadway. The emotional attraction to travel, after all, is about the love of surprise.

I have many maxillofacial surgeons and mentors to thank. The first was John Norman, AO. And then Geoffrey McKellar, Peter Vickers, and Alfred Coren. And then there was Leslie Snape and Raymond Peck. I've already mentioned them in my introduction.

But there were other surgeons too. My greatest teacher was Rohana Kumara DeSilva from Sri Lanka. There was also Teh Luan Yook from Singapore, and Ian Wilson from Australia. And also John Lowry, CBE, from England, who gave me my honorary British fellowship. I love you all.

I hope all readers of this book have their own equally excellent journey.

And of course there have been my closest peers and friends. My fellow maxillofacial surgeons who inspired and supported and pushed me. Samintharaj Kumar and Seah Tian Ee (Singapore), the brothers Arthur and Wojchiek Bilski (Germany/Poland/Australia), Jose García Piña and Alejandro Martinez (Mexico), Sergio González Otero and Antonio Vázquez (Spain), Wayne Gillingham and John Bridgeman (New Zealand), Aarnout Hoekema (Netherlands), Ericka Sánchez Zavala (Costa Rica), and Dylan Murray (Republic of Ireland).

I've had loyal referrers as well. People who never really understood my surgery, but who understood my faith. Peter Lewis and Angela Marty and Evan Stacey and Nick Moncrieff and Derek Mahony and Isidoro Ferlito and Fadi Yassmin and Andrew Nixon and Robert Bartolacci were the first among the thousands whom I have collaborated with. I apologize to the rest whom I cannot more formally acknowledge in these few paragraphs.

And I cannot acknowledge the many tens of thousands of patients, and the many more relatives and friends and supporters and co-staff except the brief few who are pictured in this book.

My engineers deserve a special unique mention. Primary is Pieter-Jan Belmans of Belgium. The other is Francisco Medina Guerra of Mexico. Both enabled many of the illustrations contained in this book, but both too contributed to many original engineering designs and possibilities especially with custom titanium. The drawings were also created by Angela Marty of New Zealand and Alessandra Coceancig (Italy/Switzerland) as well as the overall supervising excellence of Evan Stacey of Australia, my truly good friend and compatriot. The manufacturers of my devices also require mention. Razvan-Alexandru Gheorghe, PhD, (Romania/Switzerland), the inventor of the double helical bone fixation screw we use. Oliver Scheunemann (Germany), the Secretary General of SORG who first championed the idea of IMDO and who helped develop the IMDO distractor. His colleagues Karl and Christian Leibinger (Germany), who first helped develop IMDO as a concept. Heiki Kyöstelä and Jouko Nykänen (Finland), who involved me with their early developments into cone beam technology. The original imaginists who developed the segmentation software we use, Wilfried Vancraen and Hilde Ingalaere (Belgium), deserve special mention too.

In creating history, you need writers as well as generals. Joseph Allbeury (Australia) always pushed me to write. Sonia Piskorowska with Christian Haase (Germany) introduced me to William Hartman (USA). Finally, Bryn Grisham and then Leah Huffman (Chicago), who condensed and directed everything into readable treacle and honey. Leah was particularly wonderful. Truly.

My regret with all of this was only one thing: My mother was 84 when she died in May 2020. She did not read this book. But my father did. This book is dedicated to them both. I thank you both with all my heart and mind for the ideas and for the discovery of them that you started in me.

INDEX

Page numbers followed by "f" denote figures.